Butterfly Miracles with Homeopathic Remedies

LaRee Westover
butterflyexpressions.org
butterflymiracles@hotmail.com

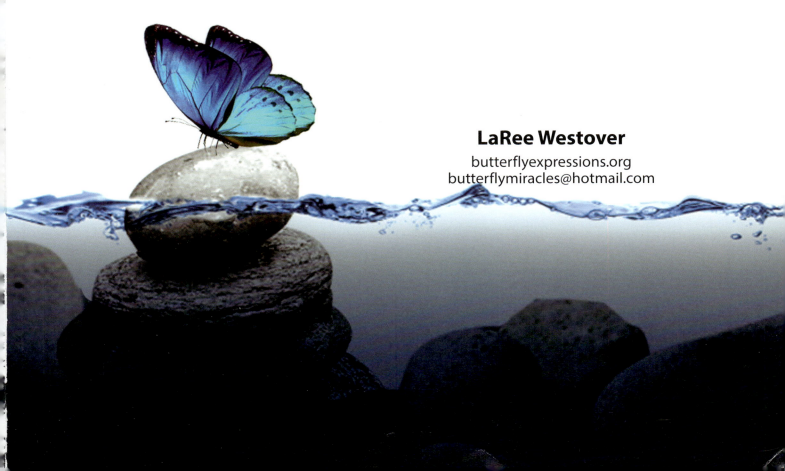

Hope Renewed

Homeopathic theory and practice differ greatly from any other healing modality, past or present, in several very basic ways.

First: Since the beginning of time, mankind has attempted to find methods to restore good health and proper functioning of the body following accidents or illnesses. Healing without causing harm has always been the goal of good men in medicine. Homeopathy can be, for everyone who is willing to make an effort, the answer to that quest.

When Samuel Hahnemann (considered the father of homeopathic theory) created his first remedy according to homeopathic protocols, he showed us a way to heal without side effects. He, and others like him, illuminated the path to the utilization of the many diverse substances found on this earth, even very toxic ones, to bring about positive changes in health without the destruction of delicate tissues or negative effects on the mind or emotions.

Second: Followers of homeopathic theory believe that every ailment of the physical body had its beginning in the vital energy of the body. Homeopathic theory also teaches that because the systems of the body are so interconnected by the vital energy, ailments cannot confine themselves to only one area of the body at a time. It is impossible to have just a pain in the head (or just a break in a bone) without having symptoms which range over many, if not all, of the systems of the body and into the emotions and mental processes. A corollary of this understanding is that all substances utilized for healing purposes (or for any other purpose) also affect a variety of body systems and go into the energy itself to reestablish (or disrupt) health.

Homeopathic remedies are studied and their effects recorded in this manner. When a remedy is given, symptoms throughout the whole body and mind are observed and the remedy is chosen to care for and restore balance to all of these areas.

Last and very important: In homeopathy, its history as well as its present-day usage, we have a graphic illustration of the goodness of God in inspiring and providing for His children. From the variety of substances whose healing properties have been discovered and utilized in homeopathy, a person can see that every creation of God found on this earth must be of benefit for the use of man. We can see that God has provided methods by which healing can be accomplished without destructive side effects.

What more could a loving Father have done for His children? Every time I reach for a homeopathic remedy—whether it is plant, animal, mineral, or noxious substance based—I feel touched by Heaven's concern and caring for me. As the remedy brings health to my physical body or perspective to my mind or emotions, I feel the additional healing benefits of gratitude and reverence.

It takes some study and effort to become proficient in the use of homeopathic remedies. It is well worth whatever effort is required! In addition, the accepting of responsibility for our own and our family's health, coupled with gratitude to the Creator, blesses and strengthens us in a myriad of ways.

May you find as much joy and success with homeopathic remedies as I, and many others, have done!

The "Butterfly Miracles" Bookshelf

ESSENTIAL OILS
History of Essential Oils
Schools of Thought
Tests and Standards
Shelf Life
Safety Guidelines
Women and Children
Methods of Use
Plant Families
Meridians and Chakras
Single Oils
Blended Oils

HERBAL REMEDIES
Nutrition and Your Body
Vitamin Absorption
Food and Nutrients
Vitamin Bandits
Drugs and Nutrition
Sub-clinical Malnutrition
Herbs as Nutrition
Doing a Cleanse Right
Use of Herbal Remedies
Basic Herbal Knowledge
Recipes: Tinctures, Teas, Salves

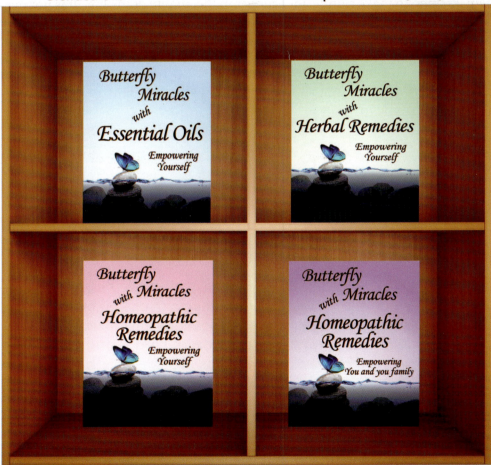

HOMEOPATHIC I
Principles of Homeopathy
Types of Remedies
Dilution and Potency
Taking Homeopathic Remedies
The Symptom Picture
Taking a Case History
Biochemic or Cell Salts
Flower Essence Remedies
Energetic Remedies
Remedies by Classification

HOMEOPATHIC II
Families - Children
Pregnancy
Labor and Delivery
Postpartum
Women's Health
Infant Care
Chronic Fatigue
Glandular Support
Headaches
Weakness

Legalese

There is absolutely no substitute for caution and common sense!

This book is written for general information and education only. It is not my intent to diagnose or prescribe for any ailment whatsoever. Your use of the information contained in this book is entirely at your own discretion and is, also, entirely your own responsibility. My goal is, simply, to bring to your attention things that, when I became aware of them, seemed to make significant changes in the quality of my life. It is not meant to be training in psychology, psychotherapy or medicine of any kind. You are advised to apply the techniques and information along with the assistance of competent professionals.

You have managed this far in your life without that homeopathic remedy you are considering and you can manage another day or two while you start slowly to determine the correct remedy, potency, and dosages for your own needs. It is my recommendation that you start slowly, with a remedy or two, determining what is best for your own needs.

There are details concerning the safe use of homeopathic remedies that cannot be contained in any book. Before using a homeopathic remedy the reader is advised to seek the assistance of a competent professional.

The statements and products mentioned in this book have not been evaluated by the FDA. They reflect traditional and anecdotal usage and data from recent scientific studies.

I hope you come to enjoy and love homeopathic remedies as much as I do

Copyright © 2011, 2013, 2016 Butterfly Expressions LLC

ISBN-10

0-9835228-1-2

ISBN-13

978-0-9835228-1-2

January 2016 Printing

Printed in the United States of America

Table of Contents

SECTION ONE: Basic Principles/Lower Potency Remedies

CHAPTER 1 BASIC PRINCIPLES .... p 1
- Philosophies of the Healing Arts .... p 1
- Contraries Versus Similars .... p 2
- Origins and Basic Principles of Homeopathy .... p 2
- Poisons as Potential Medicines .... p 3
- Dilution of Remedies .... p 3
- Basic Rules of Administration in Review .... p 7
- Fundamental Principles in Review .... p 7

CHAPTER 2 REMEDIES AND RESULTS .... p 9
- Single Remedies .... p 9
- Proving the Remedy .... p 9
- Use of High Potency Remedies .... p 9
- Low Potency Combination Remedies .... p 10
- Basic Dosage Guidelines .... p 10
- General Rules of Administration .... p 11
- Words of Caution .... p 12
- Storage and Shelf Life .... p 13
- Labeling Laws .... p 13
- Terms and Definitions .... p 14
- Acute and Chronic Diseases .... p 15
- Suppression .... p 16

CHAPTER 3 FREQUENTLY ASKED QUESTIONS .... p 19

CHAPTER 4 BASIC HOMEOPATHIC LORE .... p 23

CHAPTER 5 TAKING A CASE HISTORY .... p 25
- Taking a Case History by Traditional Methods .... p 25
- Self-Prescribing .... p 25
- The Symptom Picture .... p 26
- Note Taking .... p 27
- Being Observant .... p 27
- A Rare and Confusing Phenomenon .... p 28

CHAPTER 6 TYPES OF REMEDIES .... p 29
- Basic Types of Remedies .... p 29
- Plant, Animal, Mineral Chart .... p 31
- Some Homeopathic Terms .... p 32

SECTION TWO: Lower Potency Remedies

CHAPTER 7 CELL/BIOCHEMIC/TISSUE/SCHUESSLER SALTS .... p 37
Important Nutrients for Life .... p 37
Using Biochemic Remedies .... p 38
The Prevention of Seasonal Illnesses .... p 39
Twelve Biochemic Cell Salts .... p 40
Twelve Biochemic Cell Salts (Chart) .... p 47

CHAPTER 8 FLOWER ESSENCE REMEDIES .... p 49
Case Histories .... p 51

CHAPTER 9 Energetic and Vibrational Remedies .... p 53
Vibrational Remedies .... p 54
Color Remedies .... p 54
Sound Remedies .... p 55
Similarities and Differences Between Color and Sound Remedies .... p 55
Results of Provings .... p 56
Characteristics of Color and Sound Remedies .... p 57

CHAPTER 10 COMBINATION REMEDIES .... p 61

SECTION 3: Miasms/Higher Potency Remedies

CHAPTER 11 PATTERN THINKING .... p 65

CHAPTER 12 REALMS IN HOMEOPATHY .... p 67
The Realms of the Mind (Consciousness) .... p 67
The Other Realms .... p 69
Differentiating Between the Realms .... p 76

CHAPTER 13 GENERAL MIASM INFORMATION .... p 79
Number of Miasms .... p 80
Miasmic Criteria and Definitions .... p 81
Acquired Miasms .... p 82
My Theory of Miasms and the World .... p 83
The Individual—A Microcosm of Creation .... p 85
Healing By Homeopathic Principles .... p 89
Herring's Laws of Cure .... p 90
Suppression and Acquired Miasms .... p 92
Comparison of Miasmic Traits Charts .... p 94

CHAPTER 14 NOSODES AND MIASM DESCRIPTIONS .... p 97
Nosodes and Intercurrent Remedies .... p 97
Flower Essences as Intercurrent Remedies .... p 98
Using Nosode Remedies .... p 98
Basic Nosode and Miasm Descriptions .... p 100
Vaccinosis/Vaccine, Drug, Pollution Nosodes .... p 129
Samuel Hahnemann's Concept of Drug Therapies .... p 135

CHAPTER 15 MIASMS AND PLANT REMEDIES .... p 137
Basic Concepts of Sensations, Actions, and Sensitivities .... p 137
Sensations and Actions of the Miasms List. .... p 140

CHAPTER 16 MIASMS AND THEIR PERIODIC TABLE OF ELEMENTS .... p 145
Comparison Chart—Stages/Series and Miasms .... p 146
Brief Description of Each Series. .... p 147
Brief Description of Each Stage .... p 149

CHAPTER 17 MINERAL REMEDIES BY ELEMENT FAMILIES .... p 151
Single Minerals .... p 151
Polycrest Combination Remedy .... p 156
Additional Mineral Remedies. .... p 162

CHAPTER 18 REMEDIES OF THE PLANT KINGDOM .... p 165
Remedies by Families. .... p 165

CHAPTER 19 ANIMAL REMEDIES .... p 195
Milk Remedies .... p 196
Arachnid Remedies .... p 197
Snake Remedies .... p 201
Ocean Remedies .... p 207
Insect Remedies .... p 211
Butterfly Remedies .... p 215
Miasmic Classification of Remedies .... p 226

SECTION FOUR: Remedies for Specific Conditions

CHAPTER 20 HOMEOPATHY AND FIRST AID .... p 231
First Aid Materia Medica .... p 231
First Aid Conditions .... p 236

CHAPTER 21 LEARNING AND BEHAVIORAL DISORDERS .... p 245
Chronic Anxiety Disorders. .... p 245
Panic Attacks. .... p 246
Eating Disorders. .... p 247
Grief Issues .... p 250
Suicidal Depressions .... p 250
Self Mutilation .... p 252
Violence Disorder (and Post Traumatic Stress) .... p 253
Learning Disabilities .... p 254
Social and Emotional Difficulties. .... p 255
Homeopathic Remedies and Learning Disabilities .... p 255
Labels .... p 256
Remedies for ADHD and Other Learning and Behavioral Disorders ...... p 257
Conclusion—An Interesting Study .... p 262

CHAPTER 22 CHRONIC FATIGUE SYNDROME (CFS) .... p 265
- Symptoms of CFS .... p 265
- Homeopathy and CFS .... p 266
- Stress and CFS .... p 266
- High or Low Potency Remedies .... p 266
- Combination Homeopathic Remedies for CFS .... p 267
- Single Homeopathic Remedies for CFS .... p 272
- Comments and a Final Warning .... p 274

CHAPTER 23 HEART PROBLEMS .... p 275
- Causes and Symptoms .... p 275
- Homeopathic Remedies .... p 275

CHAPTER 24 CONTAGIOUS AND EPIDEMIC DISEASES .... p 277
- Some Things to Consider .... p 278
- One Final Note .... p 279
- Statistics .... p 280
- Statistics and the Last 100 Years .... p 283
- Prevention and Prophylaxis .... p 284
- Suggestion for Treatment .... p 285
- Disease States Discussed in this Chapter .... p 287
- Common Colds, Ordinary Flus, and Headaches .... p 287
- Contagious Childhood Diseases .... p 289
- More Contagious and Epidemic Diseases .... p 296
- Polio Charts .... p 301
- Vaccinations and the Polio Epidemic .... p 303
- To Vaccinate or Not to Vaccinate .... p 304
- Being Prepared .... p 324
- Botox Injections .... p 326
- After-Effects of Serious Disease/Suggestions for Treatment .... p 330

CHAPTER 25 TREATMENT OF CANCER .... p 331

SECTION FIVE: Appendices

APPENDIX A
Homeopathic Treatment Model .... p 336

APPENDIX B
The Process of Cure .... p 340

APPENDIX C
Kinesiology (Muscle Testing) .... p 341

APPENDIX D
Remedies—A Renewable Resource .... p 346

APPENDIX E
Remedies Lists .... p 348

INDEX OF REMEDIES .... p 351

INDEX — General .... p 357

Section One

Basic Principles and Fundamentals of Homeopathy

Introduction

"The highest ideal of therapy is to restore health rapidly, gently, permanently; to remove and destroy the whole disease in the shortest, surest, least harmful way, according to clearly comprehensible principles."
Taken from The Organon of Medicine by Dr. Samuel Hahnemann.

Homeopathy, while viewed by many in the United States as completely invalid or as some kind of weird "voodoo," is in reality the second largest system of medicine in the world. Homeopathy is based on clearly delineated scientific principles and has been repeatedly demonstrated as effective by clinical trials. While the science behind homeopathy was not clearly comprehensible at its inception, modern scientific thought (quantum physics) encompasses and explains so much of why substances prepared by homeopathic principles have an impact on the body. There is no longer any need to defend our belief in homeopathy by saying, "It just feels right and it has worked for me." The science is there and is quite impressive and definitive.

HOMEOPATHIC (AND HERBAL) REMEDIES AID THE BODY IN THE FOLLOWING WAY:

1) Neutralize acute and emergency conditions such as pain, fear, anxiety, burns, bruises, blows and physical traumas, colds, headaches, etc.

2) Balance elements, temperature, fluids, vital energy, life cycles, sleep cycles, etc.

3) Vitalize the constitution in general, improving all the organs and systems as to function and efficiency.

4) Restore health and harmony on mental, emotional, spiritual, and physical levels.

Chapter One - Basic Principles

PHIIOSOPHIES OF THE HEALING ARTS

There seems to have always been, at least in documented history, two distinct philosophies of healing. As far back as the fifth century B.C. Hippocrates (considered to be the father of medicine) recorded his observations to that effect. One method he referred to as healing by the use of 'similars' and the other method he called healing with the use of 'contraries'. Sometime around 400 B.C., Hippocrates is said to have prescribed a minimal dose of mandrake root to **treat** a case of 'mania' based on the accepted knowledge that mandrake root, in larger quantity produced a manic state. He certainly favored the use of similars but his philosophies and writings on this method was, for the most part, ignored by the main stream medical profession over the next 1000 years.

From time to time over the centuries there would be a man espousing philosophies similar to that of Hippocrates and similar to homeopathic thought today. Paracelsus, (1493-1541) a flamboyant and free-thinking German doctor whose full name was Philippus Aureolus Theophrastus Bombastus von Hohenheim, is considered to be the father of chemistry. He based his work on the observation and accurate recording of practical experiences, and on experiments with plants, animals and minerals. He postulated the idea of minerals, or the lack of minerals, being the cause of goiter and other diseases. He was way ahead of his time in many other areas, also. Some of his writings can only be interpreted as predicting the germ theory of disease. He also appears, from his writings and observations, to have been highly intelligent, arrogant, and more than a bit of a rebel.

The doctors of the time were steeped in the occult and beliefs that disease was caused by spirits. Blood letting and purging were the norm and patients died more often than not! It was sometimes hard to determine whether the patient had died of the disease or as result of the treatment. Science was mostly concerned with alchemy—searching for the elixir of life or trying to transmute one substance into another. German folk medicine in the early 1500's, however, was very much based on a like cures like philosophy, especially in regard to plants.

Paracelsus took this belief one step further and postulated that the substance, even if it were a poison, that caused a disease should be looked at as a possible cure. In his experiments and in his practice he noted that a very small dose could overcome a great disease. He was often openly critical of those who believed that contraries cure.

The medical community of his day accused him of advocating the internal consumption of lethal poisons and caused him much grief. It is interesting that within a few years of his death, and certainly today, the established medical model is nearly always high-dose consumption of various lethal poisons. His observations in many areas, including the law of similars, were ignored for another 200 plus years.

What are we referring to when we use the terms healing by contraries or healing by similars?

Contraries Versus Similars

CONTRARIES AS MEDICINES

An example of healing by contraries—antidotes as they are known in today's terminology—would be the giving of a laxative to correct constipation. The underlying problem with this form of healing is three-fold. First, most of the substances prescribed, then and now, are toxic and must be given in un-healthy doses in order to bring about a result. In other words, all drugs have side effects. The second problem lies in stopping the action at the desired level without over-doing it (example: stopping the diarrhea that has ensued because of the medicine taken for constipation). The third difficulty, of course, is the development of dependency by the body on the drug in order to accomplish a normal bodily function.

SIMILARS AS MEDICINES

The law of similars, on which homeopathy is based, states that when an imbalanced state exists (given a dis-ease name today), we seek, as a cure, a remedy that would create the same symptoms of distress in a healthy body. How can this postulation possibly make sense? Put very simply, the remedy given, because of it similarity to the disease, brings that particular symptom pattern to the attention of the energy system (or immune system, if you prefer). The body then focuses on the imbalance and handles it in the most efficient manner possible. The result is often the return of the body to normal functioning, instead of just masking the symptom without any rebalancing or correcting of the underlying causes.

#1 This "law of similars" is the first and most fundamental rule of homeopathic theory and practice.

In review, any substance that can produce symptoms of disease in a healthy person, can aid in the amelioration or cure of those same symptoms in a sick person. The closer a remedy is to the range of symptoms the person is experiencing, the more likely and effective will be the cure. Homeopathic practitioners call this "the totality of symptoms." Besides obvious physical symptoms, the list of symptoms always includes such things such as the person's emotional and mental state, what conditions improve or worsen the symptoms, and how the symptoms are manifesting, to name just a few areas.

Origins and Basic Principles

Dr. Samuel Hahnemann (1755-1843), of Germany, is considered to be the father of homeopathic thought and treatment. Hahnemann was a physician and chemist. In 1790, at the age of 35, he was working on a translation into German of a report about the treatment of malaria with china bark. The report claimed that the healing effect of this bark was due to its stomach strengthening power. Dr. Hahnemann became curious and decided to test the medicine on himself. He soon realized that shortly after taking the medicine, every time, he would experience symptoms that were similar to those experienced by people with malaria. He would experience extreme thirst, intolerable anxiety, dizziness, a feeling of numbness over the whole body, and overwhelming weakness. These symptoms would last for only a short period of time and then go away. After several such experiences, he was led to conclude that china bark, when taken by a healthy person, brought about malaria-like symptoms.

Dr. Hahnemann, with his education in medicine, would have been familiar with the writings of Hippocrates on curing with similars. Perhaps this knowledge helped bring Hahnemann to the conclusion that it was the malaria-producing qualities of the china bark that stimulated the defense mechanism of the malaria-suffering patient, thereby setting the process of self-healing in motion.

From the time of his first discovery, Hahnemann dedicated his energies and his life to the search for new remedies that corresponded to particular diseases and to finding a way to administer them that was gentle, safe and effective. Hahnemann tested substances on himself, his family, friends, students, and colleagues. By his death in 1835, he had scientifically tested nearly one hundred substances. Every reaction and every symptom that these substances activated in healthy people was painstakingly recorded in what came to be called a Materia Medica. To this day, nothing of the original protocols that he recorded have been significantly changed. It is interesting to note the verbiage of the day in the descriptions as we try to interpret them today.

The Materia Medicas of today (sometimes called remedy guides by modern homeopathic professionals) are detailed descriptions of homeopathic remedies, just as they were in Hahnemann's day. These reference books still contain many of his descriptions and "provings" today still follow many of his established protocols. All in all, more than 2000 substances, all tested according to the principles Hahnemann established, have been documented and are in use today.

POISONS AS POTENTIAL MEDICINES

Hahnemann began his search, and research, by "proving" the medications of his day, most of which were highly toxic, just as they are now. Hahnemann's research led him on to documenting the effects of other substances that were known to produce drastic reactions in people. Arsenic was one of the early examples of this testing process.

Because the substances were so toxic, it was essential to administer just enough of the substance to produce symptoms strong enough to document, without killing the person doing the trial, or proving, as the trials came to be called.

Problems with toxic medicines are—and always have been—three-fold:

1) Unhealthy, destructive doses are required in order to effect a "cure."

2) How to stop the action of the cure once it is no longer needed.

3) The too real possibility of the person becoming dependent on the substance for normal function.

After much trial and error and with, I believe, more than a little bit of inspiration, Hahnemann developed a method of diluting and succussing which made the substances less toxic while also making the remedies more potent and the healing effects both more pronounced and long-lasting. Hahnemann tapped his remedies against a Bible.

DILUTION OF REMEDIES

Dilution alone eventually produces a remedy that has no side effects, but neither does it effect a cure. Succussion is a necessary part of the preparation process. This method of dilution and succussion is still being used around the world today—although without a Bible, in most cases. It seems to be equally effective just to shake them (rather than tap them against a surface of any kind). Shaking (or tapping) approximately 100 times seems to be about right. Shaking through the curved fingers of one hand seems to be particularly effective.

The remedies Hahnemann was using to obtain his cures eventually contained nothing discernible of the original substance, and yet their effects were profound. The same is true of today's remedies; there are not discernible molecules of the original substances. In this day and age, however, we have technologies that can determine the electrical frequency of substances. Theories abound, based on these studies, as to why and how homeopathic remedies work. Perhaps they all have elements of the truth in them. The principles of quantum physics fill a lot of gaps in our understanding of how homeopathy works.

It is wondrous to me that Samuel Hahnemann made his discoveries without the use of these technologies. He operated very much by the scientific method of experimentation, carefully documenting each case and each remedy as he worked. As is often the case with trailblazing discoveries, his work seems to have been a combination of knowledge, intuition, and observation.

In 1828, just seven years before his death, Hahnemann published <u>Chronic Diseases and Their Homeopathic Cure</u> (it ran to five volumes). He discussed the use of higher potency remedies and introduced the concept of miasms, which we will describe briefly later in this section and discuss in more detail in section three of this book.

The fact that homeopathic remedies are effective—even if no molecules of the mother solution are present—is the most difficult principle for the medical profession (and many others) to understand. It is not surprising that homeopathy has often been dismissed with the objection, "There is nothing there; therefore, it cannot possibly work!" The technologies mentioned previously, which detect electrical frequencies, prove that something is certainly there. It is interesting to note that skilled kinesiologists (muscle testers) can determine one remedy, and even one potency, from another with great accuracy.

Let's look for a moment at another assumption that has been disproved. People have similarly dismissed the suggestion that plants and people are surrounded by an aura of electrical waves that can be seen by some people and that differ from person to person. But, with the invention of Kirlian photography it is now possible to prove to the skeptics that they are wrong about this. (The fact that there are people who can "see" this energy is also of interest but still seems to have little meaning for the scientific community.)

The most important proof of the effectiveness of homeopathy is in the dramatic results that are obtained by so many people in so many different situations.

Studies have shown that when a drop or two of a substance such as an essential oil is added to a bath, the entire volume of water then contains the anti-viral/anti-bacterial properties of the oil. In fact, certain of the effects are heightened, often being more pronounced in the dilute liquid than in the original substance. This is much like what happens with homeopathic remedies, except that homeopathic remedies are diluted repeatedly and shaken (succussed) between each dilution. Succussing emphasizes the properties.

Even if the dilution becomes so great that no discernible molecules can be found, the memory of the substance and the frequency of it are still there. Technology today can tell one remedy from another but, at the higher dilutions (potencies), instruments still cannot determine what the original substance was. (This fact is a very great blessing to the homeopathic community!)

DILUTION AND POTENCY

Homeopathic remedies, because they are **very diluted** solutions, can be made from just about anything. Except for the energetic variety (sometimes called imponderables), homeopathic remedies are created from a tincture or other form of solution derived from a plant, animal product, mineral, salt, or tissue of some kind. This solution is then systematically diluted and succussed (shaken) in order to, as Hahnemann worded it, (for lack of a better explanation) unlock the healing energy of the substance and transfer it to the carrier solution. The carrier solution is almost always pure water. Alcohol is usually added to the finished remedy as a preservative.

Each time the solution is diluted and shaken the potency is changed. The first time would result in a potency of 1. When the solution is diluted and shaken again it moves to a potency of 2. The dilution process can be continued indefinitely to achieve whatever potency is desired.

> **#2 The second fundamental premise, and the paradox, of homeopathic thought, can be stated in one simple sentence: the more dilute a solution, the more potent it becomes.**

The more times the remedy has been diluted and shaken, the higher its potency. Eventually the solution will contain no discernible molecules of the original substance. Nevertheless this high potency form will elicit very specific symptoms when administered to a person who is not ill. The symptoms created by the remedy are the symptom picture of the illness for which the remedy should be taken.

How much of the mother solution and how much water should be used? In other words, what is the ratio of the dilution? (Please see Appendix D for more information on homeopathics as a renewable resource.)

SCALES OF DILUTION

- There are several common scales of dilution:
- 1. The most common is the C scale, which is a 1:100 ratio
  This means that for each drop of the mother solution 100 drops of water are used.
- 2. D scale, which is a ratio of 1:10. This is also called the X scale, depending on what part of the world you ordered your homeopathic remedies from.
- 3. The M scale is a little bit different. It is a series of C scale (1:100) dilutions. A 1M is a 1000C remedy, a 10M is a 10,000C remedy, and a 50M is a 50,000C remedy. This M scale is the basis of constitutional, epidemic and other deep level prescribing.

The D or X scale (1:10 dilution) is the lowest potency. The C scale (1:100 dilution) is next in strength, with the M scale (series of C scale dilutions) being the highest potency.

SOURCES OF HOMEOPATHIC REMEDIES

As explained previously, the first homeopathic remedies were made from the medicines of Hahnemann's day which were, as they are today, mostly toxic. Other toxic substances were experimented with. Plants such as valerian and belladonna, which produce pronounced effects on the mind, were among the early "provings."

There are more than a thousand (nearly 2,000) remedies listed in various Materia Medicas today and they come from a wide range of innocuous substances as well as toxic and poisonous materials. The various homeopathic remedy families will be discussed, in great detail, later on in this book.

#3 A third fundamental principle of homeopathy is that any substance, prepared homeopathically, may become a potent and safe medicine.

TREAT THE PERSON — NOT THE DISEASE

It is absolutely imperative to the proper use of homeopathic (or herbal) remedies to understand that we must treat the entire patient, not just a symptom or two. It is also important that we don't treat based on a general disease pattern as indicated by the allopathic name of the disease. In treating the whole person, we must take into account emotional and mental factors, as well as inherited conditions and predispositions.

Imagine the whole person as a jigsaw puzzle. Prescribing on one symptom alone is like seeing only a small part of the puzzle. This method does not give enough information to work out what the whole picture is. If you look at only a symptom or two you will be unable to determine which remedy is really needed. Once you have located most of the pieces of the puzzle—and of the person—and have fitted them together into a complete picture, you will be better able to move the body, mind, and spirit toward healing.

A comprehensive list of symptoms will give you the overall picture but you should always ask yourself, "How is this person and their symptoms different from other people with similar complaints?" Each person has his own unique way of reacting to an illness or disease and the remedies used must reflect that uniqueness.

Always remember that the pains, and even the diseases, from which the person is suffering very often reflect the way in which the person is coping with the stresses of his life in general at this time. His unique personality and the unique circumstances of his life will combine to create a unique situation. The choice of a homeopathic remedy will reflect both his own nature and the nature of his circumstances.

#4 *A fourth principle of homeopathy is to always treat the whole person, not just a single symptom or symptoms based only on a "disease" name.*

"It is more important to know what kind of person has the disease
than to know what kind of disease the person has."
~Hippocrates~

SYMPTOMS GOVERN REMEDY CHOICE

As homeopathic remedies are "proven," a picture emerges of the symptoms that are common to the majority of people. There also emerges a list of less common reactions. All of these symptoms are collated and compiled. Eventually the remedy and its description makes its way into Materia Medicas. The symptoms listed in bold or bold/italics are the most common symptoms—almost universal—among the provers.

For a remedy to be as effective as possible, the symptoms being experienced by the person and the symptoms described in the book must match on as many levels as possible. Mental as well as physical patterns must be looked at. What is referred to in homeopathy as *modalities* is also very important. This is the homeopathic term for those things which make us feel better or worse. For example, Bryonia lists "worse for any motion" while Rhus toxicodendron will list "worse for inactivity. Any unusual patterns such as periodicity—only at certain times of the day or calendar—year may also be considered.

#5 This brings us to the 5th fundamental principle of homeopathy: The "totality" of symptoms will always govern the choice of the homeopathic remedy. It is critically important that the remedy "picture" match the person and his symptoms on as many levels as possible!

IMMEDIATE RESULTS PLUS LONG TERM BENEFITS

When the correct remedy—a remedy that was based on as complete a picture of the symptoms as you could gather—is given, the immediate results are often amazing! Better still, however, is that the remedy also creates a response deep in the person's energy system, informing and unraveling the mis-perceptions and imbalances that may exist there. The removal of these imbalances impacts the future for good as the body responds more appropriately to similar events in the future.

In one of the case histories found in Miranda Castro's book, <u>The Complete Homeopathy Handbook</u>, there is a marvelous illustration of this principle. In my own words, the case tells a story similar to the following:

> A private, introspective, and quiet eleven-year-old boy develops a bad sore throat. He complains of constant pain and says that it feels as though there is a lump in his throat. The pain is better when he is eating or drinking, which seems odd considering the feeling of a lump in his throat. He is home from school and is moping around and spending most of his time in his room. He seems very sad and has withdrawn from the family and looks as though he has been crying. When asked, he denies that anything is wrong. Eventually, when he is pressed until he becomes cross and angry, he finally admits that he is crying himself to sleep every night.
>
> This little boy had an adored pet rabbit which died last week and he has been getting increasingly more quiet and withdrawn ever since. His mother tells you that he had a similar sore throat last year when his best friend moved to another part of the country. Antibiotics were tried and did not help at all and it took him weeks to recover.
>
> There are two or three common remedies that fit the generals of this case, Natrum muriaticum and Ignatia amara among them. When *all* the symptoms, including the contradictory nature of a sore throat that feels better for swallowing something, are considered it is concluded that Ignatia amara is the right remedy. This remedy will move the child through the sore throat very quickly, most likely without the use of antibiotics, and help him to cope with grief more easily in the future. Both Natrum muriaticum and Ignatia amara personalities generally handle grief in increasingly difficult and destructive ways as they grow older.

#6 The sixth principle of homeopathic treatment: The correct remedy, chosen using "wholeistic" principles will produce immediate results and, at the same time, impact the future for good.

DISCONTINUE THE REMEDY UPON IMPROVEMENT

#7 Once you see a marked improvement from the administration of a remedy, the taking of the remedy should be discontinued. This rule can be considered the 7th—and possibly the most important—principle of homeopathic treatment.

A homeopathic remedy is a catalyst. It stimulates the body to begin healing itself. A muscle test is the best indication of frequency of dosage and of when to stop giving the remedy altogether. If you don't muscle test, be sure to follow the traditional rule of giving a remedy only until the person begins to show signs of improvement. Repeat the remedy when symptoms return or the improvement you were seeing stalls out. If returning symptoms have altered in any way, a different remedy based on the new symptom picture will need to be used. The administration of homeopathic remedies without using the muscle test is an intuitive judgment call based on the knowledge that you have acquired. The more knowledge—and intuition—you have, the more accurate you will be. Follow the norms outlined below but be sure to pay attention to your common sense and intuition.

Always check back with people if you have recommended a homeopathic to them. People have become so accustomed to taking medications until the bottle is empty that they often do this with the homeopathic that you gave them! This can be a rather serious mistake. If they report that they felt better for a time but now the same symptoms are back—worse than ever—they have probably taken the remedy for too long a period of time and/or have taken it too often.

BASIC RULES OF ADMINISTRATION IN REVIEW

- Always stop on improvement.

- Start again if the same symptoms return and then repeat dosages as needed.

- If you have given several doses and have had no response, stop and reassess. It is very likely that you have chosen the wrong remedy entirely. In reality, this rarely happens.

- Change the remedy if the symptom picture changes. If the same symptoms return, repeat the remedy you have given or move to a higher potency for a dose or two.

- An improvement in mood and feelings of well-being is often the first and most accurate indication that you have the right remedy and it is working.

I think of a homeopathic remedy as a pebble which, when thrown into a pond, simply goes plop. It is the ripples created within the body that are the healing responses. The closer the person's symptoms match the remedy picture, the closer you have come to hitting the center of the pond with your rock and the more beautiful—and beneficial—will be the results.

FUNDAMENTAL PRINCIPLES IN REVIEW

#1 The Law of Similars, simply stated, is "Like Cures Like." The symptoms that a substance creates in a well person are the symptoms that the substance will ameliorate in a sick person.

#2 The more dilute the remedy, the more potent it has become.

#3 Prepared homeopathically, any substance may become a potent and <u>safe</u> remedy.

#4 Always treat the whole person, not just a single symptom or symptoms based only on a "disease" name.

#5 The totality of symptoms govern the choice of a remedy.

#6 The correct remedy, chosen "whole" - istically, will produce immediate results and, at the same time, impact the future of the person for good.

#7 Stop giving the remedy at the "first sign" of improvement. The "first sign" will usually be an emotional one.

Chapter Two - Remedies and Results

SINGLE REMEDIES

Hahnemann, in his day, used only a single remedy at a time, in low potency. Many people still consider this to be the most effective method. It would certainly make it easier to gauge the results and know exactly what is being accomplished when only one single remedy has been given.

The main drawback with the use of single remedies is accuracy of prescribing. The totality of symptoms must match well the picture of the remedy for results to be obtained. This is especially true when using higher potencies. Since we are treating the entire person and not just this particular disease or set of symptoms, a clear picture of the person's life in general must be considered. This is called "taking the case." Personality, likes and dislikes, what makes the symptoms worse, and many other details must be determined.

A correctly done case history takes time and skill. Choosing the remedy, based on the details, can be difficult unless you are very experienced with homeopathics and have a phenomenal memory. If the correct single remedy is given, in any potency, the results are often amazing. **Muscle testing can be a great help here.**

PROVING THE REMEDY

A homeopathic remedy, if not well-chosen, can produce energetic symptoms similar to the picture of the remedy. Remember, a remedy will produce the symptoms in a well person that it will help eradicate in a person who is ill. The creation of these energetic symptoms, which match the symptom picture of the chosen remedy, is called proving the remedy. They are an indication that a better remedy might have been chosen.

The symptoms created by an incorrect remedy can range from mildly annoying to quite extreme The duration and severity of this reaction is worse at higher potencies or when the remedy was taken inappropriately many times. Typically, any symptoms will subside quickly once the remedy has been discontinued.

Sometimes a remedy is given because it is the closest match available and any newly emerging symptoms can be tolerated until they go away. This is an acceptable, although not the best way to give homeopathic remedies. Most of us, unless we have a large collection of homeopathic remedies, lots of experience, and good muscle testing skills, have used a less than perfect remedy when it was the best we could manage.

There is a new school of thought emerging among homeopaths. Some experienced practitioners are coming to believe that homeopathics only produce aggravation of *previous* symptoms—***symptoms not being experienced right now but that were present somewhere in the person's past.*** If this new theory is correct, you can't produce new symptoms by giving the wrong homeopathic. Only symptoms that existed in the person before will be seen and the person will be benefited by having them cleared from his energy system.

This is very good news. The remedy reaches into the energy system, brings the pattern—if it exists—on-line so that it can be corrected, but does not 'prove' the remedy in a well person or in a person who does not need that pattern cleared! This theory makes sense with some things I have seen working with people.

THE USE OF HIGH POTENCY REMEDIES

Higher dosage prescribing is divided into two areas, acute and constitutional, and will be discussed in detail in another section of this book. The premise of higher potency prescribing is to stimulate the body's healing mechanism to eradicate the problem entirely and permanently. Higher potency remedies are believed to act on the mental/psychological underpinnings of a malady and, thus, bring about a deeper, more permanent cure. I believe that all homeopathic remedies act in a 'whole person' manner and I have had success with both methods. I am often astonished, however, at the healing capacity of the higher potency remedies. People who have suffered for a long time with a chronic condition, in my experience, often do not respond at all to lower potency remedies, but respond rapidly to the higher potencies.

LOW POTENCY COMBINATION REMEDIES

Because of the knowledge and skill (or muscle testing) required in the use of single remedies, combination remedies have become popular in modern use. A combination remedy is made up of several remedies whose symptom picture includes, for example, headaches. These remedies are placed together in a single bottle. There is no attempt made to determine whether the headache is worse for hot or cold, movement or stillness, or whether the person prefers to be left alone or likes people around to whine to, etc. In fact, care is taken when creating the combination to assure that many differing, even opposing, symptom pictures are included.

This approach seems to work quite well and is an excellent starting place for learning homeopathic theories and principles. The drawback is that combination remedies can only be used at very low potency levels. At higher potencies, the person taking the remedy may begin to experience some of the symptoms that were not clearly indicated. In other words, they develop symptoms similar to the remedies that were not part of their original symptoms. For example, if one of the remedies had, included in its description, "frontal headache centered over the right eye" but the headache the person is experiencing right now is occipital in nature, they may develop an additional headache over the right eye, hopefully for only a short time.

It has never been adequately shown that mild symptom pictures are not produced by the unnecessary single remedies in a combination, even at these lower potencies; however, I don't believe I have ever seen one of any seriousness or deep discomfort. Because the potencies are low, the body seems to be able to cope with the energy of the unneeded remedies.

MAKING USE OF BOTH HIGH AND LOW POTENCY REMEDIES

Among homeopathic practitioners there is still a bit of a split between those who use low potency remedies given in quick succession for several doses, and those who use a single remedy in higher potencies only once or twice. I have found that there is a time and a place for both methods. With practice, study, and pondering, (and the muscles test) you can become proficient in the use of both types of remedies.

Higher potency prescribing is often left to experienced practitioners. I believe that the development of good muscle testing skills, combined with some practical knowledge of homeopathic principles and remedies, makes these amazing remedies amazingly effective for us. Higher potency single remedies seem to go more deeply into the system to eradicate the original causes of the problem and then prevent future occurrences. Be a little more cautious and conscientious when using higher potencies. Always read the literature of a remedy to determine if it is a match to the person and the problem. There is no substitute for careful study and thought. When done properly, high potency single remedies have no more potential for problems—perhaps are even less problematic in some ways—than do the low potency combinations.

With that opinion expressed, I must tell you that there are many combination remedies that I have used on a regular basis for many years with great results. Low potency combination remedies are especially useful for acute situations and where time (and energy) for choosing the exact single remedy is simply not available. Whenever a low potency remedy is used with success, it is a good idea to take the time later to look up each individual remedy. Try to determine which one matched the symptoms best and was most likely responsible for the improvement experienced. If this is done, a great deal can be learned about effective homeopathic treatment at the higher potencies. Following up with the single remedy identified in this way, if another dose is needed, will carry the healing to a deeper level.

Basic Dosage Guidelines

COMBINATIONS AND LOW POTENCY SINGLE REMEDIES

Combination remedies are very low potency. These remedies are meant to be taken several times a day for 3-5 days, followed by a break of not taking the remedy for the next 2-4 days. Often this cycle is repeated at least one more time. Taking a break is essential. The homeopathic remedy brings the symptoms to the attention of the vital force. In low potency, it takes several doses over a period of time to keep the energy moving in the right direction. When the progress of the healing slows, the cycle of administration is repeated.

In acute cases, where pain or symptoms have come on suddenly, giving the remedy (low potency only!) every 5 minutes for up to an hour will give you the best results with the least chance of any adverse reaction.

30C remedies are slightly higher in potency and strength. They are usually administered only 1 time per day for the same 3 or 4 days that is suggested for the low potency remedies. Sometimes they will need to be given more often and more frequently, depending on the severity of the symptoms. This is a judgement call, made based on the overall health and strength of the person. Until I learned to muscle test, how often and at what strength to administer a homeopathic remedy was always guesswork and I was never completely sure that I had gotten the dosage exactly right.

HIGHER POTENCY SINGLE REMEDIES

200C remedies are usually taken only once per day, and it is even generally advisable to skip a day between doses. For some people a 200C remedy acts as a higher potency. A repeat dose should be given when progress toward wellness has halted or slowed.

In the standard literature, 1M remedies are taken at 3 week intervals and 10M remedies about 3 months apart. However, following the muscle test paints a much different picture. In dramatic situations such as spider bites or severe burns, I have used (and seen others use) 1M and 10M remedies in succession at intervals of only a few minutes. Anything less than this would have not have produced sufficient or rapid enough results. It was necessary in each case, eventually, to antidote and start over with a clean slate. Good muscle testing skills take the guesswork out of homeopathy and make it much more effective and certainly easier.

50M remedies are meant to be used in deep level constitutional programs. They are administered at 5 to 6 month intervals and, typically, only 2 or 3 times.

GENERAL RULES OF ADMINISTRATION

A good rule of thumb in the use of homeopathic remedies is to give the lowest potency needed to accomplish healing. A 30C given 3 or 4 times a day for 4 or 5 days can be as effective as using a 200C less frequently. However, some people are not faithful about taking the remedies. You might choose to give one dose of a higher potency right then, one time while they are with you, as the most effective method for them.

Sometimes your decision to use a lower potency remedy will be based on how far you can trust the person to follow your instructions, whether they will be careful to keep the remedy out of the hands of children, and whether or not they can understand that they should not take the remedy continually until the bottle is empty as they would an allopathic antibiotic. The number one mistake made in using homeopathic remedies is continuing to take the remedy after the body has taken over the healing process as the result of the stimulation/message provided by the homeopathic remedy.

At other times you will choose the lower potency remedy because it just seems better to nudge the vital force a little bit rather than to bowl it over with the stronger remedy. This is especially true of very small children or people whose ailment has made them quite weak and debilitated. Many times small children do not need anything stronger than a 6X or 30C simply because they are not old enough to have any complaints of the long-standing variety, except the ones they have inherited from their parents. Dealing with these inherited complaints and tendencies will be discussed later in the third section of this book.

When using pellets, tip the pellets into the lid of the bottle and then into your hand. It is acceptable to touch a remedy you intend to take yourself, but never touch a remedy before giving it to someone else. Do not put any remedy you have touched back into the bottle. If any pellets fall onto the floor or onto any other surface, discard them. Returning them to the bottle can spoil the whole batch. If using a liquid remedy, never allow the dropper or bottle top to touch fingers, mouth, or anything else.

Pellets should be dissolved in the mouth, preferably under the tongue. If they are swallowed immediately, they become mixed with stomach acids before being absorbed. This makes the remedies less effective. Sublingual administration (under the tongue) is thought to send the frequency directly into the blood stream and bioplasm of the body. Sublingual administration is not necessary with homeopathics in liquid form.

Some homeopathic practitioners believe quite strongly that it is important not to eat, drink, or brush your teeth for at least 20 minutes before and after any remedy is given. Personally, I have not found this to be as crucial as the literature suggests. I have put low potency remedies in a small child's bottle or sippy cup filled with a mild juice with excellent results, time after time. I have used homeopathics in birth and emergency situations where food, or even medications, were taken right along with the remedy. The homeopathic remedies have never failed to work as I needed them to.

The size of the dose of a homeopathic is irrelevant. This is true regardless of what it may say on the bottle you just bought at the health food store. Adjusting the dose according to age or the body weight of the person is illogical by homeopathic principles. Homeopathics work by energetic frequencies; there is not a measurable quantity of the original substance in the remedy so it does not matter how much is taken at a time. How often the remedy is taken is what matters most. I usually instruct people to take 2-3 tablets if using pellets or a few drops if using a liquid remedy. Many people, however, are only comfortable when being given instructions to take a specific amount of the remedy. It is usually best to give them a quantity until they have more understanding of the principles involved.

If you use a glass or a spoon to administer a remedy, be sure to scour it out thoroughly, immediately. If you leave the energy imprint of the remedy in the glass or spoon someone may inadvertently receive a dose of a homeopathic they have no need for and then won't understand what is wrong with them as the remedy produces symptoms in their body and mind.

Very high potency remedies that need to be sipped (this is called plussing and is explained in a later section) need to be put in a container with a lid. I have had instances where people standing in the vicinity of such a high potency remedy developed clear symptoms of a remedy that was sitting on someone's desk when they passed by. In each case, the person affected was particularly weak and susceptible, but that is all the more reason to be careful. They do not need to borrow trouble from your remedy.

WORDS OF CAUTION

Problems and extreme adverse reactions to homeopathic remedies are rare. If any kind of problem does occur, it is usually the result of:

(1) Taking the wrong remedy entirely.
(2) Taking the remedy in a higher potency than the constitution of the person could easily tolerate.
(3) Taking a remedy for too long, or after the symptoms have already begun to improve.

Problems do not arise from taking too much of the remedy at one time. Since homeopathic remedies are not based on a material dose (there is almost none, or none at all, of the object the remedy was originally made from in the remedy), how much is given, or taken accidentally, is irrelevant. If your child takes a whole bottle of a remedy at one sitting, he will have no more effects than if he took 1-2 pellets or a few drops.

The higher the potency, the more potential there is for accidentally creating symptoms. Experience, developing good muscle testing skills, working carefully, and always matching the remedy to the person on as many physical and emotional points as you can will insure that you are both effective and safe in your work.

Homeopathic remedies can be antidoted by looking up the specific antidote for the remedy you have used at the back of the symptom description in a Materia Medica. Antidote remedies are usually given in 30C or 200C potency. Camphor (found in Vicks-Vapo-Rub) antidotes most homeopathics, as do large quantities of caffeine. Some toothpastes which list peppermint on the label really have a form of camphor in them. These toothpastes may affect homeopathic remedies.

ADDITIONAL NOTES

Never rush into giving a homeopathic remedy, and don't think that you have to give a remedy just because someone asks. This should apply to anything you do for anyone, but is particularly true of homeopathic remedies. If you don't know the person well, or you don't feel they will use the remedy wisely, or you feel unsure or uncomfortable in any way, then don't do it.

Always stress to people that a homeopathic remedy is a means of stimulating the body to balance itself—and, sometimes, time and patience may be required. Often we are too quick to rush in with another remedy or to give up on the one we are using. God already gave us what we would need when he provided us with an immune system. If we have maintained our body properly, it may handle the problem very nicely all on its own. This is not to be interpreted as an excuse to put off until tomorrow what should be taken care of today. If you need a homeopathic to stimulate your vital defenses, the sooner you take it the more effective it will be.

Give a remedy only when the person asks you for help (and then only if you feel comfortable doing so). If you run where you are not called without sufficiently educating the person, they will quite likely antidote the remedy accidentally; if they don't and they see an improvement it will likely be attributed to a coincidence. This is not to say that just because they are skeptical you should not help them, it is saying that giving people something they are not ready for often slows down their learning and deprives them of their right to look after their own health in their own way.

It is often difficult to admit to or even see your own emotional patterns, and emotional patterns are a very important part of identifying the right remedy. Use muscle testing or a good friend to double check your remedy choice when self-prescribing. If you test for a remedy, it is often very educational and enlightening to read the emotional patterns if you can do so with an open mind and a determination to learn and grow.

STORAGE AND SHELF LIFE OF REMEDIES

Remedies can come in several different forms. You will probably develop a preference for either liquids or pellets, or you may decide to have both for use in different situations—if storage space is not a problem for you. Liquid remedies can be applied nicely to the skin, where they absorb and are often just as effective as taking them internally. Liquids are also easier to administer to babies and small children.

Homeopathic remedies in liquid form will keep their strength for years and years without deteriorating. They must be stored in reasonably cool, relatively dry places and their tops must be screwed on tightly. It is preferable to keep remedies in dark glass as light can affect them negatively.

Remedies should also be kept away from strong-smelling things such as mothballs and synthetic essential oils. Strong magnetic fields alter their frequency, as well. When using a remedy that has been sitting idle for a long time, shake it a few times against the palm of your hand to "fluff" it back up to full strength.

Pellets also store reasonably well. You must keep them tightly sealed as any moisture will cause the pellets to clump together or disintegrate into powder. Since the quantity of the remedy taken doesn't really matter, this is only an inconvenience, not a complete disaster.

LABELING LAWS AND HOMEOPATHIC REMEDIES

Labeling laws for homeopathic remedies at this time require that both the English and Latin name of the original substance be on the label, if at all possible. Homeopathic remedies made from tissue salts are exempt from this ruling because the Latin name is often the common name. The law also requires that the potency be displayed on the label and that the condition for which it is recommended be indicated also. Since a homeopathic will be effective for an entire list of things, this requirement is not very helpful and is extremely annoying and inconvenient to the manufacturer. Further, no homeopathic remedy may claim to cure any life threatening condition.

The label must also specify how often, how much, and for how long the remedy should be taken—even if this information is irrelevant and will vary from person to person and case to case.

So, how did these laws come to be enacted (other than obvious government bumbling)? In an atmosphere of fear of what was not understood and in the face of impending legislation that would have driven homeopathic medicines underground or taken them from us altogether, a group of dedicated homeopathic practitioners and manufacturers made the best of a bad situation. They spent a great deal of time and money (and must have gotten very frustrated for their efforts) in working with the FDA and legislators to have laws implemented that would cause the homeopathic industry (and those of us out here using them) no major inconvenience.

I have read the transcripts of many of the sessions. They make amusing reading. These wonderful men were more concerned with getting rules established that would allow homeopathics to be available to people than in convincing the members of the committee of the efficacy of homeopathic treatment or trying to educate them on the finer points of homeopathic theory, although some education must have occurred.

These men somehow managed to keep homeopathic remedies, which are taken internally, from being labeled as a food supplement (which they are not, of course) by pointing out that there is no material dose of any substance in a remedy. Labeling the remedy as a homeopathic (or prana or energetic) remedy avoids prosecution for fraud since the very basis of homeopathic theory is that there is nothing there and there is no claim being made that there is! I am not sure why, having arrived at the conclusion that there is nothing there, the committee required that the label include what symptoms the remedy is for. Fortunately, it is a requirement that is easily met. Just understand that what is recommended on the label is only one thing the remedy is useful for. And remember, too, that dosage is too individual a thing to be explained adequately on any label. Don't take the label, or the accompanying literature, too seriously. Using homeopathic remedies well requires more study and responsibility than perusing labels at a health food store.

TODAY

The atmosphere for the sale of homeopathic remedies changed again a few years ago. There was a movement to place the sale of homeopathic remedies only in the hands of "qualified" (I use that term facetiously) medical personnel. Chiropractors volunteered. I am hesitant to call them qualified, although some of them surely are, because many of them have not put forth the effort to learn all that they should about homeopathy before prescribing. Many of us "lay" people are far more educated on this subject than some chiropractors are and many of the people I work with are putting forth a great deal of effort to educate themselves and become adept and self-sufficient. The prices of homeopathics in chiropractors' offices are often prohibitive.

Very recently, as homeopathic remedies become more and more popular, the federal government is beginning to show an interest in regulating homeopathic remedies by requiring licenses and specifying the conditions for education and licensing. If this occurs, it will follow the pattern that has occurred in India, England and other countries where homeopathic medicines were recognized as effective and became recognized as having a great money-making potential.

The new laws, in the various ways they have been proposed so far and are likely to be proposed should regulation go forward, would certainly keep the general population from stocking these amazing healers and sharing them with each other. The goal of Butterfly Express has been in the past to get as many homeopathics into the hands of people as possible so that, in the times of trouble, should they ever come, there is a people prepared to take care of themselves and their families using these amazing healers.

HOMEOPATHIC TERMS AND DEFINITIONS

CONSTITUTION AND SUSCEPTIBILITY

Constitution is defined as "genetic inheritance modified by environment," or "the combination of state of health and temperament as it relates to life-style and environment." A strong constitution can withstand considerable pressure without falling ill. A weak constitution has an increased susceptibility to disease. Susceptibility can be inherited, created by past or current stress, and be aggravated by poor nutrition.

VITAL FORCE

Homeopathic people believe there is a balancing mechanism that keeps us in health, provided that the stresses on us are neither too prolonged nor too great. Hahnemann called this balancing mechanism the vital force. Eastern healing philosophies refer to it as chi, prana, and various other terms. Familiar expressions such as immune system are a more western way of referring to this vital force. The body continually sends us signals about how it is coping with its environment. Some examples might be shivering when cold, perspiring when overheated, or feeling hungry or thirsty. Homeopathic philosophy, and many other philosophies, believe that disease prevails only when this vital force has been weakened in some way.

SYMPTOMS

Symptoms are those things that are going on in our lives that are not (or should not be) considered normal. Symptoms include physical things, such as itching, sneezing, pain, stiffness, and other such things. Symptoms also include mental and emotional aspects of our lives as well as the things which make us feel better or worse. Symptoms indicate that the vital force is trying to get your attention.

Symptoms, in my mind and in the minds of many homeopathic people, are looked upon as limitations to our freedom to do the things that we want to do when we want to do them. Aches and pains, fever, headache, etc., slow us down, keep us at home, and otherwise limit our lives and keep us from accomplishing the things that we would like to.

Symptoms are just what the name implies; they are the symptoms of what is really going on in the body physically, mentally, and spiritually. They are never considered to be, or confused with, the actual underlying disturbance to the energy system and body that is the real problem. Repairing or eradicating this underlying energy disturbance is what we need to focus our treatment on. Relieving symptoms is wonderful and a marvelous humanitarian gesture, but it is often only the first step. It is likely not the whole cure!

DISEASE

Disease refers to a combination of symptoms that are occurring together. In traditional homeopathic thought, symptoms are ***never*** piled together and given a disease name. A homeopath may speak of diseases as a way of communicating with the rest of the world (those people who think in the western medical model), but he thinks in terms of the totality of symptoms. This totality always includes physical, mental, emotional, better for, and worse because of, symptoms. A homeopath decides which remedy to suggest to a person based on symptoms in all categories; he does not worry about what disease a person has been labeled as having.

In modern repertories you may find disease names. If you don't take these too literally, they can be helpful in narrowing the field of possible remedy choices. Remember, each disease manifests differently in each person. You must find a remedy that matches both their "disease" and the symptoms that are unique to them.

ACUTE AND CHRONIC DISEASES

ACUTE DISEASE

Acute Diseases are self-limiting. This means that usually, given time and a little bit of care, the symptoms will usually clear up on their own. Some acute illnesses, such as pneumonia or meningitis, can become extremely serious very suddenly and need to be watched closely and remedies given. Homeopathic remedies are especially effective in the convalescent stages following the actual illness.

An acute disease has 3 definite stages. They are: 1) The incubation period. In this stage there may be no actual physical symptoms of the disease. 2) The acute phase. Here is where the recognizable symptoms surface and worsen. 3) The convalescent stage. This stage is where the person is supposed to be improving and regaining their strength, but often do not get completely well again. Well-chosen homeopathic remedies will speed up recovery, alleviate pain, and ensure that there are no long-term complications.

CHRONIC DISEASE

Chronic disease develops slowly over a period of time, often continues indefinitely with little change no matter what is tried, and is often accompanied by a general deterioration in over-all health and vitality. The development of the disease does not take a predictable course with every person as to speed or severity of developing symptoms. It is usually not possible to say how long it will last. ***An acute illness that is followed by complications can develop into a chronic, long-term illness.***

Arthritis, heart disease, high blood pressure, and chronic fatigue are examples of chronic illness. These types of illnesses certainly appear to be on the rise today. Perhaps this is due, in part, to the chemical pollution of our environment and our food supplies. I believe we must also consider the over-use of orthodox medicines as a major contributing factor in this increase of severe chronic illnesses.

CURE AND PALLIATION

A cure is the complete and permanent removal of both the symptoms and the underlying factors. A cure never relieves a symptom by "chasing" it to another part of the system. A cure should remove the necessity of any further treatments. For example, an underlying disturbance in the immune system may create a lymph drainage problem. This is manifesting in the right foot at the present time. The use of homeopathics, essential oils, or other modalities may clear the swelling and inflammation in the foot but if the immune system is not strengthened and the lymph fluid cleared, inflammation and swelling will inevitably occur somewhere else in a very short time.

A complete cure should remove the necessity of any further treatments on that issue. A complete cure is always what is being sought for, of course. Anything less is considered palliation. If you have a long standing, chronic, and very debilitating disease and you remove most of the symptoms and dramatically improve your quality of life, you are much better off than before (and, probably, very happy). Nevertheless, by definition, this is palliation rather than cure. Relief of suffering is something to be very grateful for, always. You are now in a better state of health and a better frame of mind to continue searching for the other pieces of the puzzle.

I quite often have people I am working with keep a progress or gratitude journal so that months later when they say to me, "I really haven't made much progress. I think that I will discontinue treatment," I can send them back to look at what they have written as they went along and they can remember (and be grateful for) all of the progress that they have made. This almost always gives them enough enthusiasm to get back to work until the problem is completely dealt with.

SUPPRESSION

Homeopathic treatment, like any good herbal or energy treatment, is concerned with the person as a whole. As discussed previously, all of the symptoms are considered, not just those that involve the one thing the person is focussing on at the moment. Treating just one presenting symptom often causes that symptom to go away, only to manifest somewhere else—and even as something else that looks unrelated. This happens because the underlying problem in the energy system has been ignored. Because the actual cause of the problem still exists and needs fixing, the body deepens the problem and presents another symptom somewhere else, almost always more serious and more internal to the vital organs of the body, in an attempt to get our attention that it still needs assistance with something. This process of only fixing the symptoms is called suppression in homeopathic terms.

By the very way that traditional western medicine thinks and functions, it is often suppressive. The medical profession, and people in general, do not usually recognize that the so-called successful treatment of eczema with cortisone often results in the disease being suppressed to a deeper level which will later manifest as asthma, for example. There are medical studies, however, that show a definite link between cortisone treatments and asthma, especially in children.

It is possible to suppress with homeopathic remedies if you treat only one symptom at a time instead of taking the time to make sure that the remedy you give matches the totality of all symptoms. Incorrect use of homeopathics chases the symptoms around and around and will never result in a cure. Sometimes, the result isn't even a reasonable amount of palliation.

Always treat the whole person and not just one symptom.

MIASMS

A miasm, as originally defined, is an inherited or acquired predisposition to certain diseases. The inherited miasms are the genetic weaknesses within the constitution that have been passed down from generation to generation. A family history of certain disease patterns helps to confirm the presence of a miasm. Just as we inherited our eye or hair color from our ancestors, we can inherit a tendency to temper or particular types of illnesses. Later Hahnemann and others came to believe that miasms could be spread by physical contact and acquired in a variety of other ways. Some of these theories make sense to me; some not so much.

There were three major miasms identified by Hahnemann. These were psora, syphilis, and sycosis. Polio, cancer, and tuberculosis, along with the very recent arrivals called AIDS and Alzheimer's, have been added to most lists. Recently published information by homeopathic theorists have developed the list of miasms even further. This research makes a fascinating study. (See section three for more information.)

Miasms can be a complicated topic, but miasms are the best way that I know of to understand and explain the underlying factors relating to our health. No other modality that I know of even attempts an answer to the hardest of these questions. The discussion of miasms in the third section will attempt to help you recognize and work with miasms by utilizing nosodes and high potency remedies in conjunction with Flower Essences.

DEEP IMPACT ISSUES

Deep impact issues are the traumatic events that have taken place in our lives in the past. These events leave behind discomforts or ailments that are referred to as something from which we have "never been the same since." Often these conditions are referred to in homeopathic literature by the designation NSS (never the same since).

Some examples of life events that might create a NSS situation include a serious illness, accident, surgery, or the loss of a loved one through death, estrangement, or divorce. Any traumatic event at all may be the catalyst for a NSS situation. Many chronic illness begin in just such a way. Like miasms, deep impact issues are often difficult to treat effectively with traditional medical practices.

GENERATIONAL ISSUES

A generational issue could almost be considered another name for a miasm, although the term is most often used in reference to an emotional state or psychological problem rather than a physical issue. A generational issue is usually quite easy to spot because other family members share the same mis-perceptions. Working with generational issues, just like any other homeopathic regimen, is based on matching the known symptoms produced by the remedy with the symptoms that the person is displaying at the present time.

CONSTITUTIONAL REMEDY

A constitutional remedy is the one remedy whose symptom picture (found in the Materia Medica/remedy guide) most closely matches a person on all levels. This remedy matches the person's basic personality type, the way they react to disease, what things make them feel both better or worse when they are ill, their basic body build, inherited tendencies, and emotional and psychological issues.

The constitutional remedy matches who a person was before the occurrence of traumas in their lives. It reflects who they would be if the effects of traumas, miasms, and generational issues could be eliminated.

The constitutional remedy is not the remedy that is needed for every ailment a person is currently suffering from, except in the sense that their constitution has predisposed them to certain types of illnesses. It can appear that you have found your constitutional remedy and it is being effective for most things when what you really have identified is the correct remedy for a miasm, generational, or deep impact issue.

These terms can sometimes be quite confusing. It can be difficult to tell exactly what the symptoms you are seeing represent. It doesn't really matter, however, since you are matching the remedy to the presenting symptoms regardless of the classification those symptoms might best fit into.

Miasmic, chronic disease, deep impact, generational, and constitutional work is usually done using single remedies in the higher potencies. Treating these situations will be covered in more depth in the third section of this book.

ENDEMIC

This term refers to a disease or condition that is specific to a certain group of people or to a certain locality. To be called endemic, the condition must be widely prevalent, chronic, and ongoing.

DYSFUNCTION
A term favored over disease as a description of a malfunction of the physical, mental, emotional, or energetic levels of the body.

PANACEA
This is a word, from Greek mythology, that has come to mean something that is a cure-all. Homeopathic remedies are amazing things, but they are not panaceas.

Materia Medica OR REMEDY GUIDE
The Materia Medica (remedy guide) lists the symptom picture of each remedy as discovered in the provings and by use over the years. Hundreds of remedies are arranged alphabetically, and the symptoms of each remedy are arranged according to area of the body. New remedies are continually being added with each revision of these reference books.

REPERTORIES
The repertory is an index of symptoms in alphabetical order. The remedies that have that particular symptom in their picture are listed. This narrows the field from hundreds of choices to a few remedies. You must then go to a remedy guide (Materia Medica) to determine which of the listed remedies most nearly fits the person and the symptom picture that is currently presenting.

REPERTORISATION
The process of arriving at the remedy which most closely fits the symptoms the person is experiencing at the present time. This is done by referring to each symptom in a repertory and determining which remedies are common to the symptoms you have noted. The remedies are then studied in the Materia Medica until the best possible match has been determined.

RUBRIC
This term refers to the symptoms listed in a repertory. The rubric (Hands: itching, discolored, twitching, etc.) is followed by the list of remedies that have brought out this symptom in a proving or relieved this symptom in a clinical trial.

Chapter Three - Frequently Asked Questions

QUESTION:

**If there are no molecules of the original substance present in the diluted and succussed homeopathic remedy, is the healing action only a placebo effect at work?
Do I have to believe in homeopathics for them to work?**

These two questions apply to homeopathic remedies only if you assume that homeopathic remedies operate on the principle of a material dose. Material doses, such as found in herbal preparations or food supplements, are meant to provide nutrition, anti-bacterial properties, pain relief or some such physical change for the better. Homeopathic remedies work on an energetic, not a molecular level. While many homeopathic remedies have plants as their original source material, just as many do not.

Homeopathic remedies work effectively on babies, animals, and people who are unconscious, none of whom are capable of believing or not believing in them at the time. Critics (or people who just don't understand homeopathic principles) are often quick to assume that homeopathy in general is ineffective if a remedy did not work miraculously the first time and every time. If it did work, it is often attributed to the placebo effect. This is a bit unfair, and allopathic medicines are not held to the same standard, but that is the way people often react.

Once again, it is always essential to individualize the remedy to fit the patient, not to fit the disease. Success depends on matching the person and their symptoms to the symptom picture of the remedy which will be given. Success arrived at any other way is more luck than management and will not provide any deep level and permanent results.

QUESTION:

**Is there any scientific basis for the practice of homeopathy?
It seems a bit mysterious and unscientific.**

Homeopathic medicines are prepared using a particular technique that has evolved into precise and clearly stated protocols. The protocols have been the same for many years and are the same the world over. In any other setting, this would be enough to get the results classified as scientific.

The homeopathic philosophy, with its set of rules and practices, has been around now for 180 years. There has been much knowledge added as to how and why it works because of more advanced technologies and the opportunity to conduct and report studies. But, overall, the best way to test homeopathy is to learn the principles and rules and see what it does for you and people that you know. There is a great book, <u>Homeopathic Science and Modern Medicine: Healing with Microdoses</u> by Harris Coulter. This book describes many of the trials that have been conducted over the past fifty years using plants, animals and humans to prove the effectiveness of homeopathic medicines.

QUESTION:

What is the difference between homeopathic remedies and herbal preparations?

You often find that a person who is interested in herbs is also interested in homeopathic remedies and is using both, as well as other alternative therapies at the same time. The principles that govern the two therapies are completely different, however.

Herbalism concerns itself with either the nutritional value of plants or the healing properties of the known constituents of plants. Personally, I think that these two ideas are more often than not the same thing. The plant heals because it fills a nutritional deficiency which, when filled, leads to the correction of the problem. Homeopathic remedies, on the other hand, do not contain a material dose of the substance (in fact, it may or may not be a plant at all—quite probably not). Each remedy has been shown to produce—and, therefore, cure—a specific range of symptoms. This is the remedy's symptom picture. This symptom picture determines what remedy should be used.

QUESTION:
How Safe are Homeopathic Remedies, Really?

Homeopathic remedies are the gentlest, least harmful cure possible if used following the established principles which govern their use. The quote by homeopathy's founder, Samuel Hahnemann, on page 1 of this book describes it best. He said, (remember) that "The highest ideal of therapy is to restore health rapidly, gently, permanently; to remove and destroy the whole disease in the shortest, surest, least harmful way, according to clearly comprehensible principles." This is exactly what properly chosen remedies do!

Nevertheless, James Tyler Kent, who is considered the founder of high potency homeopathic theory, is supposed to have said that he "would rather share a room with a nest of vipers than be subjected to the administrations of an inexperienced homeopath!" Why would he say such a thing? Because, in the same way that homeopathy can cure—dramatically and permanently, in many cases—it can also create distress (not enough to warrant such a statement, in my opinion) if used improperly.

POTENTIAL TROUBLE SPOTS ARE:
PROVING THE REMEDY THROUGH CARELESSNESS OR LACK OF KNOWLEDGE

If a remedy has been chosen based on only one symptom and its symptom picture includes many other symptoms which the person does not have at this time, it is possible to create an energetic version of those symptoms.

Taking too high a dose of a homeopathic or taking it for an extended period of time can also result in proving the remedy. Some of your symptoms may improve initially, then the symptoms may worsen again as you continue to take the remedy. Worse still, if the remedy was poorly chosen and did not match the symptoms (was not just right for you on a whole body level at this time), you may experience symptoms you never had before. These symptoms will be a part of the chosen remedy's picture.

The following story (or a similar one) has been told many times. I have personally seen (and even done) something similar myself on occasion.

> *A remedy was given to a child with the intent to alleviate the symptoms of a head cold and congested ears. The symptoms initially abated nicely and the child was given more of the remedy over the next few days. As the symptoms returned and worsened (proving the remedy), more doses at more frequent intervals were given. It was assumed that, since it had worked in the beginning, more was needed now and would be helpful. Eventually, the child seemed extremely ill. The congestion in the ears was so severe that hearing and sense of balance were affected.*
>
> *It was recommended that the remedy be stopped entirely and the child was rubbed down thoroughly with Vick's Vapor-Rub. She didn't care much for that treatment, and was then put into a tub and the Vick's scrubbed off. By the time she got out of the tub she was much improved in all symptoms. In a few hours she was playing and showing no signs of either head cold or ear congestion.*

A six-month-old baby was treated at a local hospital emergency room in a state of collapse. It was ascertained that the mother had been giving her baby Chamomilla 6x several times a day for colic since soon after birth. As soon as the homeopathic remedy was discontinued for a period of time the muscle tone returned but the colic did not.

It is important to understand, and always remember, the basic rule of homeopathy which indicates that a remedy is taken only until improvement begins and retake the remedy only when the symptoms begin again. Take the same remedy again only if the symptom picture is the same. Always match the remedy to the symptom picture.

CREATING A HOST OF SYMPTOMS

If a remedy has been given based on only a symptom or two, rather than on the whole person, it will work in a limited way and cure a limited number of symptoms. In these cases, it is possible to end up giving one remedy after another in order to try to get rid of the remaining symptoms. Added to this is the possibility that new symptoms have come on-line as the result of the poorly chosen remedies. The result is that the entire picture becomes so changed and jumbled that it is difficult to find the single remedy that was needed at the very beginning, and it is certainly difficult to decide what to do next. If you have created this situation, it may become necessary to antidote the remedies you have given and start over with treatment in a day or two.

SUPPRESSION

A homeopathic remedy can ameliorate a single superficial symptom such as a skin eruption in the same way that a topically applied pharmaceutical cream can. This only happens if the remedy has been chosen on a single symptom (the skin complaint - a NO NO!! - don't do it) without considering the whole person and the original causes of the problem. This creates a situation known as suppression, where the ailment is cleared superficially by driving the problem deeper into the energy of the body where it will eventually erupt in a different and more deadly form.

Suppression is uncommon in homeopathy, but is possible. If you take a remedy and the specific complaint disappears but your moods and your energy levels feel worse, then you have probably chosen the wrong remedy. You can try another remedy, but be careful of trying more than 2 or 3 and setting up a garbled picture as described above. Please remember this—it is important. Drugs suppress illnesses, setting up these garbled pictures and creating deep non-inherited (acquired) miasms (discussed further in the third section).

QUESTION:
Are homeopathics similar to vaccinations and can they be used as a substitute for vaccinations?

I considered, as I re-wrote this book, toning down my abhorrence for vaccinations. I believe, however, that it is important for a teacher to teach honestly from where he or she stands. My study of vaccinations has led me to believe that they have never been adequately proven either safe or effective and have, in fact, been repeatedly shown to have nasty side effects. As a result, I find any comparison of vaccines to homeopathic remedies to be very offensive.

There are homeopathic nosode remedies for all of the diseases treated by standard vaccination programs. If your state or school district accepts, with a minimum of fuss, the substitution of homeopathic vaccines for shots I would certainly recommend that you follow whatever homeopathic program is necessary. Antidoting the energy of the homeopathic is far easier than undoing a vaccine reaction. And even if you are lucky enough to avoid a vaccine reaction, what 3-month old (or school age child, for that matter) needs to be exposed to, and get sick enough from, major diseases like mumps and rubella in the middle of the winter cold season in order to form anti-bodies against the diseases in case they should accidentally become exposed at some future time?

In addition, every vaccine comes with a built-in immune suppressant to prevent the body from over-reacting to the serum. Suppressing the immune system at any time seems like a risky business to me. You get no such side effects from homeopathic remedies.

Homeopathic remedies do not cause the body to create antibodies. They stimulate the body's vital energy to heal itself—the definition of heal here being to return to normal, healthy functioning. Homeopathic remedies are given in diluted (safe or easily antidoted) doses, as opposed to being introduced directly into the bloodstream or muscles, as is the case with vaccinations. Vaccinations bypass the body's natural defense system in ways which are not fully understood at this time, even by their proponents.

QUESTION:
If homeopathic medicines are so effective, why isn't homeopathy more popular and more accepted in the world and, especially, in America today?

Actually, homeopathy is quite popular in many countries and is, by some reports, the first most popular form of medicine in the world. Homeopathy was, in the past, very popular here in the United States, also. In fact, in the early 1800's, 15% of physicians were homeopathic physicians. These homeopaths were graduates of respected medical schools with credentials and diplomas.

The American Medical Association came into being in 1847. Many historians—and not just "radical" unorthodox ones—believe that it was predominantly formed to eliminate the competition to their practices from inexpensive, natural remedies and the skilled administration of midwives and many people of native American heritage.

From the inception of the A.M.A., only "conventional" practitioners were accepted into this organization and "unconventional" methods and doctors were systematically ostracized and persecuted by the steadily growing A.M.A. membership. Between the 1860's and the early 1900's, even a recognized "conventional" doctor would be denied membership or his membership in the A.M.A terminated if he even consulted with a homeopathic physician on a personal health matter.

In addition to denying membership to homeopathic school graduates, the increasingly powerful A.M.A applied pressure on various funding sources so that homeopathic schools had difficultly remaining in operation. With few funding options and unable to assure their graduates of membership in the A.M.A, most homeopathic schools were forced out of business. The rest were legislated against, little by little, until the practice of homeopathy in the United States very nearly faded out of existence.

A similar pattern, a little more recent in timing and slightly different in scope, has recently been seen in India. India was one of the first countries to really grasp and utilize the principles of homeopathy and the healing provided. The use of homeopathic remedies was very widespread and completely accepted in India for nearly 150 years with knowledge and remedies passed from generation to generation. As drugs as medicines became more profitable and the success of homeopathy more publicized, pressure was brought to bear and legislation passed to regulate and control it. To practice homeopathy in India today requires graduation from one of only a very few schools recognized by the government and a government issued license. Remedies must be made by established and government recognized homeopathic houses. The price of remedies and of homeopathic treatment reflects these changes in manufacturing requirements and the increases in government control of homeopathy on all levels.

Homeopathy has conducted an amazing come-back in the United States in recent years and, I believe, we are seeing the "pushing back" of the A.M.A. as new legislation is being proposed. As in India, these regulations are being promoted as "for the safety of the public" when, in reality, they will only keep these amazing healers out of the hands of people and protect the interests of "conventional" physicians and the drug industry.

QUESTION:
Is it possible to make use of homeopathic medicines and conventional drug therapies at the same time?

Homeopathic remedies often work so fast and so well that there is no need for the conventional drugs by the time a doctor's appointment can be made and a prescription filled. However, some conventional medicines are so strong or work in such a way that they interfere with the action of the homeopathic remedy. Unfortunately, there is no research that I know of to guide us in knowing which drugs interfere with homeopathic remedies.

The decision to use homeopathy and conventional medicine at the same time must be left entirely up to the individual who is taking the medication. Most medical doctors have insufficient experience with homeopathy to provide any useful guidance whatsoever.

Chapter Four - Homeopathic Lore Hahnemann Style

This information is taken from *The Organon of Medicine* by Samuel Hahnemann and is paraphrased by me for use here. Like The Organon, these comments are not set out in any particular order. Dr. Hahnemann recorded his thoughts as they occurred to him throughout his years of work with homeopathic remedies.

As stated several times before in this book, homeopathic practitioners do not do their work based on the names of diseases. They work with each person according to his presenting symptoms and the person's basic personality. Because people are accustomed to thinking by disease names, you will sometimes find remedies grouped in modern repertories in that way. This can be useful to help you narrow the field in finding the remedy that you need. Nevertheless, the name of the ailment is irrelevant from a homeopathic standpoint. Disease names make little difference in ascertaining the correct remedy. The important things to know about any illness is the specific ways in which this individual is manifesting the disease. Disease names are part of the allopathic world. They have come into modern use in homeopathy in an attempt to make homeopathy more understandable to people who have, from childhood, been conditioned to think in disease names.

Because of the prevalence of allopathic drugs, much of what we are treating (and what has been given names as diseases) is nothing more than the manifestations of the negative effects of the drugs the person has taken during his lifetime. Hahnemann described drug side effects (remember he died in 1835) as

"The most tragic and most incurable of all the chronic diseases." He also said that "when they have gone beyond a certain point it is probably impossible ever to discover or imagine any means of curing them. In homeopathy benevolent Providence has given us relief only for natural diseases."

HAHNEMANN ALSO WROTE,

"No human means can ever repair those innumerable abnormalities so often produced by pernicious allopathic treatment. Their prolonged use always adds a new disease condition to the old ones."

I don't know if drug side effects can be totally eradicated by either herbals or homeopathic remedies, but the only course I can see as maybe even having a chance of working against them would be to treat homeopathically, according to the symptom picture that the drug has produced in the person. Perhaps the gentle nudging of the immune system by continually treating homeopathically will eventually stimulate the vital force to throw off the effects of these poisons which were deliberately introduced into the body. Some liver cleansing herbs, combined with clay foot soaks, also seem to have some effectiveness.

When a person takes a drug which is given allopathically (meaning the giving of the opposite or contrary rather than the giving of a similar), they often believe that the drug is meant to eradicate the entity which is causing the disease. According to Hahnemann, this is impossible because the drug temporarily hides the symptom from the vital force. The body does not recognize either the disease state nor the foreign medicine that was introduced because they are opposites and present contradictory messages to the vital force. In effect, they cancel each other out or, put more accurately, they hide each other from the vital force.

Since the body, for a time, does not realize that it has a problem (or two problems, if you count the toxic substance taken as a medication), it does not manifest symptoms. It may not even manifest pain or discomfort since pain is simply the body's way of bringing our attention to the need to correct something. The body doesn't call for help, because the body doesn't recognize that it needs help.

An illusion is created; the person thinks he is getting better because he feels better. With no signal being sent to it, the vital force does not activate itself against the disease. The medical world, and the patient, view this as a cure—but it is no such thing! When the medicine is removed or the bacteria has become immune to the medicine, the original disease surfaces once again. It is unchanged, or even worsened, because it has not been effectively dealt with during this time.

Since the medicine which was given is usually toxic and a fairly large dose was required, eventually an opposite counter-reaction follows from the vital force. Organs of the body such as the liver are stimulated to scoop up these poisons and take them out of circulation. This can only be done by linking the poisons to nutrients in order to allow them to pass through the kidneys and intestines without damaging these vital organs. Drug side effects are often the symptoms of deficiency of whatever vitamin or mineral was used up in the excretion of the drugs. This topic is covered more deeply in the book <u>Butterfly Miracles with Herbal Remedies.</u>

Hahnemann also believed that, "It is possible to create a very grave disease by acting on the vital principle through the power of imagination and to cure it the same way." This seems to me to be another way of saying that what goes on with us emotionally, mentally, and psychologically can make us sick or can aid us in becoming healthy and well.

"As long as there is marked, obviously progressing, improvement during treatment, no more medicine of any kind must be given." Homeopathic remedies are designed to stimulate the body's own defenses. As long as this is happening, the body should be allowed to continue its work unaided by any new remedy or by repeats of the remedy you just used so successfully. When the action stops, another gentle nudge is given by giving another dose of the remedy. *This principle is one of the most important things to understand about homeopathy! It is referred to as principle #7 on pages 6 & 7 in this book.*

The length of action of a homeopathic remedy is usually a combination of the strength of the dose and the overall health of the person. As the symptom picture changes, a different remedy which more nearly matches the new set of symptoms should be given. Protocols found in the literature for both dosage and frequency are estimates at best. If you know how to muscle test, follow the muscle test to fine-tune both the potency and the frequency of the dosage for the individual.

A wise homeopath will be careful to avoid making favorites of certain remedies that he has happened to have found indicated rather often and has had the opportunity of employing with good results. Many times less well known and less frequently used remedies might be more suitable and, therefore, more effective and should not be overlooked.

When in doubt as to which of several remedies should be used because the physical symptoms of the remedies closely resemble each other, a choice should be made based on the mental and emotional patterns. In fact, the mental and emotional patterns should be given the heaviest emphasis.

The smallest disturbance in normal balance and wellness—a hangnail or a whitlow or anything else—is an indication of a disturbance in the entire person that will worsen and become more obvious if left untreated. If there are only one or two such disturbances, many times a slight adjustment in diet, sleep, or exercise patterns is all that is required to put things right again.

Chapter Five - Taking a Case History
(By Traditional Methods)

Even if your muscle testing skills are very good, it is well worth the time and effort to learn how to take a case properly and learn to work out the right remedy by traditional methods. Information and education "inform" your muscle test and enable it to be more comprehensive and accurate. Understanding homeopathic principles, learning to observe well and to think in the patterns of homeopathic thought will improve your grasp of homeopathic principles and make you more effective than you otherwise would be. It is too easy to fall into the trap of testing based on a single symptom, rather than on the whole person or their entire symptom picture. Of course, you can make this mistake with a more traditional approach than muscle testing, also, if you allow yourself to.

You only get the answers to the questions you ask with a muscle test. If you don't have enough knowledge to ask the right questions, you will get poor answers that are responsive only to the questions that you asked. There are many books on the market that take a 'name-of-disease' approach and the FDA rules which apply to homeopathy require a statement on the label indicating what single symptom the remedy is for. Following the guidelines of these books or operating according to the labels on the bottles will keep you from being effective and cause you to make serious errors unless you temper them with a good look at the entire symptom picture and some skill at traditional repertorising (matching the presenting symptoms to a remedy description).

For the next few pages, we are going to discuss the classical approach to homeopathic prescribing, including repertorising. This is a fairly complex process and takes time, patience, and practice. Our goal here is not to make you an expert overnight. It is to teach you how repertorising is done, and give you enough information to make your muscle testing, if you use it, as accurate as possible.

A WORD OF CAUTION HERE ABOUT SELF-PRESCRIBING

It can be difficult to be objective about your own symptoms, especially mental or emotional ones. If you do not maintain objectivity, both muscle testing and repertorising can be colored by your own perceptions. Here is an example for you to think about:

> You have a particular physical symptom but you feel quite normal and calm emotionally. However, everyone around you seems to be seeing you as increasingly irritable and touchy. You have already forgiven and forgotten (according to you) that your husband left you standing in the rain in front of the grocery store a few days ago. You got thoroughly chilled that day but seemed to throw off the effects of it as soon as you got warm again.

Being perceived by others as irritable and touchy and getting chilled, both of which you may be overlooking, could be vital elements in the overall picture of your ailment. It can often be useful to talk through your case with someone else or, at the very least, to take a few minutes to interview yourself just as you would someone else. This is especially important when you are first learning. If you don't feel comfortable with the remedy that you have decided on, or the muscle test checks and balance statements "anything else?" and "anything different?" do not give you satisfactory answers, don't take the remedy. Be patient for a day or two, study it out, and don't hesitate to ask for help.

Some people are very good at knowing what their own symptom picture is—much better than anyone else would ever be—but some of us are not, or at least not at particular times in our lives. Sometimes a mis-perception of reality about our moods and emotions is part of the out-of-balance pattern that needs correcting and we simply cannot see it. On the other hand, many people have an innate sense of what they need—at least they do once they learn to trust themselves instead of their doctors. If you don't have this sense already, it would be worth any effort to get it. If you are temporarily out of balance, however, be sure to get some help from a friend in determining what homeopathic remedy you need.

THE SYMPTOM PICTURE:

As complicated as I have made repertorising sound, there are really only two parts to classical prescribing: The first is getting a firm grasp on the entire symptom picture. The second is deciding which remedy matches that picture best.

Homeopathic practitioners try very hard not to think of people in terms of the disease they are suffering from The word complaint is often used instead. For example, a homeopathic practitioner may list sore throat, cough, or headache, but stop short of calling it Bird Flu.

Symptoms are the visible signs of the complaint. For example, your child is complaining of a barking cough that is worse at night and better from sitting up. The complaint is the cough and the symptoms are barking sound, worse at night, and better from sitting up. This complaint and its symptoms are much different—and require a different remedy—from a complaint of a deep, moist cough accompanied by high fever and chills, and better for lying on the right side.

The symptom picture is a detailed list of the symptoms that you are having at present. Symptoms, especially mental and emotional ones, are considered in light of what is usually normal for that person.

Your symptoms are a form of expression and a call for help from your body. In order for a remedy to work well you need to match, as closely as possible, the person's symptoms to a remedy picture. The remedy picture is the list of symptoms produced by the remedy in its provings and in the experiences of homeopathic practitioners. These symptoms can be found in a Materia Medica (sometimes called a remedy guide). The remedy guide lists all of the symptoms that were seen when the remedy was taken for a long time. They indicate a very out of balance, serious state. Hopefully, you will never see a person with all of the listed symptoms. They would be in a very serious state of ill health, if you should.

Observations are very important. You are not simply looking for aches and pains. You will need to understand who the person is when they are healthy and then look for the symptoms that are particular to this illness and this time in their life. Vague, sometimes present and sometimes not symptoms don't count for much, except with certain remedies where vagueness of symptoms is part of the pattern. In these remedies, the symptom pictures include a "changeableness" of the symptom picture in their description.

Every labeled disease or complaint, whether it is cystitis, arthritis or eczema, is also accompanied by symptoms peculiar to the individual who is suffering from it. It differs in significant ways from another case of the same disease. If you think about your own children, you know that each of them reacts to the supposed same illness in a way that is totally unique to them. It is these individual characteristics that guide us to the right remedy.

Simply to prescribe for headache or cough is not nearly enough. If you look up either of these symptoms in a repertory you will find many remedies listed for each of them. It is the particular symptoms of the person's headache or cough that lets you begin to narrow down the choice of remedies. If you have become proficient at it, you can sometimes use muscle testing to help you narrow down the choices.

For homeopathic purposes, symptoms are divided into three categories: general, mental/emotional and physical complaints. The general category includes such things as what makes the person feel better or worse during this illness, and a host of other unusual things that don't fit anywhere else. Before deciding on a remedy, you should be able to match at least 3 or 4 symptoms in each of these areas(mental, physical, and emotional). Looking for symptoms in the various areas will keep you from focusing too much on just one or two symptoms.

NOTE-TAKING:

When working with homeopathic remedies (or any type of alternative modality, really) it is the responsible thing to do to keep good notes. With homeopathy your notes should include the symptoms that you observed, and the remedy and the potency you decided on. You should make detailed notes as to the instructions you gave concerning the dosage and the length and number of times the remedy should be taken. You should follow up with the person and include in your notes what kind of results were obtained. All of this takes time, but it is absolutely essential to responsible homeopathic treatment. I cannot over emphasize this! A scatter-gun in the dark approach will not be as effective as if you had taken the time to document your work and follow-up properly. Furthermore, if a problem arises you will have a clear record of what was done and a better idea of where you want to go next. Keeping records does not automatically obligate you to share them or to make them public in any way.

BEING OBSERVANT

When making observations to obtain a list of symptoms, pay attention to your first impressions. For example; your child wakes up in the night, crying out and calling for you. You go quickly into her room. What do you immediately smell and see? Does she seem to be in pain or just frightened? Does she want to be held? Does she want the light on or off? These impressions are sometimes all that you will get from a sick child—or an irritable or lethargic adult, for that matter. Even if you use muscle testing to choose the remedy, you will want to have noticed some basic symptoms so that you can verify your choice.

WHAT IS IT YOU SMELL?

The smell is often the first and most dramatic thing that you notice when you walk into a sick person's room. If the smell is strong and you can describe it clearly, write it down and use it as a symptom. Particular odors, and reactions to odors, are listed in most remedy pictures.

WHAT IS IT YOU SEE?

Note the general color of the person's skin. Are they pale or flushed? Are their eyes glassy or pain filled. ?Do they look as if they are feverish? Look around the room for other clues. These might include such things as bed covers that have been kicked off, agitation or restlessness, or groaning or annoyance if someone sits on the edge of the bed. Your observations will often tell you far more than the person will be able to.

WHAT IS IT YOU FEEL?

This feeling refers both to what you feel about the temperature of the various parts of the body and what you feel intuitively about the situation. Be thorough about physical symptoms of sweat, clamminess, or dry skin but do not discount the more subtle things that you sometimes sense.

WHAT IS IT YOU HEAR?

Some sick people are stoic, others feel better for complaining a little. Some children want to be held or stroked. Others want to just lie there looking pathetic. Are they discouraged, anxious, sad, angry? Often a sick person's behavior changes when observed—they either want attention and sympathy or they want to be left alone. All of these ways of responding to the illness are symptoms and you will find them in the descriptions of the various remedies.

Be sure to factor in everything else that you know about the person and everything that you know about what has been going on in her life lately. Include any information that has been provided to you by other people, such as members of her family. Consider remedies that she has previously taken and ascertain the results she obtained by taking them.

The asking of pertinent questions is a necessary skill in determining the correct remedy. Keep your questions general. The goal is to elicit a response in which the person describes in some detail her particular symptoms. Questions such as "Are you feeling sad?" or "Is it a stinging sort of pain?" often generate a simple yes or no and really does not give you much information at all. Try not to put words into the person's mouth with your questions. Sometimes talking about the illness is a form of healing. Learn to be still and just listen.

There is an excellent case-taking questionnaire and symptom check-list in *The Complete Homeopathy Handbook* by Miranda Castro on pages 227-229. This is a book that I would recommend for beginners in the art of homeopathy, although if you are serious about learning homeopathy, you will soon outgrow it. It contains a small remedy guide which includes many of the most basic—polycrest—remedies as well as a small, but quite nice, repertory section.

The point of both observation and questioning is to discover at least one symptom in each of the three categories mentioned earlier—physical, mental/emotional, and general—and what makes the person feel better or worse. These better or worse symptoms are sometimes referred to as modalities. As I have said before, and really want you to understand, you should never choose a remedy based on a single symptom. Doing homeopathy this way is rarely successful, and if it is, it will have been either luck or good intuition (and there will be those wonderful times when your intuition astonishes you). The more symptoms that fit the picture, the more effective the remedy will be and the less likely you are to create any false symptoms, make even a little mistake, or miss something.

Once you have your list of symptoms you are ready to repertorise. This sounds much more complicated than it really is. Simply look up the complaint, or any one of its symptoms, in the repertory. Then look at the remedies that are listed and match the brief descriptions with the rest of the specific symptoms you have noted. If you have done a good job of observing and asking questions, you should be left with only 2 or 3 remedies to finish choosing between. This is where muscle testing can save you much time and effort and prevent you from choosing a remedy that does not match as closely as it should have.

The next step is to confirm that your choice of remedies is the best one. Whether you have arrived at only one remedy, or two or three, go to the Materia Medica (remedy guide) and look closely at the longer description of each remedy and see if it fits. Occasionally, more than one remedy will have all your symptoms listed in its description. If so, you need to search for another clue or two that will differentiate the remedies. It is very rare to find all of the symptoms listed and, here again, being able to muscle test is very comforting. I have worked with homeopathic remedies for years, with fear and trembling (not to mention spending large amounts of time), and I have had much greater success since I learned to fine-tune my choices with muscle testing.

If you can't seem to pick a remedy that fits, you need more information than you have at the present time. You must return and observe or ask more questions. This whole process becomes easier and simpler every time you do it, until it becomes almost routine. It was interesting, as I wrote this, to realize that I no longer really even think about the steps or the categories. I just automatically look for symptoms that will set the case apart. You, too, will learn to do this with practice.

A RARE AND CONFUSING PHENOMENON:

Your general and emotional/mental symptoms may point to a remedy that does not even list the physical complaint in its picture. For example, you have the flu and are feeling restless, irritable, hot and bothered, and extremely thirsty. You find that sulphur comes up strongly for all your symptoms but isn't listed under flu at all in the repertory. The next closest remedy is *Bryonia* but *Bryonia* isn't restless or irritable. Read through the remedy pictures again to see which one fits best; the best choice will often be the one that matches the mental/emotional symptoms rather than the physical complaint because it covers more of the whole picture and the whole person. If the strong general and emotional/mental symptoms point to one remedy, then give it, even if it doesn't have your physical complaint listed in its picture. You will get better results by following this advice.

A remedy that has a good reputation for any physical complaint is always more likely to work well if there are general and/or emotional/mental symptoms that match to go along with it.

Chapter Six - Types of Remedies
(Based on Original Substance)

Homeopathic medicines can, potentially, be made from anything and everything in existence. As you glance through a Materia Medica, it may seem to you that someone has already made a homeopathic remedy from every thing possible, and that a great many of them are made from rather nasty substances. I am quite sure that there is a use in healing for all of God's creations and that everything has a frequency and its own place in the universe. I am very grateful to all the wonderful and dedicated people whose work over the years has made the knowledge of so many of them available to each of us.

Some of the substances used for the original tincture should not—as you will observe as we discuss them in more depth—ever be administered to a person in anything but homeopathic form. I am referring here predominantly to the nosode remedies, remedies based on poisonous substances, and remedies based on drugs or vaccines. Many of these remedies, however, are among the really important healers of the homeopathic world.

BASIC TYPES OF REMEDIES

FLOWER ESSENCES
- BACH
- NORTH AMERICAN
- SIERRA RANGE OF LIGHT
- MANY OTHERS

GEM ESSENCES

ENERGETIC AND VIBRATIONAL
- ENERGY SOURCES
- COLOR AND SOUND

TISSUE/CELL SALTS (biochemic)

SARCODES

NOSODES

METALS/ELEMENTS (MINERALS)

ANIMAL KINDGOM

PLANT KINGDOM

LOW POTENCY COMBINATIONS

BIOCHEMIC CELL SALTS:
There are 12 important inorganic salts that are part of the composition of the cells of our bodies. If these salts become depleted or out of balance with one another, our cells deteriorate rapidly and become vulnerable to attack by pathogens. The cells salts are made from these mineral salts. These remedies can help us with the uptake and proper balance of these mineral salts in our cells and tissues.

FLOWER ESSENCES:
These are very low potency remedies that address issues of emotional well-being, the development of character and spirituality, and mind/body health. The removal of emotional responses to certain triggers, the recognition that some ways of responding to certain situations are more appropriate and healthier than others, and the changing of negative attitudes such as fear to faith and anxiety to peace, can have profound effects on both mental and physical health.

Originally there were 36 of these remedies. They were created by Dr. Edward Bach using flowers native to Great Britain and are still referred to as Bach flower remedies. There have been hundreds of additional flower essence remedies created from flowers native to various continents and countries.

ENERGETIC:

These are a small group of homeopathic remedies that are made from energy sources. Energetic remedies are referred to in some texts as the imponderables. Some examples of these remedies are: Sol (sunlight), Luna (moonlight), Radiation, X-ray, Electricity, Neon, the individual colors, and the notes of the scale, etc.

VIBRATIONAL:

Vibrational is a more specific term used to refer to energetic remedies made from color or sound. The concept that the various wavelengths of different colors and sounds have profound effects on our minds and bodies is well recognized. Frequency is based on the vibratory rate of wavelengths. These homeopathic remedies are created in a process designed to capture that frequency. The technology of today can measure the frequency of different colors and sounds and can also measure the frequencies of these remedies. This is a relatively new field of homeopathy and is quite fascinating!

SARCODES:

This is the term used for remedies prepared from healthy tissues and organs, usually from animals. These remedies are used to stimulate the organs of the body to accomplish their various tasks efficiently. Sarcodes are sometimes used in convalescent treatments. Remedies that are prepared from human blood, urine, mucus and other discharges are referred to as auto-nosodes and are considered a part of this grouping. Some of the sarcode remedies include Adrenalinum, Carbo animalis, Cholesterinum, Colostrum, all of the ones that begin with Lac (Lac caninum, Lac defloratum, etc.), all of the various ovary and ovi remedies, Pancreatinum, Pepsinum, Pulmo rulpis, Saccarum lactis, Thyroid, Thymus, and sometimes Uricum acidum, and Lac maturnum humanum.

NOSODES:

The word nosode comes from a Greek root word for disease. This is the term used for remedies prepared from either tissues or secretions containing a specific bacteria or virus of a disease. Certain other nosode remedies are made from bacterias or viruses grown in laboratory cultures.

Some nosode remedies include Anthracinum, all of the Bacillinum or Bacillus remedies, Carcinosin, Diphtherinum, Malandrinum, Medorrhinum, Ocillococcinum, Psorinum. Pyrogenium, Staphyloccoccinum, Secale cornutum, Streptococcinum, Syphilinum, Tuberculinum bovinum, Vaccininum, and Variolinum.

METALS/ELEMENTS (MINERALS):

Most of these remedies are found on the periodic table (remember basic chemistry classes). There are also some remedies that are man-made combinations of the elements found in nature. Mineral remedies, emotionally, deal with organizational skills and difficulties with structure and our role in some area of our lives. These emotional patterns are often seen manifesting in the physical body.

ANIMAL KINGDOM:

These are remedies made from such things as the venom of snakes, poisons that are associated with bees and other insects, the ink secreted by the cuttlefish, and the milk of various mammals. Animal remedies share characteristics of competitiveness (or compliance), fitness, and defining our role in the hierarchy of life.

PLANT KINGDOM:

These are the remedies which have been made from herbal preparations of various plants. Plant remedies share the characteristic of emotional sensitivity to people. They often are very much affected by their perception of what other people think of them or expect from them.

The classifications in this section group homeopathic remedies according to the substances from which they are made and from the way in which they are prepared. Flower essences are, of course, made from members of the plant kingdom. The cell salts are prepared, in a slightly different manner, from some of the same minerals used in other homeopathic preparations. There are many other terms used in homeopathy that reflect how the remedies are used in different circumstances and applications.

The brief descriptions and general characterizations on the previous pages are too broad to be of much use in determining a remedy for a particular person and situation. A great body of work exists, done by intelligent and dedicated people all over the world, that identify underlying sensations and symptoms for different types of minerals, different kinds of animals, and members of the various plant families. Many of the remedies in each kingdom have been analyzed and matched with the miasm that they address. We will discuss each remedy family in more depth using the work of these dedicated individuals.

Below is a chart comparing the 3 physical kingdom classifications. This chart highlights some of the most notable emotional and mental aspects that the remedies in each kingdom have in common. It also allows you to see at a glance the different focus of each kingdom. This table is meant to be a learning tool to give you a sense of the general direction in which you may find yourself going.

Thinking homeopathically has become such a habit that I sometimes find myself analyzing new clients, potential employees, and just about everybody else according to which general category their predominant personality characteristics place them into. This can be a good thing or a not so good thing according to the circumstances. As a practitioner, this information can help you sort deep impact and constitutional issues from the symptoms of a current illness. This will often bring clarity and help you focus your initial efforts.

PLANT	ANIMAL	MINERAL
General: Sensitive - affected by everyone and everything, easily influenced by the opinions of others tends to be moody, quiet, and introspective	*General: Competitive* - enjoys conflict and sparring, usually possesses excellent reflexes, concerned with issues of survival and their place in the hierarchies of life	*General: Disconnected from self, structured type thinking* - difficulty thinking in holistic terms, has problems with structure or organization in some areas of his relationships or profession
Basic Disposition: soft / sensitive emotional adaptable influenced by others irritable often whiney and full of complaints artistic ability and temperament	*Basic Disposition:* alert / quick to react aggressive movements quick and sudden playful / affectionate deceitful / mistrusting jealous / malicious expressive	*Basic Disposition:* strong organized systematic calculating fastidious / neat guarded / careful all or nothing
Heard to Say: I am affected by. . . I am sensitive to . . . I can't bear. . . I felt so happy this morning but now . . . . hurts me so badly . . . . really touches me	*Heard to Say:* I'm not good enough I'm better than them I don't accept myself I will fight them on that I will beat them, outsmart them People are so cruel—but I am not	*Heard to Say:* (as though separate, but theirs) My relationships. . . My family . . . My health . . . My job . . . My skin . . My nerves . . .
Interests and goals nature plants art music changeable with life's daily events	*Interests and goals* animals pursuit and winning fighting and competing flying man/woman relationships	*Interests and goals* work intense efforts relationships matters relating to house & home concerned with money issues

SOME TERMS USED TO REFER TO REMEDIES

SINGLE AND COMBINATION REMEDIES

A single remedy contains only one remedy, rather than a combination of several remedies. These remedies can be made in any potency. Combination remedies must, of necessity, be made in low potencies. The merits and differences between these two classifications are discussed in more detail in Chapter 2, *Remedies and Results*.

CONSTITUTIONAL (FUNDAMENTAL) REMEDIES.

These are remedies that are being given, not because of a current illness or imbalance, but because the remedy's symptom picture closely matches the person's basic personality and general health. These are given at higher potencies to reach more deeply into the energy body. There is a list of common constitutional remedies in the appendix section of this book. The proper use of these remedies is discussed in later sections of this book.

ACUTE REMEDIES:

These are remedies that are prescribed for sudden onset conditions or accidents. The 30C and 200C remedies are most often used for acute and emergency prescribing. In certain situations a 1M remedy is what is needed. When indicated, follow the acute with a deeper acting chronic remedy or a constitutional remedy to help restore health and prevent relapses.

EMERGENCY REMEDIES:

These remedies are used much like acute remedies, except they usually refer to trauma from accidents or surgeries.

CAUSATIVE REMEDIES:

The cause of the disorder (called the etiology in some texts) is sometimes important in determining the most similar remedy for an emergency, acute, or chronic situation. Etiologies include shocks, traumas, injuries, excesses, mental and emotional stress, heat, cold, and vital energy or fluid depletion. These causes can be looked up in a homeopathic repertory just like any other symptom. The remedies listed are then studied for the best possible match.

The following is a list of some of the major causes of disease and suffering: abuse, accidents, alcohol, allergies, anger, bad news, blows, burns, cuts, depletions, diet, drug side effects, emotional shocks and traumas, environmental influences, excesses, being forsaken, frights, genetic weakness, greed, grief, head injuries, humiliation, infections, injuries, meat-eating, miasms, perceptions, physical traumas, poor hygiene, poisons, pride, sexual excesses, sleep, surgical side effects, work, worry, tobacco, toxins, vaccinations.

EPIDEMIC REMEDIES:

Homeopathic physicians have compiled lists of remedies to use in treating various epidemic diseases. The choice of remedies to list is based on two things. Whenever possible, the lists are compiled from successful treatment protocols accomplished more than once in homeopathic practices around the world and reported in trade journals. Other remedies, whose symptom picture matches the symptoms that commonly appear at different stages of the diseases, are also listed.

Because people are different and their reaction to illness and stress are different, it is impossible to say, "Use this particular remedy in all cases of a particular disease." It is always necessary in homeopathy to prescribe based, not on the disease itself, but on that particular person's reaction to the disease. These lists are invaluable in giving us a place to start in our search for the right remedy, and in giving us basic pictures of these diseases that we may have never yet seen in person.

Epidemic conditions are acute diseases; they are just overwhelming in their suddenness and ferocity. An epidemic remedy is given in repeated doses for a short period of time, a few days or longer, as needed. 30C, 200C, and 1M potencies are used according to the severity of symptoms. It is important to remember that the symptom picture changes as the disease progresses; the remedy used must change to meet each new symptom picture. It is also important to continue on with treatment through to the end of any convalescent stages of the illness.

INTERCURRENT REMEDIES:

Intercurrent remedies are used when a well-indicated remedy fails to sustain improvement. Improvement is said to have stalled out. Intercurrent remedies are usually given a few doses a day for a day or two, then the other remedy in the pair is given for a few days. This is much like acute prescribing except there are two remedies in play. 30C and 200C potencies work well here. Occasionally a 1M will be used for one remedy or the other. Muscle testing is a very great help here.

ISOPATHIC REMEDIES:

Isopathic means the giving of something that is exactly the same as the disease or imbalanced state. Nosodes are isopathic remedies. Giving something that is exactly the same varies a little from giving something that is a similar. Isopathic remedies are especially useful for eliminating toxic chemicals and heavy metals from the body. A person who suffers from lead poisoning from bad water, for example, may take Plumbum metallicum (lead) in its homeopathic form to help eliminate the poison. Isopathic remedies are usually administered with another remedy that closely matches the person's symptoms in the intercurrent pattern described in the previous paragraph. The isopathic remedy is almost always the second remedy given and it is given for shorter periods of time than the companion remedy.

SOME BASIC PRINCIPLES FOR ISOPATHIC USE ARE:

- Do not give it as the first remedy (typically)
- Do not repeat it too often or for too long a time. It has been found that giving the remedy too often or for too long causes the person to relapse. This is typical of all remedies. If the problem has been cleared by the treatment, continued use can create a proving and subsequent symptom picture.
- Continue any remedies that were interrupted by the isopathic/intercurrent treatment.

Isopathic and nosode remedies are meant to be used as intercurrent remedies, to jolt the energy system and jump-start the healing process once again. Another remedy is chosen that matches the totality of the symptoms and the two work together to accomplish a deep level of healing.

MIASMIC REMEDIES:

Some homeopathic remedies have symptom pictures that are very similar to certain aspects of one miasm or another. These remedies are referred to as a miasmic remedy for those particular sets of symptoms. Miasms are discussed in detail in the third section of this book. In that chapter are lists of homeopathic remedies matched with particular miasms.

Many remedies of the plant, mineral, and animal kingdoms are applicable to each miasm. Insect remedies, in the animal kingdom, are almost always useful in the tubercular miasm. Most miasms also have a nosode remedy or two that matches many of the symptoms. A nosode remedy is often the most effective way to treat a miasm but it must be administered with a intercurrent remedy. Flower Essences are proving useful here.

ORGAN REMEDIES:

Some homeopathic remedies have a strong affinity for certain organs or systems of the body. Examples of these remedies are Chelidonium majus for the liver, Crataegus oxyacantha for the heart, Avena sativa for the brain, Lobelia inflata for the lungs, Echinacea angustifolia or purpurea for the blood, Ceanothus americanus for the spleen, and Equisetum hyemale for the kidneys. A good reperatory can help you find one whose overall picture is just right for particular situations.

PATHOLOGICAL REMEDIES:

Pathology is a term used by homeopathic physicians and medical doctors alike to describe a chronic disease state. Pathological homeopathic remedies are used to combat various chronic conditions. Often, if destruction to tissues, organs or nerves has not progressed beyond repair, these remedies can help return the body to a more normal state. The similarity to the chronic condition is the primary (but not the only) factor in choosing a pathological remedy. Fundamental/constitutional remedies (the remedy that matches the person most closely without the chronic condition) are often used intercurrently with the pathological remedy. The constitutional remedy can be pursued when the chronic condition has been cleared or is in remission.

Pathological states are not limited to physical ailments only. Mental and emotional conditions such as depression, violent behavior, and personality disorders can form chronic, pathological layers. These layers may require giving several different remedies in succession over a period of time. Always move to a new remedy as the symptom picture changes, and match your remedy closely to the symptoms that are on-line at the moment, and not on remembered behaviors from the past.

Low potency remedies, in repeated doses, are considered more effective for severe pathologies like cancer and for cases in which the patient is taking allopathic drugs. You will need to take any allopathic drug history into consideration when choosing a potency. You will probably want to start with a low potency, moving higher or going to an intercurrent remedy if the cure stalls or improvement begins to fail (a relapse situation occurs).

POLYCREST REMEDIES:

This is the name given to a group of often used remedies. "Poly" means many and "crest" means time. The symptom picture of these remedies describes things that are common to human experience. The polycrests are the most often prescribed remedies, and are a good place to start in learning about and acquiring your own homeopathic remedies. Polycrest remedies are used for acute, chronic, emergency, fundamental/constitutional, and pathological conditions.

Section Two

Lower Potency Remedies

In order to work competently with higher potency, deeper acting remedies it is necessary to have a working knowledge of the basic principles of homeopathic philosophy. It is also helpful to have had a little bit of experience with the low potency remedies discussed in this section.

Chapter Seven - Cell/Biochemic/Tissue/Schuessler Salts

Important Nutrients for Life

The word *biochemic* is derived from a Greek word—bios— which means *life*. Biochemic, therefore, means the *chemistry of life*. According to biochemic theory, there are 12 major inorganic salts that make up the composition of our cells and our blood. Blood is to the body what soil is to a plant. Poor, exhausted soil that is lacking in essential nutrients produces weak and sickly plants. Poor, exhausted blood that is lacking in essential constituents will produce weak, sickly bodies that are prone to disease and unable to provide the quality of life that we would like to have. By enriching the soil, plants can be made to thrive. By enriching the blood and ensuring that the proper nutrients are being carried to the cells, a healthy balance within ourselves can be maintained or recovered.

The strength of our cells and, as a result, the strength of our organs and tissues depends on our having the necessary quantities of these important salts. If they become depleted in our tissues or cells, or if they become out of balance with one another, proper function is lost. In fact, biochemic theory maintains that *every* disease of the human family is due to a lack of one or more of these organic building blocks. I don't know that I agree with the *every*, but it is an interesting hypothesis.

ARE CELL SALTS HOMEOPATHICS?

These remedies contain no material dose of the inorganic salts and minerals from which they are made. They can not be considered supplements in any sense of the word. Although they are prepared in a manner quite similar to other homeopathic remedies, *they work by somewhat different principles*. These remedies ***do not*** create in a well person any symptoms of ill health, which is part of the basic premise of homeopathic symptom pictures. Like homeopathics, however, they bring a certain energy pattern to the attention of the body.

It seems that by highlighting and focusing our energy system on the pattern of a deficiency, these remedies encourage our bodies to look for and uptake needed nutrients until proper quantities and balances are achieved. Since these salts are the building blocks out of which our entire bodies are made, there is nothing that deficiencies of these vital minerals cannot be connected to. The corollary to this statement is, of course, that since any ailment of the body may have a connection to a cell salt deficiency, they should be used whenever the physical or emotional symptoms indicate their need.

MINERALS

The minerals represented and balanced by the cell salt remedies have many and varied uses in our bodies.

Calcium: Strengthens bones, elastic tissues, veins, arteries, teeth, joints, and aids the assimilation of other nutrients.

Iron: Oxygenates the blood. Improves the hemoglobin. Strengthens arteries and veins. Reduces inflammation, and controls fever.

Potassium (Kali): Nerve and brain health and function. Hair and skin health Dries or increases mucus secretions as needed. Aids stomach and bowel functions.

Magnesium: Relieves pain and is an anti-spasmodic. Strengthens the nervous system. Ensures the rhythmic movements of muscular tissues—including those of the heart and the uterus.

Sodium (Natrum): Effective for nerves, muscles, joints, and digestive organs. Establishes better water balance in tissues. Aids assimilation of fats and other nutrients.

Silica: Beneficial for bones, nerves, skin, hair, and connective tissues.

USING BIOCHEMIC REMEDIES

Cell salts are completely safe. They may be used by infants, children, pregnant and nursing women, the sick, and the elderly. They may be used (usually with success) by anyone at just about any time.

Cell salts may be purchased in small pellets with a lactose or sucrose base. They may also be purchased in a liquid form. If you have the pellets and you want a liquid, simply dissolve the pellets in water. How much water and how many pellets is not really important. The success of these remedies lies in their frequency and energy pattern, not in a material dose.

Cell salts may be taken internally in either liquid or pellet form. They may be incorporated into sprays, creams, lotions, or soaps. They may also be added to baths for absorption by the skin. In liquid form they may simply be placed on the body. This is one of my favorite ways to use them on babies and small children.

Biochemic remedies are usually low potency remedies, usually 6X to 30X. They are very effective at these potencies and, in these low potencies, they certainly fit Samuel Hahnemann's description of a remedy that restores health rapidly, gently, and permanently without causing harm. These remedies, perhaps because they encourage the blood toward a more balanced condition, do not seem to set up negative symptom pictures by over-use as homeopathic remedies sometimes do.

Biochemic cells salts are administered and stored in much the same way as homeopathic remedies. Be careful not to contaminate your remedy by touching it with either your fingers or your mouth. They should be stored at moderate temperatures, away from direct sunlight. Keep them away from magnets, computers, TVs, microwaves, and any other source of energy that might alter or overpower their own frequencies.

Avoid, as much as you can, products containing camphor or menthol while using these remedies (as with all homeopathic remedies). Products containing camphor or menthol can slow the action of the remedy, or antidote it altogether. Caffeine, in more than moderate quantities, can also affect these remedies negatively.

Do not be afraid to use more than one cell salt at the same time or to use the 12 salt combination, bioplasma. These salts exist in combination in the body and taking them that way makes good sense.

BIOPLASMA

Bioplasma, a combination of all twelve of these homeopathic tissue salts, is certainly one of my polycrest remedies. (Remember, a polycrest remedy is one that is useful for many people.) Bioplasma, because of its effect on blood chemistry, will slow even heavy bleeding. I have used it many times to control bleeding from injuries. As a midwife, it has been valuable to me in the control of hemorrhage on more than one occasion.

Deficiency of these minerals can be seen by looking at the face, or even at the tongue. There is a book by David R. Card, *Facial Diagnosis of Cell Salt Deficiencies,* that I would highly recommend. The book is full of information about each mineral salt. The book includes pictures and artwork which clearly show what deficiencies of the 12 inorganic minerals look like.

Cell salts often require the presence of other cell salts in order to be absorbed. Because of this, the deficiency of one mineral sometimes leads to the deficiency of another one, even in the presence of sufficient amounts of the second mineral in the diet.

RECOMMENDED BOOKS

Facial Diagnosis of Cell Salt Deficiencies, by David Card (referred to above)
Deficiencies of the cell salts can be seen by looking at the face or even the tongue. This book has some wonderful insights and includes pictures and artwork that clearly show what the deficiencies look like.

Twelve Essential Minerals for Cellular Health, by David R. Card:
This is an inexpensive and compact reference book. In this book Mr. Card has placed, in user-friendly charts and lists, the best information from his many larger books. This book is an excellent resource for both the novice and skilled practitioner alike.

THE PREVENTION OF SEASONAL ILLNESSES

Some of these remedies are beneficial for the prevention of seasonal illnesses. The following protocol is based on recommendations by J.B. Chapman, M.D., in the book <u>Dr. Schuessler's Biochemistry.</u>

Since Nat mur and Mag phos are often necessary precursors to all of the other remedies, consideration should be given to adding them to the protocol in the beginning, especially if the tissue salt remedies have not been used before by the person or not used for a while.

I have found, for myself at least, that the best dosage pattern is to take the remedies 5 days a week for 3 weeks, take a week off in which no remedies are taken and then repeat the pattern if you feel the need or an illness has occurred

The winter months in areas of the world with a seasonal climate are noted for the increase of coughs, colds, pneumonia, bronchitis and similar troubles of the nose, throat, and lungs. Colder and more moist conditions, coupled with exposure to drafts and wind, can contribute to deficiencies of Kali mur and Ferrum phos. The first illness of the season further depletes these minerals in the body. A regimen of these two remedies at the beginning as winter begins may strengthen the immune system and prevent, or at least minimize, the severity and frequency of illness during these months.

If such an illness does take hold, remember to administer these remedies for a few days during the recovery period as well. A few drops of Ferrum phos in the mornings and Kali mur in the evenings is generally recommended.

During the winter months we tend to eat more warm foods and fewer vegetables and green salads. This produces, coming into spring, a mild anemia in most people. This anemia is experienced as fatigue, lack of energy, difficulty concentrating, possible leg cramps, insomnia, and a general sense of restlessness and unease. This condition was referred to as "spring fever" in previous generations and was a direct result of the lack of the availability of fresh vegetables during the winter months.

Ferrum phos and Calc phos are the missing salts which are believed to contribute to this condition. Ferrum phos, also used during the winder months in the recommendation above, is once again given in the mornings with Calc phos given in the evenings during the months of March, April, and May.

The warmer months of summer, and perhaps the food we eat as we travel and picnic, seems to breed bacteria that disrupt our digestive and intestinal systems. Kali mur should be taken in the mornings and Natrum phos in the evenings throughout the months of June, July, and August.

In the fall, as temperatures again become erratic and then turn chilly, Ferrum phos and Kali mur should be taken. Please note that these are the same remedies which are recommended for the winter months.

By following this regimen, many of the seasonal ailments from which we too often suffer can be avoided altogether or, at the very least, greatly reduced and minimized. Energetic remedies have a positive effect on the immune system, on the blood, and on the general strength and stamina of the body.

"An ounce of prevention is worth a pound of cure."

Of course, any time an illness or imbalance occurs the appropriate cell salt remedy should be taken. The choice of the remedy is made based, as always with anything homeopathic, on the symptom picture. The descriptions of the symptoms of deficiency provided on the next few pages and in the books referred to in this chapter may be helpful to you in determining which remedies are needed.

The Twelve Biochemic Cell Salts

#1 CALCAREA FLUORATA (Calc flour.)
(Fluoride of Lime)

BODY PARTS AFFECTED Bones, periosteum (covering of the bones), elastic fiber of muscle and connective tissues, veins, arteries, tooth enamel and joints.

FUNCTION Maintains the elasticity and contractive power of muscles, arteries, and veins. Vital to the ability of the periosteum to cling to the bones. Helps maintain connective tissue integrity.

DEFICIENCY SYMPTOMS Cracks in the skin, loss of elasticity in muscles and tissues, relaxed condition of veins and arteries (leading to hemorrhoids, varicose veins and aneurysm), sluggish circulation, loose teeth, spinal injuries, hard lymph nodes in the neck, ganglion cysts, bones spurs, fibrocystic breast disease, cracks and fissures in the hands, depression, ringing in the ears and conjunctivitis.

MENTAL DEFICIENCY SYMPTOMS Great depression, indecision and fears about money.

COMMENTS Nat phos is always needed in order to absorb Calc fluor. Kali mur is also recommended to be taken along with, or just before, Nat phos.

FOOD SOURCES alfalfa, kelp, eggs, whole grains, raw green vegetables, beets, fish, apples, mushrooms, apples

PRECURSORS/FOLLOW-UPS Kali mur, Nat phos, Calc sulph → **Calc fluor** → Kali sulph

#2 CALCAREA PHOSPHORICA (Calc phos.)
(Phosphate of Lime)

BODY PARTS AFFECTED Bones, muscles, nerves., brain, connective tissues and teeth.

FUNCTION Aids normal growth and development. Restores tone and strength. Necessary for injury repair. Aids digestion. Aids bone and teeth formation. Essential for recovery from and prevention of anemia

DEFICIENCY SYMPTOMS Anemia, low blood volume, tendency to bruise easily, blood coagulation problems, imperfect circulation, bone weakness, poor assimilation of nutrients, shriveled, wrinkled, or pasty looking skin, chronic sore throat., enlarged tonsils, inability of the body to maintain warmth particularly in the tip of the nose, the hands, and the ears. General feeling of chilliness.

Pregnant women often suffer from a lack of calcium and, to a lesser degree, phosphorus. This contributes to the mysterious cravings of pregnancy. A craving for pickles and ice cream makes perfect sense since the vinegar in pickles aids in the assimilation of the calcium in the ice cream and fills the craving for cold food and drink at the same time. Calc phos deficiency sometimes manifests as pica, a craving for indigestibles.

MENTAL DEFICIENCY SYMPTOMS Impaired memorym inability to concentrate and increased anxiety.

COMMENTS Symptoms are worse at night when calcium receptor sites open. Deficiency creates cravings for the salt found in ham and bacon and for ice cold drinks or ice. Calcium, given at the beginning of labor, is a good idea, especially for night labors. Nat mur and Nat phos are often needed for optimum absorption of Calc phos. Protein, magnesium, sodium (from sea salt), and potassium are also required.

In the past, it was recommended that pregnant woman avoid salt. I suppose this *might* be advisable if the salt you use was processed to death and man-made nutrients added back in. The exact opposite is true with a good sea salt. In fact, sea salt added to the diet helps prevent both toxemia and anemia!

FOOD SOURCES Vegetables, herbs, almonds, cucumbers, oats, soybeans, white beans, dandelion greens, cherries, spinach, squash, pumpkins, and dairy products.

PRECURSORS/FOLLOW-UPS Nat mur, Nat phos, Kali phos, Kali mur, Silica → **Calc phos** → Nat sulph

#3 CALCAREA SULPHURICUM (Calc sulph.)
(Sulphate of Lime)

BODY PARTS AFFECTED Blood, skin, gallbladder, liver and spleen

FUNCTION Blood purifier and healer that removes waste products from the blood. Aids in the production of bile and is particularly helpful in the proper digestion of fats.

DEFICIENCY SYMPTOMS Pimples, sore throat, cold, all conditions arising from impurities in the blood, abscesses of any sort anywhere in the body, pneumonia, croup and acne.

MENTAL DEFICIENCY SYMPTOMS Changeable mood, sudden loss of memory or consciousness, being absent-minded, increased irritability, discontented, full of fears, anxiousness that is better for being outside.

COMMENTS Calc sulph should be given whenever there is a wound or a sore with potential for infection. This remedy is excellent for boils and for infected areas of the skin that just won't seem to heal. Silica hastens the expulsion of infection and foreign materials while Calc sulph encourages the closing of the wound and the processing of the infection through the eliminative organs of the body.

It is usually advisable to administer both Calc sulph and Kali mur should a Calc sulph deficiency occur.

FOOD SOURCES Oats, almonds, cucumbers, lentils, peanuts, soybeans, cauliflower, onions, garlic, radishes, asparagus, celery, parsley, and green leafy vegetables.

PRECURSORS/FOLLOW-UPS Nat phos, → **Calc sulph** complete Kali mur

#4 FERRUM PHOSPHORICUM (Ferrum phos.)
(Phosphate of Iron)

BODY PARTS AFFECTED Red blood cells, muscles, nerves, hair, eyes— retina, irritation and inflammation., blood vessels and arteries.

FUNCTION First-aid, oxygen carrier, supplementary remedy.

DEFICIENCY SYMPTOMS Anemia with accompanying symptoms of fatigue and the need for abnormal amounts of sleep. Dizziness, rapid heart beat, shortness of breath and headache with slight amounts of exertion, difficulty concentrating, leg cramps, insomnia, craving for unusual foods and cracks at the corners of the mouth.

Lack of red blood corpuscles. Nose bleeds, inflammatory pain, high fever, quickened pulse, conjunctivitis., varicose veins, constipation as intestinal walls become too relaxed.

MENTAL DEFICIENCY SYMPTOMS Indifference to the details of daily life, loss of hope and courage, small things seem like huge difficulties and create extreme annoyance, delirium, maniacal mood swings, dizziness as a consequence of anger, inability to find the right word.

COMMENTS Redness in the face or ears, with or without a fever, is an indication of iron deficiency. Sufficient iron in the blood is necessary to keep a beneficial fever from burning too hot and a high fever burns up iron in the blood very rapidly, making matters worse still. It is essential during periods of prolonged fever that iron levels remain up. Since vitamin C is required for the utilization of iron from food sources, the folk remedies which include rose hips and other high vitamin C herbs are very much based on scientific principles. The giving of Ferrum phos cell salts at the beginning of a fever is advised.

FOOD SOURCES Green leafy vegetables, green vegetables in general (good sources of the calcium and Vitamin C that is necessary for the absorption of iron), onions, grapes, apricots, nuts, rice, and other whole grains, sesame and other oil seeds, tomatoes, oats, red and blue berries, blackstrap molasses, brewer's yeast, eggs, and meat sources including liver.

The bio-availabltiy of iron from plant sources is lower than that from meat sources due to the presence of phytates and oxalates in some raw vegetables. Phytates and oxalates can interfere with iron absorption. Steaming the vegetables eliminates, to a great extent, the presence of oxalic acid and the addition of even a small amount of meat to the diet increases the absorbability of the iron from plant sources. The reverse is also true; the calcium present in vegetables and herbs is necessary for the absorption of iron from animal sources. It should be noted, however, that vegetables are the most important sources of iron in the diets of the majority of people in India. There is, even in the poorest of areas, the addition of small amounts of meat.

PRECURSORS/FOLLOW-UPS Kali mur → **Ferrum phos** → Kali sulph

Other possible companion cell salts when needing to uptake iron by using Ferrum phos include Calc phos, Nat phos, and Nat mur.

#5 KALI MURIATICUM (Kali mur.)
(Chloride of Potash)

BODY PARTS AFFECTED Muscles, blood, saliva.

FUNCTION Aids in the treatment of burns, ids digestion by increasing bile which is needed to process fats and fat soluble vitamins. Cleanses and purifies the blood.

DEFICIENCY SYMPTOMS Sluggish conditions, atarrhs and mucus discharges that are white in color, sore throat, torpidity of the liver, gall bladder problems, white colored tongue, light colored stools, cough, colds, anemia, restless sleep, ingrown toenail (supplement Silica also here) and seizures.

Kali mur deficiency promotes the swelling of tissues throughout the body. Examples include: Swollen ankles, enlarged ovaries, swollen arthritic joints, enlarged lymph nodes, inflammation in eustachian tubes and nose, increased swelling after sprains and fibromyalgia (also a magnesium deficiency).

MENTAL DEFICIENCY SYMPTOMS Great sadness alternating with cheerfulness, irritable and angry at trifles, often sits in silence, and intense fear of evil.

COMMENTS Has been shown to reduce obstructions in the heart, liver, gall bladder, kidneys, and bladder. Aids in the removal of heavy metals from the body. Kali mur is necessary for the utilization of fatty acids. Fatty acids are vital to the absorption of minerals and the functioning of basic body systems and organs.

FOOD SOURCES: Peanuts, hazelnuts, lentils, potatoes, spinach, blackstrap molasses, ginger, coren, asparagus, celery, peaches, cauliflower, pineapple, kale, squash, red beets.

PRECURSORS/FOLLOW-UPS Kali sulph, Nat mur, Calc sulph → **Kali mur** → Calc phos, Silicea, Calc fluor, Nat sulph, Ferrum phos **Kali mur prevents stores of Nat phos from becoming depleted.**

#6 KALI PHOSPHORICUM (Kali phos.)
(Phosphate of Potash)

BODY PARTS AFFECTED Nerves, muscles and skin.

FUNCTION The primary function is the maintenance of the nervous system through movement of nutrients through cell walls and from cell to cell. Lack of function in any aspect of the nervous system involves a deficiency of Kali phos, among other things.

DEFICIENCY SYMPTOMS Nerve problems include the whole spectrum of emotional issues, some of which are listed here. Muscle fatigue, muscle spasms, menstrual cramping, general weakness, nervous headaches, lack of energy, sleeplessness, all symptoms associated with exhausted adrenal glands, poor vision, gums that bleed easily, poor digestion and elimination, diarrhea/constipation, vomiting, skin problems, nervous asthma, low blood pressure, heart palpitations and arrhythmias.

Mental symptoms include irritability, memory and concentration issues, instability of emotions and thought patterns (unable to connect cause and effect where personal actions and choices are concerned), depression, dark forebodings, looking only at the downside of situations, timidity, tantrums, over-sensitivity to noise.

A key-note of Kali Phos deficiency is the omission of letters or words when writing, the use of wrong words, and the confusion of ideas and thoughts when making a presentation or explaining something.

comments   Periods of extreme stress or illness, as well as prolonged less severe stress, deplete the body's stores of Kali Phos. Kali Phos is often deficient in elderly persons. Nat Sulp is a necessary preliminary treatment for Kali Phos.

food sources   White beans, cucumbers, cauliflower, pumpkin, orange juice, bananas, potatoes, tomatoes, dates, figs, olives, apples, almonds, peanuts, lentils, nearly all fruits and vegetables, ginger.

PRECURSORS/FOLLOW-UPS Nat sulph → **Kali phos** → Calc phos, Silica

#7 KALI SULPHURICUM (Kali sulph.)
(Sulphate of Potash)

BODY PARTS AFFECTED Skin, mucus membranes, intestines, hair, stomach, and tissue cells.

FUNCTION Oxygen carrier, maintains hair, benefits perspiration and respiration.

DEFICIENCY SYMPTOMS Intestinal disorders. Stomach catarrh. Inflammatory conditions. Eruptions on the skin and scalp with scaling. Shifting pains.

MENTAL DEFICIENCY SYMPTOMS Feelings of being boxed in physically or emotionally. Extreme irritability, always being in a hurry but unable to get everything that is wanted done, anxiety in the evening, timid in crowds, any mental exertion aggravates all symptoms.

COMMENTS Viral infections, colds, and flus deplete Kali sulph. This deficiency must be corrected in order for the patient to fully recover. Never-the same-since (NSS) symptoms from any cause usually indicate aKali sulph deficiency.

FOOD SOURCES Almonds, spinach, peas, nuts, parsley, flaxseed, watercress, cottage cheese, green leafy vegetables, apples.

PRECURSORS/FOLLOW-UPS Calc fluor → **Kali sulph** → Nat mur, Kali mur

The body may also need a round of Kali mur before Kali sulph if the discharges are whitish in color. Whitish discharges are often found in the very beginning stages of an illness. Kali mur administered at this point can be very effective in lessening the severity of the illness or even stopping it altogether. If the infection is persistent, Calc sulph should be administered.

The oxygen carrying capacity of red blood cells is a function of Ferrum phos but once the oxygen has been delivered by the blood, Kali sulph is responsible for moving it into the interior of the cell body. Kali sulph completes the work begun by Kali mur.

#8 MAGNESIA PHOSPHORICA (Mag phos.)
(Phosphate of Magnesia)

BODY PARTS AFFECTED Muscles, nerves, bones.

FUNCTION The outstanding function of Mag phos is on the nervous system, particularly as it communicates with muscles, including the heart muscles. Mag phos affects the elasticity of muscles and prevents or eliminates muscle spasms and muscle fatigue throughout the body.

MUSCLE SYMPTOMS Coronary arteries—chest pain, heart muscle—mitral valve prolapse, fallopian tubes—infertility, uterus—menstrual cramping, blood vessels in the head—headaches. Mag phos also benefits the nervous system and helps ensure rhythmic movement of muscular tissue.

DEFICIENCY SYMPTOMS Menstrual pains, stomach cramps, flatulence, bloating, constipation, neuralgia, neuritis, sciatica, headaches with darting stabs of pain, cramps, muscular twitching, exhaustion, night sweats., sleep and memory problems, resistance to new ideas, hiccups of babies (even in utero), water retention, swelling of tissues, restless leg syndrome, tourette's syndrome, depression, lack of self-esteem, asthma and Reynaud's syndrome.

MENTAL DEFICIENCY SYMPTOMS Nerves are on edge with the inability to relax emotionally (showing as anxiety, nervous disorders, depression); susceptible to stress, pain, anxiety, and depression.

During pregnancy, lack of magnesium can contribute to morning sickness, elevated blood pressure, and toxemia. The baby may arch its back during delivery, causing a brow presentation. After birth the baby arches backwards when held or dislikes being cuddled. These babies are usually colicky and very irritable.

KEY NOTES Craving for chocolate, low blood sugar and insulin resistance.

COMMENTS Magnesium is one of the minerals that binds with heavy metals and other toxic substances so that they can be eliminated from the body safely. Since heavy metals and other toxins are so prevalent in our environment and in our food supply, chronic deficiencies of magnesium are common.

FOOD SOURCES Green vegetables, chlorophyll, chocolate (dark is best), nuts, seeds, whole grains, sea salt, corn, peas.

PRECURSORS/FOLLOW-UPS Mag phos and Nat mur are precursors to all the cell salts. They should be taken together before, or along with, any cell salt regimen.

#9 NATRUM MURIATICUM (Nat mur.)
(Chloride of Sodium)

BODY PARTS AFFECTED Cartilage, mucus cells and glands.

FUNCTION Water distribution, nutrition and glandular activity, cell division, growth and aids the digestion process.

DEFICIENCY SYMPTOMS Weakness bordering on collapse if the deficiency is severe enough. Headaches with constipation. Runny stools, thin and watery blood, heartburn, toothache, hay fever, constant sore throats with a nose that is running clear liquid, abnormal appetite with thirst, sense of coldness, low blood pressure that is alleviated by adequate intakes of salt and wate, excessive perspiration with exertion, inability to digest meats, pale and waxy looking complexion, and neuralgic pains.

MENTAL DEFICIENCY SYMPTOMS Low spirits, feeling of despair about the future, dwelling on depressing subjects or events, continually bringing up the past and dwelling on it, feeling like a good cry for no reason but consolation from others aggravates and annoys, angry irritability with passionate outbursts, excessively excited and fast moving, mental exhaustion—mental exertion causes fatigue.

COMMENTS Natrum muriaticum is the Latin name for salt and is vital for the proper functioning of our bodies. The body will go to extreme lengths to protect its reserves of salt since depletion results in serious dysfunction of organs and systems and can result in death. Sodium (Nat mur) is used by the body to produce the hydrochloric acid needed for digestion.

The relationship between sodium and potassium creates an osmotic tension that maintains the integrity of cells and the flow of nutrients into and out of the cells. Much of our caloric intake is used to run this mechanism. If the mechanism is not working properly we gain what is known as "water weight" and we utilize fewer calories each day. The result is unwanted weight gain and feeling miserable all over.

Salt regulates the amount of moisture in the body. Depending on the availability of salt, the tissues of the body will have too much water (edema) or too little water. Too little water results in the non-conduction of necessary electrical impulses to the heart and brain as well as many other serious conditions. Salt is also necessary for the uptake of calcium.

It is possible to have adequate amounts of salt in the diet and still be deficient due to assimilation issues. A few doses of the cell salt, Nat mur, can aid the body in breaking down and utilizing salt.

There are a great many drugs which create disturbances in the sodium levels of the body!

FOOD SOURCES **Sea salt,** red beets, lentils, radishes, tomatoes, dairy products, celery and celery seeds.

PRECURSORS/FOLLOW-UPS → Kali sulph, **Nat sulph** → Calc phos, Kali mur

#10 NATRUM PHOSPHORICUM (Nat phos.)
(Phosphate of Sodium)

BODY PARTS AFFECTED Nerves, muscles, joints and digestive organs.

FUNCTION Acid neutralizer, promotes liver and gall bladder functions which aid in the breaking down of fats and the assimilation of nutrients, disperses lactic acid which can build up in muscles causing stiffness and paralysis,

DEFICIENCY SYMPTOMS Stiffness and swelling of the joints, acidic blood conditions, rheumatism, lumbago, worms, golden-yellow coating at the root of the tongue, indigestion, poor sleep, waking up with indigestion, and gout.

MENTAL DEFICIENCY SYMPTOMS include irritability, tension, crabbiness, argumentative tendencies. Argumentative, irritable children are often benefited by this remedy.

COMMENTS The function of Natrum phosphoricum is to keep the body more alkaline than acidic by absorbing carbonic acid and eliminating it through the respiratory system. The tissue salt, Nat phos, promotes this function.

FOOD SOURCES Lentils, spinach, rose hips, oats, olives, carrots, rice, celery red beets, apples, peaches, apricots, lemons, papaya, grapes, watermelon and the spices coriander, cumin, anise, and ginger.

PRECURSORS/FOLLOW-UPS Nat phos and Mag phos are precursors to all the cell salts. They should be taken together before, or along with, any cell salt regimen.

#11 NATRUM SULPHURICUM (Nat sulph.)
(Sulphate of Sodium)

BODY PARTS AFFECTED Liver, liquids inside the cells, and digestive system.

FUNCTION Eliminates excess water. Ensures adequate bile. Removes poison-charged fluids from the interior of cells, treats rheumatic ailments.

DEFICIENCY SYMPTOMS Influenza, asthma, malaria, liver ailments, brownish-green coating of the tongue, bitter taste in the mouth, urinary incontinence, bed wetting, water retention, type 2 diabetes, parasites, tendency to excessive bleeding, post-partum hemorrhage (use with Calc phos here).

MENTAL DEFICIENCY SYMPTOMS Poor short term memory, stumbling over words, inability to recall the word wanted.

COMMENTS Nat sulph, both as a cell salt and as a homeopathic in deeper potency, is a leading remedy for head injuries because of its ability to remove waste materials, damaged cells, and regulate to fluid levels. One indication of the need for this remedy is drowsiness after the head injury or dizziness even weeks after the injury occurred.

Like Kali sulph, Nat sulph is rapidly depleted during viral illnesses. Attention should be paid to a possible deficiency and Nat sulph, in cell salt form, should be considered.

FOOD SOURCES lentils, spinach, oats, garlic, parsley, celery, dandelion, chillies, horseradish, broccoli, cabbage, brussels sprouts, kale, onions, red beets, pumpkin, green peppers, cucumber, bananas, apples

PRECURSORS/FOLLOW-UPS Calc phos, Kali mur → **Nat sulph** → Kali phos, Silica

#12 SILICA OXIDE (Silica)
(Pure Silica)

BODY PARTS AFFECTED Connective tissues, skin, nerves, bones, mucus membranes, joints and lymphatics.

FUNCTION Cleanser and eliminato, initiates the healing process, insulator of the nerves, restores the activity of the skin.

DEFICIENCY SYMPTOMS Smelly feet and arm pits, pus formation, abscesses, boils, styes, clogged tear ducts, tonsillitis, brittle nails, stomach pains, diseases affecting bone surfaces, whitlows, gout, enlarged thyroid, cracked nipples in nursing mothers, suppressed perspiration, difficult wound healing, ingrown toe nails, falling out of the hair, and spinal irritation.

MENTAL SYMPTOMS Firmness of purpose but lacking the physical stamina to carry through. Inability to focus or maintain attention for even short periods of time, over sensitivity to noise, anxiety, great irritability, gloomy and despondent.

COMMENTS Silica helps to expel foreign objects from the body (slivers, bits of glass, and brings abscesses to a head, opening an exit so that infection and foreign objects may leave the body.

FOOD SOURCES millet, brown rice, whole grains, peas, carrots, cucumbers, strawberries, parsley, stinging nettle, dandelion, horsetail, comfrey, bamboo shoots, spinach, nuts, seeds, lemons, guavas.

PRECURSORS/FOLLOW-UPS Nat sulph, Kalli phos, Kali mur → **Silica** → Calc phos

The Twelve Biochemic Cell Salts

BIOCHEMIC CELL SALT	DESCRIPTION	BODILY PARTS AFFECTED	FUNCTION	DEFICIENCY SYMPTOMS
CALC FLUOR #1	Calcarea fluorata (Fluoride of Lime)	Bones, elastic tissues, veins, arteries, teeth, joints	Gives tissues the quality of elasticity, preserves contractive power of elastic tissues	Cracks in the skin, a loss of elasticity, relaxed condition of the veins and arteries, piles, sluggish circulation, loose teeth
CALC PHOS #2	Calcarea phosphorica (Phosphate of Lime)	Bones, muscles, nerves, brain, connective tissues, teeth	Aids normal growth and development, restores tone and strength, aids digestion, aids bone and teeth formation	Anemic state of young girls, blood coagulation problems, blood poverty, imperfect circulation, bone weakness, rickets
CALC SULPH #3	Calcarea sulphuricum (Sulphate of Lime)	Blood, skin	Blood purifier and healer that removes waste products from the blood	Pimples, sore throat, cold, all conditions arising from impurities in the blood
FERRUM PHOS #4	Ferrum phosphoricum (Phosphate of Iron)	Muscles, nerves, hair, crystalline, blood vessels, arteries, red blood cells	First-aid, oxygen carrier, supplementary remedy	Congestion, inflammatory pain, high temperature, quickened pulse, lack of red blood corpuscles
KALI MUR #5	Kali muriaticum (Chloride of Potash)	Muscles, blood, saliva	Treats burns, aids digestion, cleanses and purifies the blood	Sluggish conditions, catarrhs, sore throat, torpidity of the liver, white colored tongue, light colored stools, cough, colds
KALI PHOS #6	Kali phosphoricum (Phosphate of Potash)	Muscles, nerves, skin	Nerve nutrient, aids breathing, contributes to a contented disposition, sharpens mental faculties	Nervous headaches, lack of pep, ill humor, skin ailments, nervous asthma, sleeplessness, depression, timidity, tantrums
KALI SULPH #7	Kali sulphuricum (Sulphate of Potash)	Skin, intestines, hair, stomach, tissue cells	Oxygen carrier, anti-friction, maintains hair, benefits perspiration and respiration	Boxed-in feeling, intestinal disorder, stomach catarrh, inflammatory conditions, eruptions on the skin and scalp with scaling, shifting pains
MAG PHOS #8	Magnesia phosphorica (Phosphate of Magnesia)	Muscles, nerves, bones	Anti-spasmodic, benefits the nervous system, helps ensure rhythmic movement of muscular tissue	Menstrual pains, stomach cramps, flatulence, neuralgia, neuritis, sciatica, headaches with darting stabs of pain, cramps, muscular twitching
NAT MUR #9	Natrum muriaticum (Chloride of Soda)	Cartilage, mucus cells, glands	Water distributor, aids nutrition and glandular activity, aids cell division and normal growth, aids digestion	Low spirits, headaches with constipation, thin and watery blood, heartburn, toothache, hay fever
NAT PHOS #10	Natrum phosphoricum (Phosphate of Soda)	Nerves, muscles, joints, digestive organs	Acid neutralizer, aids in the assimilation of fats and other nutrients	Stiffness and swelling of the joints, acidic blood condition, rheumatism, lumbago, worms, golden-yellow coating at the root of the tongue
NAT SULPH #11	Natrum sulphuricum (Sulphate of Sodium)	Liver	Eliminates excess water, ensures adequate bile, removes poison-charged fluids, treats rheumatic ailments	Influenza, asthma, malaria, liver ailments, brownish-green coating of the tongue, bitter taste in the mouth
SILICA #12	Silica oxide (Pure Silica)	Connective tissues, skin, nerves	Cleanser and eliminator, initiates the healing process, insulator of the nerves, restores the activity of the skin	Smelly feet and arm pits, pus formation, abscesses, boils, styes, tonsillitis, brittle nails, stomach pains, diseases affecting bone surfaces, whitlows

Section Two

Chapter Eight - Flower Essence Remedies

EMOTIONAL WELL BEING

Flower essence remedies are very low potency remedies that address issues of emotional well-being, the development of character and spirituality, and mind/body health. The removal of emotional responses to certain triggers, the recognition that some ways of responding to certain situations are more appropriate and healthier than others, and the changing of negative attitudes such as fear to faith, and anxiety to peace, can have profound effects on both mental and physical health.

Dr. Edward Bach, an English physician and the creator of the original 36 Bach Flower Remedies, wrote in the early 1930's that, "Behind all disease lie our fears, our anxieties, our greeds, our likes and dislikes. True healing involves treating the very basis of the cause of the suffering. Therefore, no effort directed to the body alone can do more than superficially repair damage. Treat people for their emotional unhappiness, allow them to be happy, and they will become well." While the idea of emotional underpinnings to physical ailments is finding acceptance today, this was truly revolutionary thinking in Dr. Bach's day.

ARE FLOWER ESSENCES HOMEOPATHICS?

Flower essences, while considered by many to be homeopathics, are created a little bit differently and work by slightly different principles. In addition, there are no poisonous, unhealthy, or inorganic substances used in their creation. They are made from flowers, considered to be the crowning achievement and highest frequency cycle of plant life. These remedies are prepared from a sun infusion of wildflowers or garden blossoms in natural and very pure water. This solution is then diluted following homeopathic protocols. They are used only in the first 1 to 3 dilutions, making them very low potency, mild remedies.

HOW DO FLOWER ESSENCES WORK?

Flower essence remedies do not seem to follow the homeopathic law of similars, which is the very foundation of homeopathic theory. To work by the law of similars, these remedies would have to create within us negative feelings and emotions in order to draw these imbalances to the attention of our psyche and the innate healing abilities our minds and bodies possess. Flower essences do not do this. Instead, as Dr. Bach described the process, they "flood our natures with the particular virtue we need, and wash out from us the fault that is causing the harm." Flooding our natures with the opposing virtue is the way to eradicate any fault, in my opinion. Focusing on the fault only feeds the negative and gives the fault more power.

Perhaps Dr. Bach's explanation is an oversimplification, but it does explain the action of these remedies quite well. For example, Holly flower essence does not create feelings of envy, jealousy, or hatred in persons to whom it is given, even in large quantities or over long periods of time. Instead, Holly flower essence brings a feeling of connection and love into our hearts, even if we have been troubled in our lives by jealousy, envy, lack of connection to others, and even strong feelings of hatred.

Flower essences address our emotions. In fact, flower essence literature contains no reference to physical ailments at all. The descriptions of the states that the remedies address concern themselves completely with emotional and mental health.

Dr. Bach advised, "Think of the patient, not the disease. . . . The main reason for the failure of modern medical science is that it is dealing with results and not causes." To Dr. Bach the cause of the body's vulnerability to disease lay in the emotions. Physical ailments were the result of these emotional misperceptions and imbalances. Many Eastern philosophies and even Christianity believe much the same thing.

Flower essences remedies are so gentle that often a person will not have a sense of having had an emotional problem. Only in retrospect will the person be able to see what attitudes have changed, softening into a more positive and healthful perspective. I have found that keeping a journal, where the intuitions and insights stimulated by the remedies can be recorded, is both helpful and enlightening. There is much to be learned about oneself this way.

EMOTIONAL HEALTH AND OUR PHYSICAL BODIES

The scientific community, over the last two decades, has confirmed that our psychological and emotional state influences many of our bodily functions—far more than most of us realize. Our immune system, adrenal glands, hormone levels, and the neurotransmitters of our brain and nervous systems are known to be affected by our thoughts and the state of our mental and emotional health. While there is very little in the literature about physical ailments, and physical states are not the focus of flower essence remedies, flower essences remedies bring about profound physical changes.

Flower essence theory recognizes, more than most modalities, that the underlying emotion behind a physical problem may not be the same for one person as another. For example, two people may suffer from chronic headaches. For one, fear may be the overriding emotional cause, while for the other, loneliness may be the issue. (Perhaps the loneliness is tinged with a fear of being alone and fear is the underlying emotion, after all.) The flower remedy will act by flooding the person with the positive emotions of faith and connection to others until the negative emotions give way. The remedy opens a door, allowing us to see an alternative way to think and react. We still must choose between the old dysfunctional pattern or the new, more life giving, healthier one.

EXPECTED RESULTS

In most instances, change in emotional patterns come quite quickly, within a few weeks. In some instances of deeply rooted psychological patterns or beliefs, it may take longer or require follow-up with other remedies as the perception changes. The remedies do not create any kind of emotional or physical dependency. In fact, the remedies have a self-limiting effect. The need for the remedy diminishes as the person makes discoveries about his psyche and perceptions and moves toward a more balanced and healthy emotional state.

J. Herbert Fill, M.C., a psychiatrist and former New York City Commissioner of Mental Health, used flower remedies almost exclusively over tranquilizers and psycho-trophic drugs. He found flower remedies to have a profound and long-lasting effect on his patients, and they were free from any side effects. "I deal with emotional problems as well as physical ones," says Dr. Fill. "In my observations, these remedies appear to work on a much deeper level apparently assisting the individual in resolving deep-rooted conflict, as opposed to simply relieving the symptoms."

Dr. John Bolling, a specialist in behavioral and drug abuse problems and former Assistant Professor and Chief Resident in Psychiatry at New York University's Bellevue Medical Center, found significant health improvements in 80% of the patients he treated with flower remedies during a clinical study. Although other types of treatment were used simultaneously (meditation and hypnosis) Dr. Bolling found the most impressive part of the study "was the dramatic improvement shown in the overcoming of blocked emotional patterns by 20% of this group who prior to the study had been deemed resistant to any form of treatment."

Dr. Bolling stated, "Clearly Dr. Bach's remedies were the primary factor here. In addition to the marked improvement in their emotional state, these patients are now more open and receptive to other treatment modalities which had not been effective before."

Case Histories

#1. Harold Whitcomb, M.D., of Aspen, Colorado, uses flower remedies, especially in his treatment program for chronic fatigue syndrome. He finds that deep-seated, buried emotions are common in people with chronic fatigue and that the flower remedies help to bring these emotions to the surface, allowing them to be seen, acknowledged, and changed.

#2. A forty-year-old man suffering from chronic asthma since age three came to see Dr. Susan Lange, O.M.D., of the Meridian Health Center in Santa Monica, California. The man's long treatment history included inhalants and prednisone (a steroid hormone with effects similar to cortisone). Dr. Lange ascertained that the initial outbreak of the man's asthma coincided with the onset of his parents marital difficulties. The man's parents fought openly in the home, and his mother eventually committed suicide.

Dr. Lange performed acupuncture to open blockages in the man's chest and treated him with Fuchsia, a flower essence native to America that addresses the repression of deep-seated emotions such as anger and grief. Because the man was masking his suffering behind a cheerful facade, Dr. Lange incorporated Bach's traditional flower remedies Elm and Agrimony into the treatment protocol.

As the energy held in the man's chest released, Dr. Lange treated him for a blockage in the solar plexus and administered the flower essence Sunflower for issues of self-worth. Finally, he was treated for repressed kidney energy and was given Basil, Sticky Monkey Flower and Rock Rose. These remedies addressed his fear of intimacy. Within three months the man was able to discontinue all previous medication and was free of his asthma, reports Dr. Lange.

#3. When treating children, Dr. Lange also likes to treat the parents simultaneously. She finds that their problems often (usually) interconnect. In one case, a mother was experiencing a postnatal depression and couldn't relate to her child. Mariposa Lily, a flower essence native to America, was given to both the mother and the child to help them with parent/child bonding. The health of both mother and child improved, as did their relationship.

#4. Julian Barnard reports seeing a nine-year old girl suffering from repeated migraines who was tense, anxious and depressed. She was given a single bottle containing the flower remedies Gentian, Water Violet, Walnut and Bach's Rescue Remedy formula. Within days her mother reported marked improvement, noting that her daughter had been transformed back to her happy, outgoing self.

#5. A three-year-old child stung on the throat by a bee became frightened and hysterical, screaming in pain. He was given Bach's Rescue Remedy directly into his mouth and immediately became calm and quiet. With the stinger removed, Rescue Remedy was applied to the skin to alleviate inflammation. The entire episode was over in two minutes.

TRAUMA AND PREVENTATIVE THERAPY

"Flower remedies are particularly beneficial in helping to relieve acute trauma associated with accidents, bruises and injuries, as well as grief that would occur following the loss of a loved one," says Dr. Barnard. He also believes that using flower remedies can be a tremendous preventative therapy, and that by correcting underlying emotional problems, one can ensure that many physical problems will never occur.

I have been using flower essences for many years. I have found them to be gentle, effective, and absolutely amazing. Because they do not set up symptom pictures like homeopathic remedies do, it is impossible to misuse them or to do any harm.

Descriptions of these remedies can be found in a homeopathic Materia Medica or on the web.

Chapter Nine - Energetic and Vibrational Remedies

Energetic and vibrational remedies are homeopathics that are made from non-material energy sources. They are sometimes referred to as "imponderables." A definition that I like is "homeopathic remedies made from those substances which can be measured but not weighed." This group of remedies include Sol (sunlight), Luna (moonlight), Magnetis polus ambo (Magnet), Magnetis polus arcticus (north pole of magnet), Magnetis polus australis (south pole of magnet), X-ray, and Electricitas (electricity), to name just a few.

Are these homeopathics really anything at all? Having been exposed to, and made very ill from, exposure to electricity over a period of time, I can say, with conviction, that the symptom picture of Electricitas (electricity) is a very good description of the physical, mental, and emotional symptoms I experienced and had to recover from. I wish that I had known about this remedy at the time.

Samuel Hahnemann conducted the original provings concerning magnets and the magnetic poles. Further provings and research have been conducted over the intervening years. The major homeopathic houses now produce and distribute these remedies. If one believes that energy from these sources affects the physical body, the mind, and the emotions, then it follows that remedies made from these things can also affect the physical body, the mind, and the emotions in similar ways.

As I read through the descriptions of some of these remedies I found some common symptoms among them. Some of these commonalities are:

- A variety of symptoms in the nerves and nervous system
- Depression of various sorts (one remedy lists depression following a meal, for example, and another lists sad and depressed without reason)
- An effect on the female menstrual cycle, with scanty or profuse menses
- Heart irregularities, palpitations, and chest pain
- Headaches of various types
- Irritability
- Sleep disturbances which covered a very wide range—including sleepwalking according to the cycle of the moon, dreams, sleeplessness, and periods of agitation during sleep.
- Stiffness of limbs
- Mental confusion, memory difficulties
- Variations in appetite
- Sensations of coldness
- Various types of vertigo

MAKING THESE REMEDIES

Most of the remedies are produced by exposing milk sugar capsules to the energetic pattern chosen. Others are created using an alcohol and water solution in which to "capture" the energy pattern. (This capturing is sometimes referred to as imprinting.) Imprinting is accomplished in a wide variety of ways depending on what the source of the energy is.

Vibrational Remedies
(Color and Sound Remedies)

People are more than mechanical, physical beings. We are spiritual beings, housed in a physical tabernacle. Our spirits resonate with and are balanced by the vibratory rates of various colors and sounds.

All homeopathic remedies work in the realm of energy—they have left the physical world of the material dose behind. They reflect the energy pattern of the physical substances from which they were made. Matter is energy manifesting physically. Color and sound remedies differ from other homeopathics only in that they were already energy sources that were then captured in a slightly more physical form in order to be then potentized according to homeopathic principles.

All of us recognize that we respond differently to one color than to another, and that the different musical strains arouse different types of emotions in us. We know which things soothe us and which colors or sounds energize or balance us. That the frequencies of color and sound have been potentized as homeopathic remedies is exciting. These remedies are relatively new, fascinating to become acquainted with.

In the next few pages I will share with you what little I know about them and point you toward some other sources of information.

Ambika Wauters of Tucson, Arizona, is the creator of the color and sound remedies. Her color and sound remedies are the only ones, and the only information on these remedies, that I have seen is in her book titled <u>Homeopathic Color and Sound Remedies</u>. I was intrigued when I learned of her work with homeopathic remedies of color and sound. Her books on chakras and energy healing have been valuable to me in the past and correspond with my own experiences in these areas in many particulars.

Color Remedies

During a course of homeopathic study in England, Ambika Wauters asked her homeopathic instructor, Ian Watson, how and from what, homeopathic remedies were made. He replied that homeopathic remedies could be made from any substance on the planet. She then asked if, in his opinion, homeopathic remedies could be made out of color. He responded that, theoretically, it was possible and challenged her to try making some and see whether or not they worked. Following, she says, the impressions received in a dream, she went to work.

She eventually created 10 homeopathic remedies, which were made by exposing colored theatrical gels and Indian silks to sunlight and water. The colors used were—and still are—red, orange, yellow, green, turquoise, indigo, violet, magenta, pink, and a spectrum remedy which is made from all the colors in combination. Their creation was followed by several years of provings and clinical trials.

Samuel Hahnemann said that the best provings were those done on groups of people living under the same conditions, exposed to the same stressors, eating the same kinds of food, and drinking the same water. The first trial of the color remedies was at a Buddhist monastery in California, which certainly fit Hahnemann's criteria. The symptoms experienced by the original provers and the results of clinical prescriptions were carefully recorded.

The color remedies were first made available to the public in 1998. The response, around the world, was immediate and favorable by lay people and practitioners alike. The results of her efforts were eventually accepted by the famous Homeopathic Pharmacy, Helios, in England, who now produce these remedies for Ms. Wauters.

The strength of a color remedy is dramatically altered by the conditions under which it is made. It was discovered that remedies made in the bright sunlight of California were different and stronger, in some ways, than the original ones made in England.

Two batches of color remedies were taken to Helios labs for testing. One batch had been made during the winter solstice and the other during the summer solstice. Testing produced an interesting distinction between the two batches. The hot colors of red, orange, and yellow were strongest in the batch produced in the winter solstice. Green, turquoise, indigo, and violet were strongest in the batch produced in the summer solstice. It appears that nature gives warmth when it is needed most and reserves coolness for the hottest times of the year in some energetic fashion. Magenta and spectrum showed no difference in strength when comparing the two batches.

Sound Remedies

Sound remedies are made by holding tuning forks over pure water for a specific length of time. Students at the School of Spiritual Homeopathy were provers for the original remedies. Each prover in the group would take the same remedy, at the same time. Each carefully recorded her experiences and responded to a series of questions. This information was collated to determine the theme of each note, and to further understanding of its healing properties. These initial provings were followed by clinical trials. Initial results have been published, but understanding these remedies is still a work in progress.

Sound remedies have a strong impact on people who have become stuck in some aspect of their lives. Sound remedies shift energy, allowing us to think about the direction of our lives in more clear and focused ways.

Similarities and Differences Between Color and Sound Remedies

Color remedies work predominantly on our etheric bodies—the aspect of our energy field that acts as a conduit for energy to enter and work with our physical bodies. The previous sentence is a good description of chakras, and it would seem that color remedies directly influence our chakra centers. Chakras are very sensitive to color and produce colors which vary according to the state of balance they are in at the time.

Sound remedies act most strongly on the astral body. This body is responsible for our desires and aversions, and our mental processes. As the channel for our thinking, the astral layer of our energy has a profound effect on our souls and our spiritual lives.

Sound remedies produce almost instant and immediate reactions. Because of this, sound remedies have been kept at very low potencies. At these low potencies, the effects of the remedies do not last long and dosages must be repeated to produce long-term results. Used properly, these remedies work deeply. Color remedies work more slowly and, like most other homeopathics, have been potentized to different levels (6X to 30C).

Color remedies produced very different reactions in each prover, according to each person's personality. Some of the colors worked more physically, others worked more subtly on the emotions that were behind the physical manifestations. With the sound remedies, however, all provers experienced similar symptoms. The remedies were very distinct from each other.

The Results of the Provings

The color remedies seem to work more individually and to set people apart as individuals, strengthening their sense of self and independence. Sound remedies worked more collectively, fostering a sense of community. Each person in the group, while taking the sound remedies, experienced similar things and they coalesced as a group. They insisted on working and playing together and came to enjoy each other's company to a pronounced degree.

The color remedies have been around about 25 years now (2015). Sound remedies have been available for only about 10 years. This makes them new comers in the world of homeopathy.

These remedies fit, vibrationally, somewhere between flower essences and regular plant remedies. Like flower essences, they work on the emotions and energy states that underlie physical disease. The color and sound remedies may be used alone, but they seem to work best in conjunction with deep-acting mineral, plant, and sarcode homeopathic remedies. They also support the action of miasmic and constitutional treatments, but do not reach deeply enough on their own to handle long-standing chronic illnesses.

In provings and clinical trials, color and sound remedies have been shown to:

- Have a direct effect on body temperature and fluid retention
- Increase or release feelings of irritability
- Promote feelings of tranquility
- Assist with the expression of emotions
- Enhance levels of confidence and self-worth
- Influence our ability to give and receive love
- Restore vitality and joy
- Increase energy levels
- Influence chronic diseases
- Relieve depression
- Clarify our perceptions of ourselves and the world around us
- Help us form clear speech and rational thought
- Stimulate deep levels of joy
- Deepen our inner knowing and receptivity to spiritual guidance

Characteristics of Color and Sound Remedies

One tone of the scale and one color of the spectrum seem to share similar healing characteristics. Some of these are listed in the following charts.

RED AND MIDDLE C   ADRENAL CORTEX
Emotional Symptoms

These remedies are specific to feelings of being disconnected from or unaccepted by home, family, or community. These are excellent remedies for chronic depression, suicidal thoughts or tendencies, prolonged grief, and any inability to cope with a move, a job change, or the loss of a relationship through separation or death. Theses two remedies are good for helping a person feel more grounded to earth, better able to find and follow their purpose in life. Excellent aid for the development of organizational skills.

Physical Symptoms

Helpful with pain and irritation in joints and ligaments, particularly of the feet, ankles, knees and hips. These areas are our 'connection' to the earth. Red and middle C also have an affinity for bowel and rectal problems, circulatory problems, varicose veins, and autoimmune imbalances. One area in which these two remedies are of great value is in childbirth and postpartum care.

ORANGE AND D   OVARIES AND TESTES
Emotional Symptoms

The color orange and the D note address the polar opposites of the attitudes of poverty consciousness or an abundance mentality. Developing and maintaining the attitude that there is enough for everybody and Heaven is blessing me in particular brings great joy and peace. These remedies can moderate feelings of selfishness and greed based on the false presumption that there is not quite enough for all of our needs. These remedies can be useful for depression and states of very low energy brought on by depression. Either one, or both together, can relieve feelings of despair, especially those that accompany a feeling that nothing ever changes for the better in our world and nothing ever will. These two remedies should also be considered for the emotional drivers of any eating disorder.

Physical Symptoms

These remedies are used for sexual dysfunction of both sexes, PMS and other menstrual difficulties. They seem to have an affinity for the digestive system, the urinary tract, and the immune system. This makes them of value for allergies, constipation, eating disorders, and autoimmune disorders.

YELLOW AND E   PANCREAS
Emotional Symptoms

Yellow and E are good for times in our lives when we feel afraid, unsettled, or angry. Our minds may be feeling fuzzy and frazzled, and we lack our usual resilience and inner strength. Perhaps we have even become dependent on others in order to make simple decisions. Yellow and E can strengthen our sense of independence and personal power, helping us remember that the choice of focus and direction in our lives ultimately resides within ourselves.

Physical Symptoms

These remedies are mild and general diuretics. They are of benefit to each of the organs of the body, but particularly to the liver, gall-bladder, stomach, pancreas, pulmonary and respiratory organs. Interesting, symptom addressed by these two remedies is right eye vision problems or loss.

GREEN AND F   THYMUS
Emotional Symptoms

The thymus is considered to be the master gland of the immune system. Just as the physical thymus stands guard against attack by bacteria and germs, the emotional thymus is associated with our perception of safety or attack from people and situations around us. These remedies can aid us in our relationships with family, friends, and community members by giving us clarity about their intentions and feelings towards us. Feelings of vulnerability can lead us to avoid progress and change in our lives; these remedies can bring a resolution of conflicts within us, and help us move forward with enthusiasm and peace.

Physical Symptoms

These two remedies have an effect on the fluid levels in the cells of the body, acting as a diuretic throughout the tissues. This effect is most pronounced in cases of pulmonary or cardiac based edema. In fact, these two remedies are considered regulating and toning to the entire cardio/pulmonary system. Generally, they are very calming remedies.

TURQUOISE AND G THYROID
Emotional Symptoms

Since the thyroid is located at the base of the throat, it is often associated with issues of communication and creative expression. Turquoise and G are of benefit for those who struggle with tendencies to gossip, exaggerate, or even tell lies. They are also of benefit for those who are timid and shy in their communications.

Physical Symptoms

The range of physical symptoms controlled by the thyroid is large. Some of those symptoms include sore throats, tired or strained vocal cords, and pain in the neck or shoulders. These remedies can also be useful in programs to stop smoking, drinking, or overeating. They act as stimulants to the thyroid and parathyroids.

INDIGO AND A   PITUITARY
Emotional Symptoms

The color indigo is always associated with wisdom, knowledge, intuition, discernment, and imagination. The indigo color remedy, and the associated sound remedy of A, are helpful for balancing the opposites of these qualities. They should be used when intuition and good judgement seem to be lacking, when the thinking processes have become muddled and unclear, and when the mind seems to have become closed to new ideas and methods.

Physical Symptoms

The physical symptoms of indigo and A are predominantly concerned with congestion to the head and inflammation or other problems with the eyes, ears, and nose. They make good calmative remedies for anxiousness and insomnia. They may relieve migraine headaches and headaches brought on by eye strain. They may also be useful in reducing high fevers.

VIOLET AND B   PINEAL
Emotional Symptoms

The major secretion of the pineal gland is seratonin. People who are lacking in seratonin often suffer from depression, insomnia, and a lack of spiritual striving and connection. Because Violet and B act on the pineal gland, they may increase understanding and intuition, clear our perceptions, and foster appreciation of life while, at the same time, tempering ego and quelling prejudice and narrow-mindedness.

Physical Symptoms

These remedies act as tonics to the nerves. They have been of value in the treatment of liver conditions, jaundice, and nausea. They act as antiseptics in the cleaning of wounds and seem to speed healing. Just as yellow has an affinity for problems in the right eye, so violet has an impact on problems in the left eye.

PINK (NO NOTE OR GLAND APPLIES)
Emotional Symptoms

Pink is a remedy for the heart and is particularly appropriate where grief, disappointment, separation, and loss have robbed the person of either the desire or the ability to give love or be involved in other loving relationships. This remedy can be an aid to new mothers in bonding with their child and in avoiding postpartum depression.

Physical Symptoms

The pink color remedy may alleviate heart palpitations and arrhythmias that are the result of tension or sorrow. This remedy has a reputation for increasing milk production in new mothers. I suspect it is most effective when the cause of the problem is emotional rather than physical.

MAGENTA AND HIGH C   PINEAL
Emotional Symptoms

The symptom picture of these remedies includes feelings of unworthiness and self-doubt. These remedies can open us to receive love, happiness, health, and prosperity. They can increase our insight and creativity, make us more open to change and growth, and increase the joy and enjoyment we find in life.

Physical Symptoms

Magenta and High C remedies act as general tonics and can increase physical energy levels, focus the mind, and improve the memory.

SPECTRUM AND THE CHORD
Emotional Symptoms

These two remedies act against tension, fatigue, exhaustion, and burnout. They are particularly effective with chronic illness and pervasive discouragement.

Physical Symptoms

Any physical symptom that is evidence of overwork and exhaustion may be ameliorated by these remedies. They are specific for lack of vitality from overwork, illness, or substance abuse.

Chapter Ten - Combination Remedies

Combination remedies, as discussed previously, are made up of several individual remedies combined together. Each remedy in the combination has the general ailment as part of its symptom picture. Each remedy also has specific details that may, or may not, exactly match the circumstances.

Sometimes the taking of one of these remedies is all that is needed to bring relief. In other instances, the remedy appears to work for a while, or works to a level below what is required, and then stops working. In such circumstances, the proper homeopathic response would be to move to a deeper, higher potency. Doing this is not possible with a combination remedy. Moving to a higher potency would set in motion the symptoms of each remedy that do not match the malady closely enough.

The solution, then, is not more of the combination remedy. It is to determine which ingredient of the combination is responsible for the improvement. This will always be the remedy (or, possibly, two remedies) that most closely match the person and their symptoms. Each ingredient remedy will have to be looked at more closely using repertorising methods of analysis.

Two examples to help you see how this works follow. There is a small book, *Butterfly Miracles with Homeopathic Remedies II*, describing other low potency combination remedies available at www.butterflyexpressions.org.

EXAMPLE #1 ABSCESS REMEDY

The ingredients of this remedy are Pinus sylvestris and Cadmium oxidatum. (I choose this remedy as an example because it has only two ingredients.)

Pinus sylvestris has in its list of symptoms such things as pain, swelling, inflammation, mucus in various locations throughout the body, and glandular distress. Cadmium oxidatum also has pain and pressure from inflammation, the pain being greatly relieved at the appearance of an eruption. Cadmium is indicated for dull achiness all over, chills, and fever with great sweat.

For our example, let's say that the person has an abscess on the back of their neck, something like a boil. There is no sign of fever, sweat, chills, or body aches such as are indicated in the Cadmium symptom picture. Nevertheless, because both these remedies specify inflammation, this remedy would likely bring some relief from the pain. It may even bring the abscess to an eruption stage more quickly. Very good. The remedy has worked well.

But let's say that a new abscess forms a few days or weeks later. This would be an indication that there is still something wrong at a deep energy level. Taking another round of the Abscess Remedy might, or might not, bring relief this time. Either way, the underlying problem has not been properly addressed. A deeper acting, higher potency remedy is called for.

Since there was no fever, sweat, chills, or body aches, taking a remedy with these symptoms at a higher potency may (very likely will) create those symptoms in the person. They are not going to be happy about that! You should go to your Remedy Guide and study Pinus sylvestris more closely. If it matches the mental, emotional, and general symptoms of the person quite well, give it at a higher potency. If it does not, you will need to find a remedy that does match closely! Usually, that remedy will be one of the ingredient remedies of the combination that brought them a measure of relief at the low potency.

EXAMPLE #2 ALLERGY RELIEF #1

This is a remedy which has often brought me a great deal of relief.

The ingredients of the remedy, and some of their characteristics, are:

Grindelia robusta—typical allergic responses of lung and respiratory distress, asthma, rashes, **itchy eyes**

Urtica urens—allergic reaction creating <u>chronic gout</u>, <u>joint pain</u>, <u>burning pain in throat</u>, and <u>itching blisters on fingers and hands</u>. These symptoms may be the result of **an allergic reaction to shellfish** that was recently eaten.

Hydrophyllum virginicum—symptoms relating to the eyes, swollen eyelids, eye inflammation, itching, sensitivity to light

The person being treated in our example (me) is displaying all of the symptoms shown above in **bold** but none of the ones <u>underlined</u>. Taking this combination remedy would most likely, after relieving the eye symptoms, create the underlined symptoms.

It is possible, although not common, to take the low potency combination remedy too often or for too long and set up some of the symptoms. I have done it and felt the itching on my fingers and hands and the burning in my throat accompanied by joint pain. At this point, I was finally smart enough to think it through and take just the Hydrophyllum virginicum, which matched very closely.

Interestingly, I have taken Urtica urens with great results when suffering the listed symptoms after a reaction to shellfish.

That is how homeopathy works. There is not a remedy that works all of the time for any person. The symptoms that the person is experiencing must match closely the symptom picture of the remedy if the treatment is to be effective. That is one of the basic premises of homeopathy and the only way to obtain the results that you desire.

Do these examples mean that you should not use combination remedies. NO! I have carried Allergy Relief #1 with me for years. It has come in very handy for reactions to plants in the desert, in mountainous regions, and by the seashore. I have used it to treat reactions to food eaten in restaurants and to relieve eye strain from driving. I have used it to keep a cold from dropping into my chest and to treat several allergic rashes. I have taken it to relieve scary symptoms of a very serious allergy that I used to have until I could get to something better. But, when I returned home, I put myself on a program of deeper homeopathics and liver cleansing herbs. The result is that I no longer have all of these annoying allergies. I still carry my trusty Allergy Relief #1, just in case, but I rarely use it unless a head cold is coming on!

Combination homeopathics can be of great value. Just recognize them as what they are—a temporary relief, a band-aid, a first step in the complete process of healing. Sometimes, they are all that is needed; more often they should be followed by a more complete and deeper potency program.

Section Three

Pattern Thinking

Realms

Miasms

Miasms and Remedy Families

Higher Potency Remedies

In order to work competently with higher potency, deeper acting remedies, it is necessary to have a working knowledge of the basic principles of homeopathic philosophy. It is recommended that you re-read the material in Section One of this book before proceeding. At the very least, be prepared to turn to the index at the back of this book and look up explanations for any terms you come across in this section that you are not completely familiar and comfortable with.

Chapter Eleven - Pattern Thinking

PATTERN THINKING

Pattern thinking is a method of critical thinking that some say is becoming a lost art in the world today. The ability to look for the patterns in history to prevent repetition or to look for patterns in scripture to aid one in learning lessons about living is a valuable skill. Using this skill to look for the patterns of one's life and matching these patterns to the patterns inherent in every remedy is a valuable skill in homeopathy

It is very important to the understanding of homeopathic patterns to know that the most important patterns deal with the person's perception of reality. Reality for each person begins as perception in the emotions and in the mind. Events and relationships happen and we respond to them in ways that are individual and unique to us. These perceptions and responses become our inner reality. The more material world of physical symptoms, discomfort, and disease is only an imperfect reflection of our inner reality.

By looking for patterns in our symptoms we are able to build up a working model that allows us to see more clearly the way in which the real but invisible world—the world of feelings, perceptions, attitudes, and reactions to trauma—are being physically expressed as illness in our bodies. This understanding is vital in matching a remedy to the situation and, more importantly, matching it to the person as a whole.

HOMEOPATHIC PATTERNING

A pattern, in homeopathy, is made up of two parts, the background and the foreground. The background indicates the general type of remedy needed while the foreground symptoms will lead a classical homeopath to the specific remedy within a general remedy type and family.

The background consists of those ideas, feelings, and **reactions to stress** that are common to the person in all phases of their lives. Perhaps today those issues are being seen in the digestion, whereas last year the distress was in the respiratory tract. Wherever they are appearing at the moment, these varying symptoms show the same general perceptions and reactions to stress. They are a part of this person's pattern and can be used to determine the general type of remedy needed. The background pattern of a remedy from the mineral family is very different from the background pattern of a remedy from the animal kingdom.

The foreground pattern is those characteristics that are unique to the person at this time in their life. They may be the very specific and particular way that the body is presenting the background perceptions at this time or they may be so unique as to be out of character for that person at this time. The background symptoms and emotions are still there, some very visible with others somewhat muted. The foreground symptoms will define the particular remedy within the general grouping.

CHOOSING A REMEDY BY PATTERNS

In classical homeopathic prescribing, the presenting *background* symptoms are used to choose a general category of remedies—a mineral or a plant, for example. Then the *foreground* symptoms are sorted from the background ones and used to determine a specific remedy within the more general category.

When muscle testing for a remedy, we choose the remedy we will use from a list following the muscle test. Then we review the general characteristics of the category of that remedy. Is it a plant remedy, a mineral, a member of the animal kingdom, for example? Should I look for a remedy from the air or from the sea? Then we look at the specific symptoms of the remedy itself that do not really apply to the general description.

By pondering the various bits of information we learn more about the person and the manner in which the stresses of their life are manifesting in their physical body. The more we ponder and study the better informed and more accurate our muscle test will be the next time we use it to test a homeopathic remedy. We will also catch glimpses of and gain understanding about, the amazing science and rapidly expanding theories of homeopathic prescribing. The science and the theories of homeopathy expand with every passing day.

SOME PATTERN TYPES IN HOMEOPATHIC THOUGHT

Miasms, which were mentioned briefly in Section One of this book and will be developed in much more detail in the beginning in chapter thirteen, are one of the most basic and informative patterns homeopathic practitioners use to understand their clients and the remedies that will serve them well.

Types of remedies were discussed in section one and are re-listed below. Another way of finding patterns among remedies—and then matching them to individual persons and situations—is to understand the general characteristics of the various types of remedies.

Archetypes, the grouping of remedies and people according to basic personality styles is a new trend in homeopathy. The exciting piece of this type of pattern thinking to me is that the descriptions of the personalities include the attributes of a healthy state of being, not just the negative descriptions found in most homeopathic remedy pictures. These healthy personality types are referred to as *genotypes*, with the descriptions of unhealthy states being called *phenotypes*.

Realms is another method of looking at the origin of the remedy and comparing it to the basic nature of the person. The other realms, besides earth, are sky, sea, and one Peter Fraser refers to as the underworld. I have my own terms and definitions of this realm based on my Christian faith.

I do not like the term, The Underworld. It describes some, but not nearly all, of the attributes of the remedies Peter Fraser has classed here. The term is a spin on ancient mythology and almost completely discounts the views of Christianity. Nevertheless, many of the feelings, thoughts, and perceptions attributed to this class seem to be valid. Because of the narrowness of the evolutionary and mythological perspective, many other attributes (in my never-to-be humble opinion) have been missed entirely.

The name, and what it denotes from a religious point of view, is somewhat offensive to my own Christ-centered understanding of how this world works. In this work of my own creating, the underworld will be renamed and some of its descriptions will also be "tweaked" to what is closer to reality in my own mind. I will refer to Peter Fraser's underworld as the realm of death and rebirth. I just can't bring myself to use the term, underworld, to describe what I believe this realm consists of. It is just too concentrated on the negative and leaves too little room for positive personal choice.

The realms will be explored, in a little more depth, in the next chapter. My perspective differs from that of Fraser in several areas. I must, of course, teach from where I stand and from my own perspective, point of reference, and understanding, while giving credit to Peter Fraser and others for their efforts.

REVIEW OF GENERAL REMEDY CATEGORIES

In section one we discussed the groupings in a general and rudimentary fashion. In the next sections we will discuss these basic categories more fully and apply individual remedies within each group to specific ailments and symptom pictures.

BASIC REMEDY TYPES—A REVIEW

- Biochemic Cell Salts
- Flower Essences
  - Bach
  - North American
  - Range of Light
- Energetic and Vibrational
  - Energy Sources
  - Color
  - Sound

- Sarcodes
  - derived from cells of healthy tissues or organs
- Nosodes
  - made from diseased tissues or from a virus or bacteria considered responsible for a disease
  - (*to correspond to various miasms*)
- Minerals (Elements and Metals)
- Plant Kingdom
- Animal Kingdom

Chapter Twelve - Realms in Homeopathy

In identifying the overall pattern of a case, it is helpful to consider the general symptoms that a person is experiencing and their general frame of mind as it pertains to each of the realms. In order to do this, we must have at least a basic knowledge of the important features of each realm. It is helpful to have at least a basic understanding of the psychology of the mind and the differences in the psychology of the various realms.

The Realms of the Mind (Consciousness)

Psychologists, in some circles, have recently concluded that consciousness has three distinct components: the subconscious mind, the conscious mind, and the super-conscious mind. The conscious mind is defined as awareness and choice; the subconscious and the super-conscious minds as opposing environments from which we view the world around us. It is from these opposing viewpoints that we obtain our "facts" and form the rationale we use for the choices that we make.

THE SUPER-CONSCIOUS MIND

The super-conscious realm is known in many spiritual traditions as Heaven or, for those who do not acknowledge a God, the Higher Self. This part of the consciousness is described as knowing no fears, no blocks, no ignorance. The early Greeks and many other cultures, past and present, refer to this part of our subconscious/non conscious mind as the heart.

The super-conscious mind contains the memories of those times in which we acted in full awareness of our true nature as a child of the Divine and as a successful and competent being. The "facts" stored here are memories of actions taken in love, forgiveness and peace in total absence of all fear, anxiety and prejudice. This higher mind sees the interconnections and deeper meanings of the experiences of our lives and helps us make our conscious choices from a position of love, strength, and faith.

In the body, the super-conscious mind seems to be focused in the heart and the neocortex of the brain. Energetically, according to eastern philosophies, it is focused in the top four chakras and in the 5th and 6th meridians—the meridians of the heart.

THE SUB-CONSCIOUS MIND

This newer school of thought also defines the subconscious differently from the way it has been defined in the past. According to this new definition, the subconscious mind contains all the raw physical energies of birth and impending death. The outlook of the subconscious mind is colored by fear of death and fear of change.

Here in the sub conscious mind are stored the memories of all the experiences in which we were reacting from basic survival instincts—whether our survival was in serious jeopardy or not! Fear, anxiety, panic, self-protection, and lack of trust characterize these memories, and they can become the "subconscious basis" for our reactions and choices if we let them. Every subconscious memory is an incomplete experience that the soul has not fully understood and come to terms with . These paralyzed chunks of incomplete understanding create dark spots, or blocks, in our energy fields and rob us of peace.

In the body, the subconscious mind is focused in the brain stem and lower brain; energetically, it is found in the lower three chakras and in the 1st, 2nd, and 4th Meridians (Gall Bladder/Liver, Kidney/Bladder, and Stomach/Spleen). The negative states of these meridians and chakras give us an idea of what the heart/super-conscious mind is battling in order to bring peace, confidence, harmony, and perspective into our lives.

The subconscious mind contains a wealth of knowledge about our physiology, and its protective instincts are a necessary part of our psyche. We need to recognize danger when that danger is really real, and act accordingly. But the subconscious mind has a darker side because it is the home of incorrect perceptions and the negative emotions of stress, fear, and self-protection. If we choose to dwell there, this darker side can color our view of the world, impede our vision, and prevent us from moving forward to accomplish all that we would like to—and are meant to—accomplish.

THE CONSCIOUS MIND

The conscious mind, in contrast to the other two kinds of consciousness, contains no memories at all according to this new psychology. It knows nothing of itself but is best described as the "Eye of the Soul." The conscious mind is the point of awareness from which we draw on the "knowledge" in the subconscious or super-conscious realms of our minds. Here, with our conscious mind, we decide how to react and which of our life's experiences we will draw upon to make decisions, choose our actions, and form the basic premise of our lives.

The conscious mind takes the bits and pieces of our past, connects the dots and forms an opinion: "I am this" or "I am that," "people in my world are this or are that, and "the world functions like this" or "the world functions like that." The conscious mind chooses what we use to determine reality.

In the body, the conscious mind is focused in the center of the brain. In fact, neurologists have found that destroying the midbrain's limbic cortex causes complete loss of the sense of self; they can remove any other part of the brain or body with little effect on the person's perceptions of self and the experience of individuality. There is no doubt that the mid-brain defines the personality; without it the brain cannot process the pieces of memory that we use to define ourselves. It is, I think, significant that this part of our mind is found in the most protected, central area of the brain where it is less likely to be damaged from traumatic accident.

As the seat of free will and the point of choice, your conscious mind shapes your daily life. The attitudes and ideas you identify with determine the kind of person you will be and the experience of life that you will have. Only two choices exist. You can look toward the super-conscious mind or toward the subconscious mind. Your view of life, and your basic intuition and responses, will flow from the source you identify with—love and service or fear and self-centeredness.

If your conscious mind looks predominantly toward the super-conscious realm, it will bring you feelings of "I am whole and complete, full of purpose and truth, wise, loving, beautiful and harmonious." If, instead, it looks toward the subconscious, you will feel afraid, unworthy, ugly, defensive, frustrated and angry. You will feel like you have "gaps" in your understanding and will probably set yourself up in some form of the "victim" mentality.

The choices between these two realms are very dramatic and they are mutually exclusive. We can have the experience of love, light and the flow of truth, or the experience of immobility, fear, judgement, and anxiety. Life really does boil down to opposites—faith/love and fear/lack of trust-and brings to mind the scripture, "Perfect love casteth out fear."

What does all of this mean? It means that how we perceive the world is a conscious choice! The reality is that continually choosing to draw from one or the other bank of memories builds neural pathways in our brains. Our responses to the people around us and the world in which we live begins to seem automatic and our perceptions become our version of reality. We see the world as safe and our place in it as secure and worthwhile or we see the world as a hostile place where we must always be on the defensive and looking out for ourselves as best we can.

What does all this have to do with homeopathy? I believe that homeopathic remedies communicate on an energetic level with the sub conscious mind. It is almost as though they open the door to the super-conscious mind and let us get a glimpse of another and better way. We do not have to go through the door just because we caught a glimpse of the possibilities. The choice is still ours, but the homeopathic has just given us a view we may not have had before.

I believe the homeopathic remedy also provides us with a moment's hesitation in which to make up our minds. Instead of just "gut reacting" we make a choice but if we have been seeing only one choice as possible we have really had no choice at all! We must be able to access both the negative memories and the positive ones if we are to have an opportunity to make a choice at all.

Taking counsel from the super-conscious mind, whether it resides in the brain or the heart (or both), is to look through the spiritual eyes of faith. It is to be watching and praying always.

The Realm of the Earth

MAN

Man is a creature whose natural physical home is on the earth. The fact that we live and move on the ground defines much of who we are and how we think during our mortal existence. Many of the homeopathic remedies are made from substances which come from the earth. The plants grow there. Many of the minerals exist in the earth. The animals, with the exception of birds, some insects, and the snakes, are considered earth realm remedies.

CHOICE AND ACCOUNTABILITY

The earthly realm is the realm of the conscious mind. It is the point of choice in our own lives just as the earth was a place of choice for Adam and Eve.

STRUCTURE AND SOLIDARITY

Structure is the most important aspect of the realm of the earth. In the body, the parts that are important and most affected when this realm gets out of balance in a person are the parts that have to do with structure. The skeletal bones are always a part of any remedy that applies to earth, as are the muscles and the connective tissue which hold the bones in place. Skin symptoms are also often seen because of the skin's role in protecting and holding the whole together.

The structures of which the earth is formed, whether naturally occurring or man-made, are not really built for or meant to be moving about on their own. Mountains do not move and plants are rooted firmly in the ground. The movement of the structures of our bodies are often a part of the ailments connected to this realm. An inability to move may be manifested physically, as with arthritis or stiffening of muscles. Lack of movement may also express itself as an inability to accept change or to make needed changes in our thinking and behavior.

MASCULINE TYPE ENERGY

The energy of the earthly realm is predominantly masculine. It is governed by reason and by logic and the emotional has little place there. (No, I am not trying to be sexist; just trying to explain this realm as it was explained to me.) The basic impulses are to tame and explain. If that is not possible, ignoring is almost always considered an option.

HIERARCHY

The drive for position or power is very strong in the earthly realm. To be in control is of great importance. The hierarchal structure of earth is usually a patriarchal one. It tends to be competitive, especially in the animal kingdoms, and is too often based on success and worldly achievement. There is always somebody to outshine and some new level of achievement to be reached.

FEAR OF FAILURE

Feelings of insecurity, fear of failure, and feeling a need to constantly prove oneself is a powerful emotion in this realm. Social situations, or any situation really, that lack structure and organization create feelings of insecurity and fear. Power and position, safety and security, become unduly important.

PERMANENCE/CHANGE

Changes in the earth generally come slowly and for a reason. Changes are often built on the foundations of the past. The energy is progressive and cumulative. Things get bigger and better and things are judged on how much bigger and better they have become.

KNOWLEDGE

Knowledge, like structure and permanence, can be built on the foundation of what was previously known. Earth energy is scientific and mathematical in nature. It has a tendency to become too detailed, too specific, too structured and, often, less and less connected to reality and daily life.

ABUNDANCE ISSUES

Material things, wealth and possessions, which are products of the earth, become immensely important. They are, too often, the way that success is measured on this earth. The greater the emphasis placed on earthly things, the greater is the fear of losing them. Abundance issues, the feeling that there is not enough for you and me both, are very much a part of this realm and of the remedies that help us achieve balance here. There seem to be endless possibilities for having more and more and, sometimes, there is a feeling that we can never have enough, and certainly will never have a surplus.

NURTURE

Nurture, as it applies to earth, has more to do with nutrition, the digestive system, and the absorption of nutrients. Digestive issues are often found in the realm of the earth.

FATHER/SON RELATIONSHIPS

Possessions and land in this earthly realm are often passed from father to son. This is part of the idea of structure—building on the past and building for the future. The father/son relationship described in this realm is, I think, symbolic of the Savior and His Father. This relationship is very important in the realm of the earth and in earthly remedies. Everything denotes there is a God and speaks of his character and attributes.

REMEDIES OF THE EARTH

The plant remedies are firmly grounded in the earth. Although the plants extend into the other realms by either reaching for the sky or having their feet planted in water and wetlands, they have a predominant energy of earth about them. To my mind, and that of my husband, plants are messengers and messages from a loving Father who could not be everywhere. Their substance (herbs) and their energy (plant based homeopathics and essential oils), by helping us heal our physical bodies and perfect our very natures, speak to us clearly of God and creation.

The mineral remedies, of course, are often dug from the earth itself. Other minerals, such as Natrum muriaticum, have a connection with the sea because they have been dissolved and transformed there. The gases escape readily (as some of us would like to) into the realm of the sky.

The animal kingdom is even more diverse with some living out their entire lives in the sea. Others, like the insects, spend parts of their lifespan on or in the earth and another part of their time in the sky. The birds are born on the earth but spend much of their time in the sky. Some animals reside in both earth and sky.

While the energy of the earth and the remedies obtained from it are very diverse, there are underlying themes and patterns readily seen. The diversity also forms itself into fairly recognizable sub-categories and patterns—insects, plants, minerals, etc. *Bryonia, Rhus toxicodendron, Lycopodium, Thuja, Conium, Staphysagria,* and *Anacardium* are a few plant remedies that clearly show earth-like properties in their remedy picture.

The Realm of the Sea

ANCESTRY AND INHERITANCE

The realm of the sea is the realm of the pre-consciousness mind. It is the realm of those things that we brought with us from the other side of the veil of forgetfulness. It is fitting that our earthly beginnings should have been in the amniotic waters of our mother's womb. Here, we ***became***, building our own unique individuality from the composite inheritance of physical, emotional, and mental traits that were being handed to us as a genetic inheritance.

FEMININE ENERGY

The energy of the sea is usually very feminine in nature. Action and thought in this realm are ruled by emotion, instinct, and the whisperings of the Spirit. There is a sense of what is right and what is dangerous and to be feared that is a natural part of the flow of the realm of the sea. This natural order of moving away from danger and toward nourishment and good is sometimes difficult to explain in earthly terms and to people living predominantly in the earth realm.

Often that feminine energy of the sea is a maternal, nurturing type of energy. It is a realm of emotions and relationships. The relationships that are most important in this realm are the blood relationships. Nothing is more devastating to a "water" personality than disharmony in, or loss of, a family tie or family member.

BOUNDARIES

Water is an element of flow. No part of the sea is fully separate from any other part and, even on land, water flows into and over whatever is in its path. While water is fluid and described by many as "going with the flow", water is also a very strong and powerful element—strong enough to cut its way through almost anything eventually and destroy everything in its path. Water can be either an element of patience or an element of restlessness and agitation. Whatever it is, it is the basic element of life.

The endocrine system and the immune system to which it is tied belong to this realm. These systems have strong ties to the establishment of or loss of boundaries between ourselves and others.

MOTHER/CHILD RELATIONSHIPS

The relationship of mother and child, which begins in the watery world of the womb, is the primary relationship of this realm and the potential area of the greatest pain. The mother/child relationship is meant to be one of unconditional love and is the deepest of the blood relationships.

UNCONDITIONAL LOVE/INSTINCTUAL DISLIKE

The love of this realm, even outside the mother/child relationship, is one of unconditional-type love. It is based on a recognition that each person is trying to build the best they can with the materials and tools they have. In the manner of opposites, the dislikes of this realm can be just a deep—as deep as the sea—and just as unrelenting.

STUCK IN ONE PLACE

The creatures of the sea are, for the most part, caught in a place they can never get away from. The water is their world and always will be. The over-riding keynote of this realm and personality is a sense of being unable to move on, being unable to get away from or do anything about the things that are affecting us so deeply. This sense of helplessness and hopelessness can lead to resentment, brooding, mind-chatter, and an inability to put past grievances behind us. The resentment and brooding are rarely expressed. It seems unworthy and not worthwhile to the person to express that which cannot be changed or moved away from.

TIME/PROJECTS/ORGANIZATION

Time often seems to be suspended in and around the sea. There will be issues with appointments and schedules, issues of procrastination, and difficulty with deadlines and organizational skills. Time is simply irrelevant for those caught in the sea realm. Things will take the time they take and be finished when they are finished, if they are ever completely finished at all. The world of the sea is a world of continuum—one thing flowing into another and new things always added to the old.

NUTRITION

The role of nutrition in the realm of the sea is a very different role from that of the nutrient and absorption issues of the earthly realm. Nutrition in the sea realm has far more to do with emotion than with the function of the physical body that is prominent in the earthly realm symptoms. There may be dysfunction in the digestive system of a sea remedy patient but it will be tied to an emotion.

I really liked the description of the difference in Peter Fraser's book, <u>Using Realms in Homeopathy</u>. He says, "A baby that is unable to digest his mother's milk is more likely to be expressing something from the earthly realm. While a baby that is unable to latch on and suckle properly is more likely to be expressing something from the realm of the sea."

SOCIAL RELATIONSHIPS

The social relationships of the sea are usually matriarchal. There will usually be a great deal of cooperation with sisters, aunts, and grandmothers as they trade baby sitting and protect the young. Balanced water energy creates very stable groups with little competition; the opposite, of course, is also seen where problems exist and balance has been lost.

COMMUNICATION/EMPATHY
Communication is important in the realm of the sea. This communication is more about understanding and sharing than about instruction. There is a need for the continuity of information, knowledge, and skills from one generation to the next and there is a need to know what previous generations believed in and stood for. Many species of fish live in schools which move and react as a whole, rather than as individuals. There is a need, in water energy, for the family unit, and even classroom groups, to move with this type of unity.

The energy of water, the sea realm, is the way in which we came into this world. There is much of beauty and harmony in this energy. But, like the demanding days of motherhood, it is also a place from which we must move on to other levels of development. The resentments and brooding of the sea must be left behind for the growth toward the light that is the energy of the earth and sky realms.

REMEDIES OF THE SEA
The remedies of the sea include themes of exploration, trade, and communication. Underlying themes are related to survival, feelings of abandonment, betrayal, persecution, isolation, and violence. The positive aspects of these remedies include finding the stillness and calm, emotionally, of the sea and a feeling of connection with all of humanity and even with all of creation.

Water is the substance that is most vital to life and makes up the greater part of our cellular structures. Salt, which is derived from the sea, is an absolutely vital nutrient. The natrum (sodium) remedies play an important role in homeopathy when dealing with issues in the realm of the sea.

The sea also has an affinity for the generative organs. While difficulties with the male organs, testes, and prostate can often indicate a sea remedy, it is the female organs and the processes associated with them in which the pattern is the strongest. Ailments involving the ovaries, uterus, female hormones, the menstrual cycle, and the processes of pregnancy and birth have a sea-like quality. *Natrum muriaticum, Sepia,* and *Murex* are polycrest sea-type remedies.

These organs also have symptoms that are closely aligned with the underworld (or, in my terminology, with birth and death) as well as correspondences to many remedies from the earthly realm. *Lachesis* is a generative organ remedy that has Underworld symptoms. Remedies of the Earthly Realm include *Platina, Pulsatilla,* and *Chocolate* as well as any member of the Lily family. Differentiating between them is usually quite easily done.

Calcarea carbonica, although a mineral, is made of the pearl of an oyster and has the influence of its sea origins in its picture. Other sea creatures in the homeopathic world are *Sepia, Murex, Spongia, Asterias rubens, Corallium rubrum* and *Cypraea eglantina.*

The Realm of Death and Rebirth—Light and Darkness (Fraser's Underworld)

BIRTH AND DEATH
The energy of this realm is the energy of birth into this world and of the birth into the eternal world that we call death. It is the energy of the light within and it is also the energy of the darkness that is its opposite.

UNRESOLVED TRAUMA
This is the realm of the sub-conscious mind. It is here where the dark pieces of unprocessed traumas and events from our past are stored. It is these negative dark bits, called energy cysts in some modalities, whose dissolving and resolving bring us from darkness into light and give us rebirth and renewal one step at a time.

PASSIONS/SEXUALITY
This energy is the realm of the passions. These passions include love and hate, envy and jealousy, and the passions of desire. Passionate emotions that are extremely powerful are the keynote of this realm. These emotions can be as destructive as they can be beautiful. The passions of this realm seem to center around love and sexual passion.

RELATIONSHIPS

The relationships that matter in the realm of the spirit are the relationships of love and sexual connection. The choice of who we love and the way we conduct these relationships should be subject to both reason and inspiration, but sometimes they are not! Problems in these relationships are the dark side of this realm. The heights to which human love can take us is the realm of light that exists within this realm and within each of us. Families are eternal. Relationships were meant to last. This realm exists, in some form, in each of us.

LOVE AND HATE

Extreme hatred, while not the exact opposite of love that apathy is, behaves in ways similar to the negative aspects of out-of-control passionate love. Sexual perversion partakes of some of this dark energy, also.

ANCESTORS/LOVED ONES ON THE OTHER SIDE

The darkness and light of this realm comes into our lives when someone we love dies, leaves, or betrays us. In death, our loved one moves out of this world but we are undeniably connected to them and they to us. Interactions with those inhabiting the spheres beyond our own are features of this realm. Opposites are at play here, too. We may experience visits from both the realms of light and darkness. Of particular note and beauty in this realm is the experiences of guidance we sometimes receive from ancestors that have passed on.

DARKNESS/LIGHT

Within this realm are obsessions and fear of the darkness that we are afraid exists within ourselves. This darkness has its opposite in the light and tuition of the Spirit. We simply know what we know, though we may not be able to explain the knowing. Sometimes, these thoughts and feelings come to us fully formed, in whole sentences, and are accompanied by the conviction and fire of the promises of the Spirit.

COMMUNICATION

This realm is rarely manifest in physical form; it is only realized through emotion and thought. Both good and evil thoughts and intentions can be communicated without the passage of words. The subliminal discerning of thoughts and emotions is a manifestation of the intangible nature of the light and the darkness that coexist in this realm and within ourselves. These undercurrents of emotion can bring peace to one another or they can inflame the senses, bringing disharmony and unsettling emotions.

EXPRESSION OF SELF THROUGH CREATIVITY

Art is often used to express the powerful emotions of the soul. With art we can explore the nebulous concepts of desire, beauty, love, fear, and hatred without getting too close and personal. Art describes and defines the world around us and the emotions that are swirling within, helping us to better understand ourselves.

THE PHYSICAL BODY

A keynote among the physical symptoms that do exist in this realm are issues having to do with the heart, both as the center of passions and as the major organ of circulation. This affinity includes the veins and the arteries. The free flow of information from spiritual sources—or the lack of such communication—often manifests as some type of inflammatory type symptoms.

REMEDIES FOR THE REALM OF LIGHT AND DARKNESS

The realm of the underworld is a place of passing through and then going beyond. This transience is reflected in the remedies that apply here. Snake remedies are the primary remedies of the negative aspects of this realm. Snake remedies also indicate a movement between the darkness of death and the light that is its opposite.

The plant family, Solanaceae, has strong ties to this realm. This is especially true of the members of this plant family that are poisonous to one degree or another. Some of these plants are *Belladonna, Stramonium, Dulcamara, Hyoscyamus niger,* and *Mandragora.*

In the mineral family, the radioactive minerals are also of this realm. This is seen most clearly in *Plutonium*, which, oddly, was named for the mythical ruler of the Underworld. *Radium* and *Uranium* also show many of the symptoms of this realm. *Positronium*, another radiation remedy, has some features of this realm but is also an imponderable with sky qualities. Color remedies often have a place in this realm

The Realm of the Sky

SPIRITUALITY AND ASPIRATION
The realm of the sky is the realm of the super-conscious mind. It is the place where doubts and fears are left behind and faith can flourish. We feel our place as children of divine inheritance with boundless abilities and potential. The realm of the sky is a place of spiritual aspiration and striving for perfection.

EMOTIONAL PATTERNS
The emotions which belong to the super-conscious mind include unity, cooperation, wisdom, creativity, confidence, peace, generosity and receptivity to the guidance of the Spirit. The emotions of this realm are usually positive and optimistic ones, but when out of balance they can reach extremes of negativity.

FREEDOM
The most important and over-riding feeling of the realm of the sky is the feeling of freedom. This freedom is the expansiveness of infinite possibilities, the freedom to do and to be anything that one wants to do or to be. There can be no comprehension of the limits to the realm of the sky because there are no limits to the edges of space. The realm of the sky also represents eternity.

BEWILDERMENT/DESPAIR
Boundaries are an important aspect of realms. The earth is a realm of hard edges and clearly defined boundaries. The sea is softer, more flowing, but there boundaries set by the need for air that clearly govern there. The underworld represents death and life which are quite separate from each other. The boundaries between these two aspects are only breached according to the laws of heaven. The sky allows for a freedom from boundaries that can be found nowhere else.

This lack of boundaries can leave people with a sense of being lost in both time and space. No boundaries creates a sense of bewilderment. A world of boundless possibilities can be daunting and contribute to feelings of helplessness, hopelessness, loneliness, and despair.

RELATIONSHIPS
The lack of boundaries of the sky element also extends to relationships. Here, as in all things, there are positive and negative aspects. On the negative side, we can lose our personal boundaries, lose the ability to say "no" when necessary, and be much too susceptible to the opinions and influence of others.

Positive attributes of the sky realm include deep empathy and compassion and an ability to understand the needs and feelings of others. This love is love in the Christian sense, pure and unconditional. It can be the feelings between a teacher and his students and the healer and his clients, as well as the love shared by family members.

PATH IN LIFE
The realm of the super-conscious is about finding one's own special mission and calling in life. It is about the quest for perfection and the fulfilment of one's personal potential.

LIFE ON EARTH/ASPIRATIONS OF PERFECTION
Man is a spiritual being having an earthly experience. Like the creatures of the sky that must come to earth to lay their eggs and raise their young, we are bound to the earth and subject to temptations and wrong choices. The realm of the sky is one of aspiration and a seeking for perfection. It will take us from the imbalances and imperfections of this world and into the eventual perfection of eternity.

THE PHYSICAL BODY
The realm of the sky has a particular affinity for the nervous system. Neuropathies and degenerative nerve and brain diseases are often seen here. Alzheimer's, with its confusion and bewilderment, is a negative manifestation of the sky realm.

Ailments of the lungs and breathing difficulties are also of the sky realm, especially when the symptoms are restrictive and suffocative.

EXPRESSION OF SELF THROUGH CREATIVITY

Music, carried in waves upon the air, is the way in which many members of the sky realm express themselves. When there is not the opportunity to express the soaring emotions of the soul, there is always the longing to do so.

REMEDIES OF THE SKY

There are only a few remedies made from substances that are entirely of the Sky. These remedies include Sol, made from lactose exposed to concentrated rays of the sun; Luna, moon rays; and the sound remedies.

Remedies made from gases are of the sky realm but many of them have an air of expectancy and change making them remedies of transformation—moving from one realm to another—as much as remedies of the sky.

Movement Between Realms - Transformation

Most substances from which homeopathic remedies are made belong to a particular realm. There are, however, remedies made from substances, plants, or animals that move between two or more realms in some way. Whenever there is movement between realms there is some type of dynamic transformation, not just a simple change, happening—or about to happen—in that person's life.

Change and Impediment to Transformation

There are two important things to note and pay attention to with any transformative, moving between realms, remedy. The first of these is to note the path by which the change is taking place. In which body system and, therefore, in which realm did the first inklings of change occur? The answer to this question can direct you to the realms involved in the transformation.

The second important feature to watch for in transformative processes is the issues, unique to that person, that are standing in the way of or slowing the accomplishment of positive change. In what way are they sabotaging their own efforts? Where and when do the slip ups and back-slidings occur? What precedes these fluctuations in their forward progress and growth?

Changes are about moving in new directions and, since they are symptoms in motion, they will not be static or stagnant. In fact, the path and the symptoms of the issues may manifest in contradictory ways.

The background information of a case will lead you to, or confirm for you if you muscle tested to find the remedy, the right realm and/or miasm. The path of transformation will lead to the particular remedy within the general groupings.

Movement Between Earth and Sky

The transformations that occur when we move from a remedy of earth to a remedy with aspects of the sky are generally positive and reflect a growth in personal and spiritual development.

BIRDS

Birds are the most important of these remedies. They strive for the freedom of flight and the joy of the skies. The first bird remedies were proven just a few years ago but the provings were well done. The bird remedies are slowly coming into their own in the world of homeopathy. *Falco peregrinus,* the peregrine falcon, and *Haliaeetus leucocephalus*, the bald eagle, are the two primary remedies of the birds and even these two are not yet represented in current remedy guides.

INSECTS

The insect remedies such as Apis mellifica, Vespa crabro, and Cantharis have been around for some time and are polycrest remedies of great value in many areas of life on planet earth. Many new insect remedies have been proven in recent years. Among them are butterflies and other insects with a larval and a chrysalis stage. The provings of butterfly remedies, of which there have never been any in the homeopathy world, indicate transformative properties that are very pronounced.

SPIDERS

The spider remedies are indicative of a peculiar state of suspension between the earth and the sky with a very real mix of hiding in the dark thrown in. Spider remedies, therefore, have a little bit of the underworld/spirit realm in their symptom pictures. Spiders are linked to the different realms by their webs, but the web also suspends them between the realms as well.

TREES

The giant, tall, and very ancient tree remedies have particular lessons to teach us about ourselves and our ancestors. They are about striving and reaching upward while remaining firmly fastened to earth and reality.

DRUGS

These remedies take a peculiar path into the darkness. Some say they produce a transformation to the realm of the sky; others see this transformation as a hollow one, full of the deception of the dark side of the spirit realm.

Movement Between the Sea and the Earth

The movement from sea energy and sea remedies to the energy of the earthly realm and the remedies common to it are often cyclical in nature. They involve cycles such as menstruation or allergies that are tied to the seasons, for example.

Some of the ocean remedies, the amphibians, and the insects are involved in this type of transformation.

Movement Between Darkness and Light

The snake remedies are the primary remedies of this transformation. Snakes symbolize evil and darkness in our minds, even when lying peacefully coiled in the sun. Lethargy, laziness, feeling isolated and insecure are keynotes of snake remedies.

Snake remedies almost always include a negative aspect that involves using methods that are "a little bit shady" to further one's earthly ambitions and goals. Deceit, selfishness, and cruelty are often seen. Snake remedies have an affinity for and a symbolic relationship with the blood—the blood that flows in our mortal veins and the blood of Christ which was shed for our sakes. Positive aspects of snake energy have certainly not been well documented.

Differentiating Between the Realms

ATTITUDES AND EMOTIONS

One way to determine which realm a person or a case fits most closely into is to look at the basic attitudes that the person displays. This is revealed in the way they do things and in the way they relate to their world and the people around them as well as in their choice of words to express themselves.

The way the disease or discomfort are expressed through the emotions and what emotions may have triggered the imbalance are very important pieces of any homeopathic puzzle.

Earth

ATTITUDES OF EARTH

Laws and rules are very important in the realm of the earth. Careful reason, with thought and planning, usually precedes any action taken. Knowledge and learning are supreme. Their ideas are fixed because they see them as being based on reason, logic, and common sense. Explanations are required when your opinion differs from theirs.

EMOTIONS OF EARTH

The emotions of the earth are masculine in nature and center around concepts such as respect and responsibility. Emotions such as caring will tend to be shown by actions, not words. Situations that have no reasonable solution cause extreme pain. Negative emotions, such as frustration and anger, are acted out. Feelings of inadequacy, based on questioning whether they will be able to take effective action when it is needed, is a keynote. The earth is about worldly things and worldly success.

Sea

ATTITUDES OF THE SEA

Feelings reveal the attitudes of the sea and they are more important and given more credence than what has been learned with the mind. Beliefs are based on what feels right instinctively. Unique to this realm is the fact that contradictory feelings and opinions may exist at the same time without undue stress about the conflict between them. It is assumed that the understanding brought by new feelings in the future will resolve any discrepancies being noticed or felt at the present time.

EMOTIONS OF THE SEA

Positive emotions such as concern and compassion are displayed in more passive ways than in earth realm emotions. They will usually involve listening and sympathizing with occasionally bits of service thrown in.

The defining emotion of the sea is resentment and it is of a passive sort that may never be expressed out loud. Feelings of doubt and insecurity, self-criticism, and self-destructive behaviors—including eating disorders—are common.

Light and Darkness

ATTITUDES OF THE REALMS OF LIGHT AND DARKNESS

People from these opposing realms are passionate about their ideas and beliefs and, sometimes, a bit closed to the beliefs of others. One negative attitude of this realm is the exclusion from their circle of friends those who do not think as they do. Only agreement with their ideas is acceptable to them. They almost always feel a great need to express the things that they know, out loud, to others. The positive aspect of this realm is absolute faith, frequent communication with beings of light, being absolutely right much of the time, and—often—being able to see the future clearly.

EMOTIONS OF THE REALMS OF LIGHT AND DARKNESS

Passions of all varieties are keynotes of this realm. They are passionate about their chosen life partner and passionate in the furthering of causes in which they believe. They are subject to the less positive passionate emotions of hatred and vindictiveness. Insecurities and fears are most likely to be directed outward. They will take the fight to those whom they regard as enemies and to those whom they fear. Jealousy is a particularly strong negative characteristic emotion of this realm.

Sky

ATTITUDES OF THE SKY

The key attitude displayed by people living in the sky realm is the understanding that comes from communicating with other beings (people and animals) on a soul-to-soul level. They often display deep empathy. They rarely feel a need to argue with the beliefs of others because they understand where they are coming from and have a deep faith that any shortcomings of other people will eventually be worked out. Of course, when out of balance, the exact opposite of these positive traits is displayed.

EMOTIONS OF THE SKY

Since sky people are able to understand so well the feelings and troubles of others, they often feel a great need to help them. If they are powerless to do so, there can be a great deal of pain. When they are in a good state of mind, they feel great peace. When they are unable to help, the pain may drive them to disconnect from others and from the world as a whole. They feel isolated and alone. Sky realm aloneness is a particularly painful type of loneliness.

Chapter Thirteen - General Miasm Information

In section three, we will discuss miasmic patterns, the nosode remedies that match many of them, and other remedies that are used to treat miasmically. We will discuss, in more detail, the remedies from the three major kingdom classifications—minerals, plants, and animals. Finally, we will discuss practical applications of these remedies to our everyday lives, to behavioral disorders, learning disabilities, accidents, injuries, childhood diseases, and the possible use of homeopathic remedies in epidemic/pandemic situations.

The information in this book has been compiled from many sources. Of course, I have not had personal experience with all of the conditions, diseases, and (certainly) the epidemics listed in this book. I, and other people who work with homeopathic remedies, have spent a great deal of time studying specific conditions and matching remedies to them to give us all a starting place if we are ever confronted with them. Mostly this information is meant to give you enough confidence to get started thinking, studying, and working with deep level, high potency remedies.

MIASMS

Miasms, as was explained briefly in Section One, were defined early in homeopathic thought as inherited imbalances that predispose us to certain illnesses, physical weaknesses, and negative thought patterns. Samuel Hahnemann, is the originator of this theory—as far as we know, was a contemporary of the men who first defined the "germ theory" of illness—the body being invaded by a pathogen which must be eradicated and expelled. Homeopathic theory, both as it applies to remedy pictures in general and to miasms, reflects this bias. Remedy pictures and miasmic descriptions focus on the out-of-balance, destructive aspects of human nature rather than on who we can become.

The laws of nature (and scripture) teach us that there is and must be opposition in all things. Everything within and around us has its equal and opposite form or state of being. If there is a negative aspect there must be an opposing positive possibility. This opposition is absolutely essential to our growth, development, and wellness. Without opposition there can be no real choice, no agency, no real growth, and no real healing.

"No virtue can exist without its corresponding evil: without the evil of danger there could be no courage, without suffering there could be no sympathy, without poverty there could be no generosity, and so forth. Without darkness there could be no light, without cold there could be no hot, without depths there could be no heights. Thus there must be wickedness so there might be righteousness, death so there might be life, that which is satanic so there might be that which is godly.... Any therapy that purports to free men from the burden of sin by denying the existence of sin also denies to its adherents that joy and peace which can only be known by obedience to the laws of God." (Robert L. Millet, quoting Joseph Fielding McConkie)

It has long been my belief that the best way to remove a "vice", whether spiritual, mental, emotional, or physical, is to flood our beings with the opposing "virtue." I have longed for and, when possible, tried to ascertain and record the positive qualities—what we will be like when we are well in body and mind—of various remedies and of the miasms. The flower essence descriptions do this to some extent and are one of the reasons I love them so much! They give us tiny pieces of the puzzle in trying to determine the positive qualities of other homeopathic remedies and of the miasmic patterns themselves.

A miasm under this theory becomes not so much the enemy that must be driven out as an opportunity and a challenge that will provide growth and learning until it becomes another step on the road to excellence and wellness. "Alternative" medicine is a positive science. Instead of focusing on getting rid of miasmic "vices" a better approach might be to apply ourselves to replacing them with "virtues", both physical and spiritual. After all, the more we emphasize the negative, the more power we have given it in our lives.

With all that said, however, one cannot heal from one's own mistakes until one has admitted that one has made them and that they were awful and need to be repented of and moved away from.

To think holistically is to remember that disease is, in many ways, a growth opportunity. Symptoms are evidence of the body and the spirit making its best attempt to heal itself. Discomfort and limitations can be very real teachers about what needs to be addressed in our lifestyle. Illness can inform us about where change is needed in our reactions to stress, our habits, and our personal emotional patterns and resultant behaviors. As we look at illness in this way we are better able to consider and understand the ways in which we may have participated in the creation of our problems. The idea that there is something out there, or uninvited within us, that is doing bad things to us and controlling our behavior, is an invitation to participate in a victim mentality. Being a victim strips us of responsibility and limits our capacity and freedom to achieve! Please, please do not think of miasms in this way!

The original three identified miasms—psora, sycosis, and syphilis—were believed to have been the result of "disease agents" whose signatures were then passed down to subsequent generations. Hahnemann lived contemporary with the early emergence of the germ theory of contagious diseases. This theory had not yet been widely accepted but it seems to have influenced his thinking to a great degree.

According to original miasmic philosophy, every person living on earth reflects one or more of the miasms every day. They react in certain discernible ways to life. The negative reactions and the illnesses that result have been tracked and spoken of far more frequently than the opposing positive traits. While it is true that the influence of the miasm makes a person more vulnerable to specific negative emotional patterns and physical ailments *it must always be remembered and understood that a miasm is only a vulnerability, a tendency which, as it is replaced with positive change, can be a catalyst for growth.*

THE NUMBER OF MIASMS

Hahnemann's theory of miasms was relatively simple but there are so many studies being conducted and materials being published about miasms from all over the world that keeping track of it all can be confusing. Amazing material, but it is very vast and extremely varied, agreeing on some points while diverging on others.

One of the greatest variations in thought and understanding among homeopathic practitioners is about how many different miasmic patterns there really are. Samuel Hahnemann listed only three before he died—psora, sycosis, and syphilis—and these miasms had very distinctive ways of manifesting themselves. There would be either a sycotic or a syphilitic pattern seen, with psora continually underlying the other two. Psora would be in either a heightened or subdued state according to circumstances. Hahnemann believed, and I agree with him, that the psora miasm was the inheritance of every person born into this mortal life.

As time went on there began to be identifiable new patterns. The first new pattern to be identified was named tuberculosis. The symptom picture seemed to be a spin-off from the syphilitic miasmic pattern with psora manifesting predominantly in the lungs rather than on the skin. Tuberculosis has very distinctive and describable characteristics, and is now thought to be a miasm in its own right.

Along with tuberculosis, some homeopaths began listing leprosy as a separate miasm. Leprosy contains much that is syphilitic with psora manifesting predominantly in the skin symptoms instead of in the lungs. Like all disease states with a syphilitic diathesis, leprosy moves quickly to patterns of extreme destruction.

The next major miasm-like patterns seem to have occurred simultaneously with the polio epidemics of the last century, and following that, the almost epidemic increase of cancer in the industrialized nations of the world. Cancer and polio now appear as separate miasms on most lists around the world. Recent researchers and writers, most notably Peter Fraser, are delineating two more miasms, AIDS and Alzheimer's. Fraser has an interesting theory that new miasms emerge as a result of shifts in the moorings of societies. Another extensive miasmic grouping is being referred to as the vaccinosis miasm. Ian Watson, in a fascinating little book published in England in 2009, mentions the emergence of yet another miasm. He refers to it as the radiation miasm, referring to global effects of nuclear accidents. He says,

> "A nuclear explosion in Chernobyl contaminated the grass being grazed by sheep in the north of England, which affected the people eating them everywhere. We can no longer act in isolation and expect to be free of consequences. Interestingly, the internet is teaching us the same thing."

Each researcher and theorist categorizes the miasms a little bit differently, depending on their focus. The ones whose philosophies I will discuss here are well-known and well-respected in their areas of expertise.

Rajan Sankaran has done a great deal of work with plant remedies, especially with the emotions that characterize the remedies of various plant families. Sankaran lists 10 miasmic categories. I was an herbalist long before I learned about homeopathy and a lot of my life is connected with the world of essential oils which are, of course, derived from plants. Sankaran's work is particularly fascinating to me as a result. His theories will be the topic of further discussion later in this book.

Jan Scholten (and others) have worked predominantly with the remedies of the mineral kingdom. Scholten has developed his own list of miasm categories using a unique nomenclature and grading system. Scholten divides the miasms according to the columns of the periodic table, making 18 miasms in all. Each of the 18 miasms is further broken down into 7 levels of intensity represented by the rows of the table. Scholten has cross referenced his list—somewhat—to Sankaran's, which has been very helpful to me.

Still other researchers are concentrating their work on nosode remedies and on remedies made from various drugs and environmental poisons. They have created lists of possible remedies for the various miasms identified by others. Their lists are based on matching a person's symptoms with the symptom picture of the remedy (classical homeopathy), whether or not the person can identify exposure to that particular substance. This makes sound homeopathic sense since homeopathic healing depends on the use of a *similinum*, or similar, rather than the use of the exact substance or organism that created the problem.

Always determine whether an intercurrent remedy needs to be used if the chosen remedy is a nosode.

MIASMIC CRITERIA AND DEFINITIONS

To be considered a miasm by the standards of professional homeopathic practitioners, a disease pattern must meet at least some basic criteria. The criteria are listed, as far as I understand them, below:

1) There should be distinct, inherited pieces in the disease pattern. It should be possible for family members to recall similar emotional and physical patterns in their parents and grandparents and to see signs of these same traits in some of their children and grandchildren.

2) There is usually a matching nosode with a clearly defined symptom picture. A nosode is a remedy made from the bacteria or virus that was responsible for the original disease somewhere in the generational line in which the miasmic pattern is appearing. Remember, the miasm and the disease are not, at least when passed down the genetic line, the same thing at all. The miasm is a susceptibility to either the disease or a composite of symptoms that include many of the symptoms of the disease. It is also the growth obtained by conquering those tendencies and illnesses and the positive traits that have resulted. These positive traits will have also been passed along generationally and can be seen in members of the same family.

3) There must be a larger, well-defined pattern of physical, emotional and mental symptoms and behaviors. This pattern of symptoms involves the entirety of the body/mind/spirit complex and is seen and described similarly by homeopathic practitioners around the world. The opposite, positive traits can be perceived and pondered if we are to grasp the full significance—disease and potentialities—of the miasm.

Not all of the patterns of a miasm, good or bad, will manifest at the same time in a person's life. There is always more than one way in which the possible symptoms may arrange themselves. Each person's response to their life situations will be unique and the remedy needed will be individual to them. The pattern, however, will lie within parameters of their dominant miasm. It can *always* be assumed that there are unseen and non-manifesting symptoms which lie beneath what is presenting at the present time.

4) If we don't go deep enough when addressing the presenting symptoms, we run the risk of leaving behind the deeper aspects of the whole to manifest in a slightly different form at another day or time. A miasm, if not treated properly and necessary life style changes made, will relapse and will eventually deepen into a more seriously destructive miasm. This progression will occur in a predictable pattern unless there is suppression, discussed later, that drives symptoms of the disease energy deeper into the body.

5) A miasm, when properly treated, doesn't just go away. As we give up the destructive patterns, tendencies, and physical weaknesses of the "natural man" in our quest for salvation and perfection, we find our former weaknesses becoming our strengths. We don't rid ourselves of the miasm. Rather we demonstrate the positive qualities instead of the negative ones. The road and the results will be unique to each individual, just as it should be.

The cancer miasm and the newly emerging Alzheimer's pattern do not seem to stem from infectious diseases like the rest of the miasms were thought by Hahnemann to have been. Suspected causes and contributors to both cancer and Alzheimer's are many and varied, but they are not believed to be caused by infectious agents at this time. The newest members—if they are members—of the miasm family, vaccinosis and radiation, are not caused by infectious agents either.

The cancer miasm has as its foremost nosode the remedy Carcinosin. Scirrhinum, a lesser known and scantily proven remedy, is another effective cancer nosode.

Since there is not a specific disease entity recognized as the cause of Alzheimer's there can be no specific nosode for its treatment at this time. There is not even, as far as I can tell, a leading contender for a polycrest remedy. In some circles, both medical and alternative, it is speculated that aluminum poisoning plays a role in at least some cases of dementia and Alzheimer's. Certainly the remedy, Aluminum oxydata, matches many of the symptoms and should be considered as part of a potential treatment protocol.

ACQUIRED MIASMS

Some homeopathic theorists consider the new miasms to be not inherited patterns but acquired changes due to the weakening of the core energy of the human race by drugs and various environmental poisons and toxins. One doctor who conducts research involving human blood samples has noted that over the last several years the younger the person is whose blood has been drawn, the shorter is the time it will take for the blood to break down completely in a laboratory setting. The blood of an older person will be viable for tests for several hours, while the blood of a younger person will sometimes be completely broken down in 20 minutes. Years ago, he claims, blood samples were viable for testing for several days. He attributes this change to the amount of "metal debris" found in the blood sample. This is very scary if it is true!

We accumulate metals in the blood from so many sources—vaccines, the pans we cook in, the linings of the cans our food comes in, fertilizers, weed sprays, and dental amalgams to name just a few. I suspect that metal is not the only poison that we are accumulating in our bodies at an alarming rate. There is too little known about the changes these chemicals make in our body chemistry and in our genetic codes to have even the slightest idea what the risks or the answers are.

Homeopaths the world over have come to understand that there are new, perhaps miasmic, patterns developing at an alarming rate as the result of vaccinations. There is much discussion about whether these disease patterns, although not inherited as miasms usually are or the result of disease agents as the original three were, will be inherited by subsequent generations. Research seems to indicate that a tendency to certain cancers (and the cancer miasm which contributes to this susceptibility) is now, at least in part, an inherited condition.

Speculation also abounds about whether the miasmic changes that are occurring as a result of vaccinations are due to the introduction of viral and bacterial agents into the blood, or are occurring as a result of the metal alloys, stabilizers, and immune suppressants that are part of the make-up of every vaccine. Whatever the case may be, the vaccinosis miasm is not one single miasm but is an amalgam of the reactions to each and every separate vaccine. If such alterations can be passed to subsequent generations and follow the criteria listed above, which they seem to, then we are creating new miasms and new troubles for humanity at an alarming rate.

The vaccinosis heading also includes the negative impact of drugs—prescription, over-the-counter, and street-type drugs as well as every type of environmental poison known to man in this day and age. Vaccinosis is a vast category with symptom pictures showing a large range of diversity but still having a core set of common features as well.

My Theory of Miasms and the World

I have thought and read and pondered on miasms for many years now. As I have connected some previously unconnected dots and come across new philosophies, I have changed my mind on points here and there from time to time. I have come to some conclusions (subject to further change as I learn more) that provide a comfortable and workable model for myself. My working model places Hahnemann's original three miasms as the foundation on which everything else builds. This model incorporates the works of Sankaran, Scholten, and others and includes my own personal religious beliefs and the insights I feel that my faith and religious study gives me.

My study of miasms has deepened my understanding of my physical body and the relationship between the physical and the mental, emotional, and spiritual aspects of myself. It has also brought the history of the world into sharper focus for me and is providing what I believe to be a greater understanding of what the future holds, especially where health matters are concerned. My studies have helped clarify my feelings about the purposes of life on earth and strengthened my testimony of the restored gospel that I love. Hahnemann's theory of miasms, when I came across it the first time, seemed to explain so much that was at that time nearly incomprehensible to me. The more I study and ponder homeopathic theory the more homeopathy and the world make sense to me.

The following pages are my personal philosophy—what other position can I teach from?—interwoven with Hahnemann's theories and those of many others. I will give you what information I can about the theories of others such as Rajan Sankaran, Jan Scholten, Ian Watson, and Peter Fraser.

HAHNEMANN'S CHRONIC MIASMS

Samuel Hahnemann was the first to divide the sufferings of mankind into what has become known as the theory of miasms. There were three different miasms identified by Hahnemann during his lifetime. These were **psora, sycosis (sycotic), and syphilis (syphilitic).** These terms are still in use today. Sycosis and syphilis do not refer specifically to the medical conditions of the same names although those diseases are considered at least partially descriptive of the symptoms of these two miasmic states and may have originated in some way back in time from these diseases. From religious and philosophical standpoints, it is interesting to note that both diseases have a moral/sexual element. Hahnemann speculated that the miasms were the result of the suppression of gonorrhea and syphilis by the allopathic drug treatments of his day. He created nosodes of those diseases and used them in treatment. They are still in use in this way today.

MORTALITY AND MIASMS

Every branch of homeopathic theory of which I am aware believes that the Psora miasm has been inherited by every member of the human race (or every living thing, depending on your point of view). In my own mind, based on my religious conviction, the psora miasm is very much connected with the choice made by Adam and Eve in the garden of Eden to enter mortality. This is not "original sin" in the traditional Christian definition of the word but is surely based on my understanding of scripture.

Psora, to me, represents in part the changes that occurred in the physical, but not quite mortal, bodies of Adam and Eve when the choice was made to accept this mortal state. As their descendants, this decision affected all of us and provided the opportunity for us to gain physical bodies and participate in the lessons of this probationary earthly life. Other homeopathic theorists think and teach the reasons for psora underlying all according to their own understanding and belief systems.

One characteristic of psora that I find interesting to ponder on in this context is the keynote of "difficult to treat." Nothing done or given for any condition ever seems to work for long. This reminds me of the difficulty of trying to form good mental, physical, and spiritual habits. The natural tendency of man is to back-slide into former patterns, even ones that were obviously not good choices in the first place.

The psora picture also contains a focus on, and difficulty with, the acquisition and use of this world's goods. It epitomizes for me the difference between Eden, where everything desired was automatically provided and was in a perfect state, and the world in which Adam and Eve found themselves when they left the garden. In the world, they were required to earn their own bread and subdue and govern the earth. The psora struggle with the world is seen on all levels of the symptom picture. There is lack of vital heat and a desire for warm clothing, struggles with the absorption of nutrients, feelings of being forsaken (cut off from God?), anxiety and restlessness, depression, mental confusion, and—my favorite description of God's children as a whole—being intolerably self-willed and having an aversion to work!

CHOICES

As mortal beings, we each find our own way to relate and respond to the world around us. According to Hahnemann there are really only three basic choices, with each choice having extremes at both ends of the scale. The results of our choices will manifest in our emotions, in our mental state, and in all aspects of our physical bodies.

THE THREE BASIC CHOICES ARE:

1) inhibit or exaggerate all responses to stimuli

2) induration—dilate or contract, soften or harden— emotionally, mentally, physically, and spiritually

3) make a choice to heal or to completely destroy what we feel cannot be fixed, whether a single cell, an organ, a relationship, or—under extreme stress—even ourselves.

PSORA, SYPHILIS, SYCOSIS

Psora represents the first choice of the three listed above. There will be either inhibition or exaggeration. Inhibition is seen, among other symptoms, in the lack of reaction, lack of warmth, lack of energy, debility, despair, and mental confusion that is characteristic of this miasm. The exaggeration is seen in the over-reaction to some stimuli that results in allergies, hay fever, eczema and psoriasis, offensive discharges, profuse sweating, and the tendency for every scratch and cut to become infected. Psora is the opposite poles of inhibition, deprivation, and loss of function with excitability, irritation, inflammation, and hypersensitivity on the other end of the scale.

The sycosis miasm is representative of the second choice listed, that of *induration*—dilation or contraction, softening or hardening. The opposite states of this miasm are often seen in bipolar (manic/depressive) disorders. The physical symptoms of sycosis run the range from over relaxation of the muscles which leads to the prolapse of organs, to the tightening and hardening that results in stiffness throughout the entire body. The extremes of the sycosis miasm are also seen in procrastination followed by running all out to complete a project on time. Another example might be the build-up of tension inside that can only be released by exuberant and expansive shouting and movements that is typical of this miasm, especially in children and teens. Often, in a sycosis pattern, there are too few general symptoms to prescribe on effectively, accompanied by an overgrowth of such things as warts, moles, and polyps.

The third choice, above, is represented by the syphilis miasm. Syphilis is a very deep and desperate pattern. There is a perception of a weakness in oneself that cannot be fixed, or seeing problems as so bad that they can only be dealt with by destroying everything and starting over. This desperation may manifest as destruction of a group of cells within the body to save the whole person or, emotionally, the destruction of a relationship because it is perceived as broken beyond mending. There is despair of recovery from illnesses, general hopelessness, suicidal depression, as well as birth defects that include deformity of bones and missing organs or teeth. Syphilis symptoms also include great debility and prostration. The keynote of this miasm is destruction—the violence of destroying all that is not perfect or worthy in others or in oneself.

Ian Watson describes psora as the backdrop on which our lives play out. We cannot live on this earth and not be subject to struggle and survival issues of all sorts. We share these basic challenges with every living creature that God created. With psora as the pivotal point, we can see sycosis and syphilis as complementary opposites. The sycosis pattern is filled with overproduction and a tendency to excess while syphilis is characterized by despair and destruction. The energy of the sycosis miasm is expansion, including expansion to excess, while syphilis represents the inner world and the fear of the darkness that sometimes exists in our own inner spaces.

THE INDIVIDUAL — A MICROCOSM OF CREATION

It is my opinion, and that of many other people, that the structure of the cells is a microcosm of the structure of the body. Cells perform the functions of reproduction, growth, utilization of energy and nutritive resources, protection, sensory interpretation, and response to thoughts just as our systems as a unit do. The structure and organization of our bodies (along with each of our cells) is seen as a microcosm of the pattern of the universe and all of creation. That which occurs on one level (in our cells or in our bodies) is similar to what is occurring on other levels throughout the universe. What occurred in one era—or dispensation—of earth's time will prove to be a type and a pattern of what will occur in other eras and dispensations.

My husband very effectively looks for patterns in scripture and in history as a way of understanding the past, the present, and the future. Peter Fraser, in his new book, calls this type of thinking *pattern thinking*. This thinking requires that we stand back and look at things from many angles until the patterns become clear to us. Pattern thinking is becoming a lost art in this era of specialization and compartmentalization in medical, scientific, and many other fields Thinking in this way, however, is absolutely essential to understanding miasms, ourselves, and our relationship to God.

MIASMS AS A REFLECTION OF SOCIETY

Peter Fraser has postulated the theory that the new miasms such as AIDS and Alzheimer, are the result of conditions existing in our society at this time. His theories provide possible clues to what brought about some of the other miasms. His hypothesis makes sense when applied to miasms such as malaria, leprosy, tuberculosis, and cancer. Perhaps they even bring the long-standing miasms of sycosis and syphilis into clearer focus. It also raises the specter, at least in my mind, of what conditions, now lost in unrecorded history, may have created what unidentified miasmic patterns that are playing a part in the miasms of today.

Fraser's theories also do not have much of an explanation for why each new miasm seems to be destructive on more levels than the previous one. For that explanation I have had to look to my personal religious beliefs and my study of and training in various energy modalities. Please do not take offense at my religious references; just rewrite my theories of both religion and energy to fit into your own paradigms. I am trying to explain the mysterious and nearly unexplainable in my own mind, and then on paper, the very best way that I know how. (Reasoning with myself is usually how the books that I have written came about.)

THE DEEPENING OF MIASMIC PATTERNS

No matter how you choose to group miasms, psora, sycosis, and syphilis form the backbone of miasmic classification in everybody's systems. I believe that psora, as the original miasm and representative of the human condition, is both the least destructive and most stubbornly pervasive miasm. Until I came to understand AIDS and Alzheimer's better, I considered syphilis to be the deepest, most desperate and destructive of the miasms and at the other end of the scale from psora. Each of the other miasms, in my mind, fall into place somewhere in between psora at the top end and syphilis (or now AIDS and Alzheimer's) at the bottom end.

The place of each miasm along the classification scale is set by the severity of the physical symptoms, the desperation and intensity of the emotional patterns, and the depth and intensity of any destructiveness. Each new era of history produces a miasmic pattern that is deeper and more destructive than the previous one. The continual deepening of miasmic patterns, to my way of thinking, is illustrative of the deepening of the overall pathology of the earth as it moves through the ever more destructive phases that have been foretold in scripture until the times and conditions predicted for the days just before the second coming of Christ.

MIASMS AND CULTURAL CHANGES
THE CREATION AND DEEPENING OF MIASMS (ACCORDING TO PETER FRASER AND MYSELF)

In short, Peter Fraser believes that disease is a reflection of the culture, the changes that are occurring in society, and the challenges society is facing at a given time. Fraser says, "When a culture with one way of thinking is suddenly faced with (the need for) change to a new way for which it is not yet adapted a disease state is almost inevitable." New inventions bring about changes in society. These changes often "bring about the new state suddenly and completely, and this leaves no time for individuals or for the culture to adapt. The result is an immune type of reaction, a sudden and extreme disease that spreads suddenly and very quickly."

Section Three

Perhaps, the best way to illustrate Fraser's theory is to describe some of the miasms according to his thinking. I must warn you that there will inevitably be more than a little of my own thoughts thrown in. To read Fraser in the original I would suggest the book *The AIDS Miasm—Contemporary Diseases & the New Remedies*, especially the first few chapters where Fraser presents a truly fascinating philosophical discussion.

Fraser, like most classical homeopathic practitioners, focuses on out-of-balance patterns. There is very little mention of the positive aspects of any miasm in his work.

Psora: I believe, as I have indicated earlier, that psora *represents the fall of man from Eden/immortality to mortality,* a situation where one has to struggle in order to survive. Fraser describes the psoric phase as a reaction to mankind moving from a state of unawareness, through speech to awareness. That description does not fit with my personal religious beliefs as it is more evolutionary than scriptural, but it is a fair description of the prevailing philosophies of many people. Struggles to adapt to a new order of things with hypersensitivity, survival issues, and reactions to environmental stimuli are keynotes of the psoric miasm. The reactions are *restricted to the level of the skin, the appendages, and the mind and, while annoying and persistent, are not deeply destructive.*

Acute (or Hydrophobic): This miasm, according to Fraser, marks the change in man as he moved from *coping* with mortality to *going on the attack.* There is a definite and firm *spiritual and physical struggle against both illness and evil.* Sudden and dramatic fevers and illnesses are keynotes of this miasm.

Sycosis: The sycosis miasm's emotional attitude includes a comprehension of one's own weaknesses and imperfections. Attempts to preserve one's place in society (a competitive spirit) cause feelings of inadequacy. The reaction of this miasm is to *hide these weaknesses from others and from God*, burying oneself in guilt to the point of neurosis, and *putting off the day of repentance or responsibility* for the treatment of any physical illnesses as long as possible.

Leprosy: The emotional attitudes here are, not surprisingly, feelings of *persecution and isolation* and the desire to isolate oneself ever further. The destruction of leprosy is predominantly on the *skin*, indicating that under-lying psora is in an active state. The deepening destructiveness is shown in the seriousness of the skin deteriorating and falling away. Leprosy is considered to be an extremely destructive form of pure psora with the skin symptoms becoming not just itchy but truly horrible and life-threatening.

Tuberculosis: It is interesting to note that although there is evidence of TB's existence for many thousands of years on a small scale, it became epidemic in the 19th century during a time that was characterized by industrial cities, urban congestion, and pollution. The nature of the disease and the miasm includes feelings of oppression and restriction with an intense desire to escape, to travel to get away from imposed limitations. The tuberculosis miasm deepens in destructiveness from the skin to more *vital-to-life organs, the lungs.*

Polio: The emotional patterns of polio fluctuate from wild optimism one moment to deep despair and hopelessness the next and illustrate the early stages of manic depression. In trying to analyze the changes in world culture at the time (about the time I was born), I find a definite shift of more women in the workplace and fewer women staying at home with the children. There was a new attitude of "a chicken in every pot" and the entitlement mentality of every family deserves "two cars in the garage." The early stages of polio resemble a summer cold but quickly progress to paralysis of muscles, the filling of the lungs with fluid, and the eventual destruction of internal organs—a more total destructive body response than is present with any previous miasm including leprosy or tuberculosis.

Cancer: Cancer is the first miasmic pattern that is not traceable to a particular disease entity. Not all cancers are inherited miasmic conditions; many seem to be triggered by environmental toxicities, artificial hormones, exhaust fumes, radiation exposure, and many other things although it can certainly be argued that some sort of underlying weakness or predisposition exists in some people and in some families. The mental/emotional pattern of the cancer miasm includes the need for perfection in all that one does, coupled with a deep sense of never having done enough or being good enough. This miasm includes a need to please and placate others. One must always do one's very best and one must please and placate others to avoid catastrophe.

A keynote of the cancer miasm is a history of abuse or domination with a two-fold, either-or response. There is in this miasm the early stages of the confusion that becomes debilitating later on in the Alzheimer's miasm. One of the two responses mentioned above is a passive internalization of stresses. This internalization creates, first, inflammation and then, hard lumps and tumors. The second response is anxiety and worry coupled with a need for perfection in oneself that, quite literally, eats away at the body and soul. The increasing deepness of this miasm is illustrated by the fact that cancer can strike anywhere in the body and destroy any organ and so often results in death.

Syphilis: The syphilis miasm reflects the feelings of being a very small and insignificant part of the bigger machine of society. Peter Fraser considers these feeling to be a reflection of the industrial age. Suspicion and fear are key elements of this emotional pattern. The fear is often held at bay by an attitude of "I'll get them before they get me" or "I'll be so tough and mean that no one dares mess with me."

I place the destruction of Syphilis below (more destructive than) even cancer. A person caught in the cancer miasm seeks perfection and, failing that, tries to destroy herself. A syphilitic person considers himself broken beyond repair and seeks his own destruction. The deepening of the destruction is seen particularly strongly in relationship issues. A syphilitic person often sees his relationships, especially his primary ones, as broken beyond repair. The actions he takes to "fix" these situations too often results, either intentionally or unintentionally, in the destruction not just of the relationship but of themselves. Too often there is damage to the other persons as well.

AIDS: The AIDS miasm seems to be a product of the electronic age in which boundaries are cast away. Electronic friends can be anywhere in the world rather than close to our hearts. Often there is a feeling of being watched and spied on. The connection to family erodes away as we spend more and more time with electronic devices. Peter Fraser describes this miasm as "a breakdown of boundaries, a confusion on all levels of personal and collective identity." The basic emotional patterns of this miasm are disconnection, feelings that no one really knows us on a personal level any more, and an inability to connect in caring ways with one's own family.

The nature of the AIDS miasm illustrates the ever deepening pattern of destruction in the newer miasms. The AIDS miasm seeks, not just the destruction of the individual as seen in previous miasms, but the destruction of our culture's core values of monogamy and family. The result is broken homes, broken lives, and broken children. AIDS also seeks the destruction and restructuring of society as a whole.

Alzheimer's: Perhaps Alzheimer's is, as some believe, an aspect of the AIDS miasm. Fraser's description of AIDS as "a confusion on all levels of personal and collective identity" certainly describes the Alzheimer's miasm. Alzheimer's begins with a decline in thinking skills, ability to reason, and memory loss which progresses until the person becomes lost in a fog, not recognizing friends or family and no longer even knowing who they are or where they fit in the world. In my opinion, this is the deepest and most destructive of the miasms. It is interesting to note that such complete deterioration of the mind can be accompanied by so few physical symptoms. It is as though the person is already moving out of this physical world and can't even focus on the "here and now" enough to fall apart physically. Alzheimer's sufferers so often seem to be living in another realm entirely.

THE PRESENTATION OF MIASMS IN OURSELVES

In each individual and individual disease state, one miasm will usually be predominant in presentation. The predominant miasm will reflect either the hardening/softening or destruction/healing that are represented by sycosis and syphilis. Each of the other miasms contain elements of these two basic choices, in varying degrees of severity. Some of them—cancer and tuberculosis are examples—seem to combine both sycosis and syphilis at the same time. Hahnemann and others of the "old school" believed this combining to be impossible. They lived in a different world from the one we have built for ourselves in modern times.

As has been mentioned before, psora will be seen underscoring everything once one knows what to look for. There will also be stray bits of the previous, less desperate, miasm that have not been over-shadowed by the symptoms of the new one into which the person is moving.

The workings of the mind/body/spirit complex are never simple. While it is true that a miasm left unchecked deepens into another, it is not altogether true that the entire individual—every physical, emotional, mental, and spiritual aspect—is moving at the same time toward either healing or destruction. The slipping into a deeper layer almost always begins in the spiritual and emotional aspects. It is recognized in healing energy modalities throughout the world that "as a man thinketh in his *heart,* so is he" or, at least, so he will become. It is thought that leads the physical body into changes in so many instances. The mind may show symptoms of the deeper pathology while the physical body shows symptoms of the lesser miasm. The physical body will eventually follow into the new pattern. If we can learn to control our thoughts, moving constantly toward compassion, love, and gratitude, there is much that can be done to move ourselves upward on the miasmatic scale. Finding the things that balance us spiritually and emotionally is crucial.

TRIGGERS TO MIASMIC PROGRESSION

A miasm becomes an issue for us—becomes dominant in our lives at this time—when our vital force (the life energy that supports and sustains us) is weakened in some way.

What things weaken our vital energy? What things act as triggers to this weakening process? Physical trauma—through accident, injury or surgery—environmental pollutants, drugs, vaccinations, and negative emotions are often cited as stressors to our vital energy.

A complete list would be quite endless, but the over-riding factor is always our personal responses to those stressors—physical, emotional, mental, or spiritual. Responding to life with faith, patience, compassion, optimism, and enthusiasm is the best medicine ever. The effects of our personal responses are so important that many modern-day homeopaths believe that the *modalities*—what an individual is sensitive to, what makes his symptoms better or worse, especially emotionally—are the most important factors in identifying miasmic patterns in our lives.

Rajan Sankaran was the first that I know of to introduce the thought that every remedy picture is an illustration of a particular response pattern to certain life situations. The presenting picture, while often negative and out-of-balance should be seen, realistically, as a reflection of the best that the person can manage to do in the circumstances. It is hoped that, with the aid of homeopathic remedies and other treatments, they can do something both different and better in the future. The acknowledgement, by themselves and those around them, that they are doing the best that they can is essential. Forgiveness of self and the compassion of others is often the first step toward a belief that they can be well and happy. Belief is hope, and hope begets the faith required for real healing.

EMOTIONS

There is quite a debate among homeopaths and energy workers about whether negative emotions first cause a disruption in the energy fields of the body, or whether a disruption in the energy field (from drugs, environmental pollutions, trauma, etc.) creates corresponding negative emotions. I'm not sure that it really matters much. Negative emotions, whether they are the cause or the effect, certainly keep the ball rolling and deepen miasmic pathologies.

There are a couple of things that ARE important about emotions and miasms. The first is that the moving of a miasm from dormant to active far too often begins with the thoughts we allow to play on the stages of our minds. The second important thing to remember is that our thoughts and our emotions are very much under our own control. Perhaps we have not understood in the past the principles that govern the control of thoughts. Not understanding is not a workable excuse because lack of understanding in no way changes the effects of negative thinking in our lives.

Energetic modalities such as homeopathic remedies, essential oils, and energy work do not *force* a change in our thoughts or perceptions. They simply unblock the energy, opening a window in our souls which allows us to see the damage our emotions, perceptions, and responses to stress are creating in our lives. The most important aspect in any energetic based healing work is the desire to move in positive directions.

HAHNEMANN AND THE NEW MIASMS

Hahnemann is sometimes criticized by modern "thinkers" for the supposed narrowness of his miasmic theories. This is, in my opinion, unjust and unfair and, quite possibly, indicates a serious lack of understanding on the part of the critic about history and the time and place in which Hahnemann lived and did his amazing work. The man was obviously a deep thinker, connecting dots and arriving at remarkable and useful conclusions. Was he influenced by the thinking of others? Of course he was. Anyone who reads and ponders inevitably is—and probably should be. No one man can think every worthwhile thought and draw every worthwhile conclusion by himself.

Did Hahnemann miss the significance of each miasm becoming deeper and more destructive than the previous one? No he did not. He understood very well the significance of the destructive tendencies of the syphilitic miasm. From his limited access to information about the history of human suffering, he was able to identify the three most basic patterns in human suffering. Although he did not have a personal acquaintance with the industrial or computer ages and the resulting impact on mankind because he lived before they occurred, his early observations and reasonings form the foundation on which further observation of human nature have taken place. His provings of remedies and the remedy pictures he recorded illustrate a holistic thinking pattern that is a shining example to us all.

HEALING BY HOMEOPATHIC PRINCIPLES

Homeostasis is a healthy state of balance between an individual's physical, emotional, mental, and spiritual needs. True healing is the alignment of innate physical attributes with natural emotions and desires, all of which are then governed by spiritual intelligence, self-control, and Christ-like compassion. The expression of all of these aspects is unique to each individual and the remedies needed to assist the individual to achieve balance will also be unique.

A particular miasmic state in different individuals will show many similarities but there will also be aspects unique to each individual. The proper remedy must include BOTH the similarities and the unique symptoms and aspects and must reflect BOTH the current imbalanced state and the return of the physical/emotional/mental/spiritual complex to health. This return to health will almost always follow the principles of Herring's Laws of Cure.

Most of the compiled symptom pictures of homeopathic remedies in the Materia Medicas reflect only the pathological symptoms. Learn to look for the general, neutral, underlying themes of people's troubles, the themes of the remedies themselves, and the themes of the miasms that drive the symptoms. Finding the theme among the plethora of negative descriptions enables us to see what positive attributes we can expect to uncover and allows us to understand the course that their healing is likely to take.

It may take a bit, or a great deal, of pondering to discover the opposing virtues and balanced states of each remedy. These positive attributes must be kept in mind in order to understand miasmic philosophy and to recognize miasms in our own lives. Achieving the positive qualities—not just avoiding the negative qualities—is the goal of all that we do in alternative healing. Ours is a positive healing science.

Herring's Laws of Cure

Constantine Herring was a German-born homeopath who emigrated to the United States in the 1830's. He is credited with bringing Hahnemann's concepts and the healing modality of homeopathy to the United States. He is often referred to as the Father of American Homeopathy.

As a medical student at Leipzig University in Germany, he was asked by a professor to write a book disproving the legitimacy of homeopathy. He took the assignment seriously, studying the writings and observing the teachings of Samuel Hahnemann. He even conducted his own experiments, proving remedies, and soon became a personal friend of Dr. Hahnemann. During this time, he received successful homeopathic treatment for a seriously infected wound. Shortly after this treatment, Herring quit his job, left the university, and devoted his life to the study and practice of homeopathy.

One of his contributions to homeopathic philosophy was his observations on the order in which the body typically heals when undergoing proper homeopathic treatment. His writings on this topic became known as Herring's Laws of Cure among subsequent generations of homeopathic practitioners. Herring did not refer to his own observations as *laws*. It was James Kent who originally coined the term, *Laws of Cure*, at a lecture he was giving on homeopathy.

I think it is both appropriate and worthwhile to cover the pattern by which healing occurs here during this discussion of miasmic theory.

RULES FOR THE PROGRESSION OF HEALING

The body has a memory of what it is like to be whole and balanced. Perhaps it is a memory of our creation or a yearning for balance and perfection. Our bodies seem to want to return to or to achieve a more perfect state of being. Observation has shown that progress toward wellness, assisted by homeopathic remedies, occurs consistently in a specific pattern if that progress is not interrupted by such things as drugs or surgeries.

1. Emotional/psychological first and then physical
2. From the present to the past
3. From inside to outside
4. From top to bottom

(1) Emotional/psychological first: Emotional clearing, in my experience, is often the first thing that you see. This is particularly easy to see when working with acute ailments. When treating a deep miasm the progress of the healing will likely begin with the emotions but then move quickly to the organs which are vital to life. When conditions in the body deteriorate for any reason (acid/alkaline balance, drug therapies, trauma) the body does its best to protect the organs and systems that are absolutely essential to life. In most cases, these vital-to-life organs were the last systems to be affected because they were most protected. Emotional/psychological symptoms even sometimes take a back seat to the healing of the more recently acquired, vital-to life symptoms.

An example of emotional clearing first in an acute situation might be a person who has a severe cold with an intense cough. Before the physical symptoms actually begin to improve, the patient usually reports that they feel better. This can be observed most easily in children. Within a few minutes or at most an hour after taking the remedy, they seem less cantankerous and more content. The physical symptoms of fever and cough, however, will not have abated at all as yet.

(2) Present to past: The process of healing occurs exactly in reverse of the manner in which the mind/body/spirit presented symptoms as it moved toward destruction. As we heal, out-of-balance energy patterns are brought, briefly, to the attention of the vital force. Sometimes, if you are watching closely, a remedy will push old symptoms that may have been forgotten to the surface. These symptoms will clear of their own accord, usually overnight. It is important that these emerging energy signals not be treated using drugs or even homeopathic remedies given based on those symptoms alone. Doing either of these things encourages the surfacing chronic condition that is indicated by the emerging symptoms to go "back in" again. This process is called *suppression* and can seriously and negatively impact progress toward complete healing

For most of us, even if we have been herbal and alternative for years, our previous disease patterns have not been cleared from the energy matrix completely. Rather, they were suppressed in one way or another. Suppression of symptoms is discussed further in the next section. For this section of the discussion on the progression of cure, it should be noted that suppressed symptoms behave erratically, surfacing in what seems to be random times and places, creating all sorts of havoc with the body, mind, and emotions. Suppressed symptoms emerge "out-of-sync" and can confuse the orderly picture of symptoms clearing according to Herring's Laws of Cure.

(3) Inside to outside: As someone moves toward healing, symptoms clear beginning with the innermost vital-to-life organs of the body such as the heart, lungs, and digestive system. Thus true healing usually begins inside the body and then moves to the surface areas.

If an individual comes to you for help with migraine headaches and you treat it properly, targeting the entire body/mind complex and not just the headache symptom, healing is likely to occur among the internal organs first before clearing the headache at all. The person may experience stomach, bowel, or respiratory problems as the homeopathic remedy focuses on the energy of these organs and brings their out-of-balance states to the attention of the vital force. These symptoms will be mild and temporary and then these symptoms will clear as internal healing takes place.

Skin rashes, whitlows, and arthritis of joints, especially in fingers and toes, will be the last to clear. Ailments of the skin and extremities are not considered by the energy system to be as vital to the body as the internal organs.

(4) Top to bottom: Symptoms are said to "drip" off the body, starting from the head and clearing downwards. The hands and the feet are often the last to be healed. This law is very much affected by the operation of the other laws.

If a person is suffering from rheumatoid arthritis and the symptoms began in the fingers and then progressed to the knees and the hips, the hips and knees are likely to feel better first, following the pattern of the most recent symptoms clearing first. "Top to bottom" and "inside to outside" are certainly rules in the progression of cure. However, they are often trumped by the progression of the cure moving from the most recent symptoms first, backwards through time, to the original symptoms and the clearing of the original cause. The original cause was often emotional, is still present, and lies at the core of everything else.

Homeopathic practitioners use their understanding of the progression of healing to monitor treatment and to be sure that they are prescribing the best possible remedies. James Tyler Kent said in a lecture to advanced homeopathic students in 1900:

> "Every homeopathic practitioner who understands the art of healing, knows that the symptoms which go off in these directions *(meaning according to Herring's Laws of Progression of Cure)* remain away permanently. Moreover, he knows that symptoms which disappear in the reverse order of their coming are removed permanently. It is thus he knows that the patient did not merely get well in spite of the treatment, but that he was cured by the action of the remedy. If a homeopathic physician goes to the bedside of a patient and, upon observing the onset of the symptoms and the course of the disease, sees that the symptoms do not follow this order after his remedy, he knows that he has had but little to do with the course of things."

SUPPRESSION AND ACQUIRED MIASMS

The goal of any healing practice should be to clear the offending organism or pattern completely, removing all symptoms permanently. Suppression is the term used in homeopathy to describe what happens when a symptom is merely covered up or driven deeper into the body. Allopathic drugs, by their very nature, do not eliminate the causes of disease. They may eliminate the bacteria or germ and suppress the offending symptoms for awhile, but they do not remove the out-of-balance energy pattern.

The suppression of an illness with an allopathic drug alters the body chemistry, driving the disease deeper into the energy system where it will eventually manifest as something else—usually something more severe and seemingly unrelated—later on. Hahnemann explained that the drug, based on the theory of opposites rather than on the theory of similars, has the effect of hiding the illness from the vital force, the immune system in our terminology, for a time. This allows the problem to continue unchecked until it reaches the more vital-to-life areas of the body.

Suppression produces a change in the expected direction of the process of disease. It may also create alternating states—first hypo and then hyper situations, complex diseases that are difficult to treat, protracted recoveries, difficult convalescences, addictions and destructive behavior patterns, and a lack of sufficient symptoms to diagnose from.

The suppression of any disease pattern often leads to a more deep-seated illness. For example, many children whose eczema has been "successfully" treated with steroids by the medical profession suffer from asthma at a later date. Homeopaths believe that the suppression of the eczema created the asthma by driving the surface ailment deeper into the energy system. Once the homeopathic treatment has cleared the lungs, the eczema is brought to the attention of the energy system. As a result, the eczema may reappear. The resurfacing, and then subsequent clearing, of the eczema is recognized as progress toward eventual cure. The healing is moving both toward the past (#2 in the progression of healing sequence) and toward the outside of the body (#3 in the sequence).

The suppression of symptoms disrupts the core energy patterns of the system. Besides the symptoms already listed as possible results, suppression of milder symptoms can alter a person's susceptibility to their environment, lower overall vitality, and create psychological and behavioral problems. These disrupted states are thought to be the basis of some of the newly identified, non-inherited (acquired) miasmic patterns such as cancer and Alzheimer's.

Another negative impact of suppression is the periodic reoccurring, often in yearly cycles, of symptoms that were thought to have been eliminated. As you work with remedies and read about them in the Materia Medicas, particularly those that are listed for the treatment of miasms, please pay attention to how many of the symptom pictures include periodicity. If this pattern was true in Hahnemann's day when many of these descriptions were written, how much worse must it be now in our society where reaching for a drug is an every day occurrence for so many people?

The symptoms which surface as the result of the normal progression of healing are usually milder than the original disease. They can be annoying—like the temporary re-emergence of mild allergies to food and pollen that I get at each deeper level of homeopathic that I use. Energy work, such as Tao or holding meridian points, often brings relief of these symptoms and seems to speed the healing by aiding the homeopathic remedy in realigning the energy system. Energy modalities, because they complement the homeopathic remedy, do not drive the symptoms deeper as described above. That is one very good argument for learning energy work and muscle testing as a complement to homeopathy.

Other examples of the link between a milder disease state, which was suppressed by drug therapies, and a more serious condition are being made by researchers and reported in medical journals regularly. Similar examples of this type of miasm creation are being found when the physical body is exposed to chemical toxins in the environment. The connection of vaccinations to the creation of serious miasmic-type illnesses is also well-documented.

It is believed that many of the same problems that occur when drugs are employed as therapies occur as the result of toxins, chemicals, environmental poisons, and vaccinations.

TREATMENT OF ACQUIRED MIASMS

Often the most effective way to treat any problem that is the result of suppression by drug therapies or chemical poisoning is by the giving of a nosode remedy (based as closely as possible on the original poison which caused the problem). This remedy is given according to the rules for the administration of nosode remedies.

The newer miasms of tuberculosis, polio, and cancer respond to treatment in this way, as do many other situations. There are studies and statistics that support the conclusion that drugs, chemicals, vaccinations, environmental pollution, fertilizers, weed sprays, or a combination of all of the above and/or many other toxins contribute to these miasms and the disease states to which they make us susceptible.

Perhaps, as Hahnemann speculated, *all* of the miasms except possibly psora are the result of suppression by allopathic drug treatments. I believe the world is not so simple as to be made up of either/or scenarios. The miasms, as I see them, are a combination of our view of the world, the choices we make, the events, traumas, and toxins that have impacted our system, the genetic inheritance we received from our ancestors, and probably, factors that we haven't even gotten a glimpse of yet.

MIASMS—IN SUMMARY

Each of the miasms has emotional patterns unique to itself. Such misalignments in emotional energy inevitably lead to misalignments and illnesses in the physical body. Whether we like it or not, agree with it or not, all actions and attitudes have consequences.

Key emotions of the cancer miasm include poverty consciousness and the taking upon ourselves of the responsibility to make everything right for everybody and to be unrealistically perfect ourselves. The correlation of these and other emotional patterns to the eventual development of cancer is being recognized more and more in both mainstream and alternative medicine. What is it that is creating these attitudes? Are such attitudes creating the miasm or is the environment creating the miasm which then creates the attitudes?

The emotional patterns of the emerging AIDS miasm are also interesting to consider. The electronic age has created a world with the illusion of no boundaries. This results in emotional feelings of vulnerability and exposure. Other emotional patterns of this miasm are attitudes such as being deserving of or wanting to get something for nothing and wanting gratification now with little regard for possible consequences.

Each miasm, whatever its cause, has an unmistakable influence on the health and vitality of our minds and bodies, and left unchecked, drains and depletes the vital force over time. Miasms warp the body's vital force in a profound way, wide enough and deep enough to create debilitating conditions ranging from schizophrenia to rheumatoid arthritis, or they can impact more mildly and produce such conditions as hay fever or a tendency to headaches.

Most of us have inherited portions of the basic miasms and we have most likely acquired a couple of the other miasms on our journey through life. Only one or two of these miasms will be active and influencing our individual health at any given moment. Drastic events, such as head injuries, surgeries, drug treatments, and emotional trauma can often shift which miasm is in control and influencing our overall vital energy at a particular time in our lives. The clearing of a miasm often brings another, usually less destructive one, to the forefront where it can be recognized, accessed, treated for, and cleared.

The removal of miasms creates a very powerful strengthening influence on our minds and bodies, and allows us to enjoy greater health, happiness, and energy. Often homeopathic treatment for a miasmic pattern will eradicate a chronic illnesses. What is more, the removal of the miasm from one generation will affect the generations coming thereafter. Working on your own issues, physical and emotional, is one of the greatest gifts that you can give to future generations.

We can overcome the past, transform the present, and brighten the future through homeopathy.

COMPARISON OF MIASMIC TRAITS

Psora	Sycosis	Syphilis	Tuberculosis (Psora/Syph)
Mental: difficulty with deep mental concentration, impractical, full of ideas, easily fatigued mentally & physically, timid, fearful, attention span short, selfish, shrewd, deceitful, restless, hyperactive, pretend or mis-perceive in their minds and then believe what they have told themselves	**Mental:** pessimistic, hard realist, skeptical, secretive, suspicious, jealous, has fixed ideas, hidden self disgust, quarrelsome, rudeness, cruelty, easily angered, seeks for control of other's minds & lives, inferiority feelings, anger that is weather related, tendency to harm others and to harm animals	**Mental:** displays mixture of madness & genius, deep sense of irony, stubborn, destructive, feels guilty, self-destructive behaviors, cruelty, lack of affection, rudeness, obstinate, melancholy, likes solitude, lack of self confidence, does not trust others, feelings of no way left but suicide, cannot explain symptoms	**Mental:** dissatisfaction and lack of tolerance, changeableness, romantic, extroverted, erratic, intolerant, angry, judgmental, apathetic, overly optimistic yet dissatisfied and always wanting to change jobs, etc., lack of concentration, irritable, unconcerned or indifferent, absence of hopelessness, absence of anxiety
Fear: manifested as anxiety and worry; many phobias	**Fear:** shown outwardly and vocally	**Fear:** as anguish of both mind and spirit	**Fear:** of things, but wants them anyway
Physical: allergies related to food; assimilation problems; diseases linked to calender (seasonal)	**Physical:** predominantly pelvic region and lungs with symptoms such as asthma, sinus issues, joints, and heart	**Physical:** body destroying itself, problems with bones, cranium, lungs, in vitro - structural birth defects	**Physical:** combination psora/syphilis, lung complaints but very seasonal, allergies by season
Skin: usually skin disorders, injuries become infected easily, lack of something, weakness, "Hypos"	**Skin:** catarrhal discharges, oily skin, excess perspiration, growths, warts, moles, excess or exaggeration	**Skin:** open ulcerated sores with pus, eruptions do not itch but slow to heal	**Skin:** red eye-lids (sometimes psora) sweaty palms & soles of feet, translucent skin that is fine and smooth, bruises easily
Pains: itchy, crawly, tickling, burning, bruising, pressing	**Pains:** sudden, intense, spasmodic, crampy, colicky	**Pains:** not intense enough for the symptoms, or alternatively, deep, aching, agonizing	**Pains:** neuralgic, sharp, piercing, twisting, stitching, sense of great exhaustion
Made Better By: summer; warmth both internal & external; lying down; heat	**Made Better By:** motion, winter, dry atmosphere, feels better for vomiting, passing gas, the breaking of blisters	**Made Better By:** change of position, lukewarm room or climate, during winter, cold	**Made Better By:** dry weather, open air, daytime, depends on which miasm dominates
Made Worse By: cold & winter; during sleep, standing still	**Made Worse By:** rest, damp cold, moist cold, rain, change in barometer, sudden heat or cold	**Made Worse By:** night, extremes of temperature, movements, summer heat, warmth of bed covers, sweat	**Made Worse By:** thunderstorms, night, pressure in chest, milk, fruits, greasy foods, closed room
Desires: sweet, sour, fatty fried, spicy, oil, hot foods	**Desires:** nuts, peppers, pungent, salty Aversions: meat, milk, spices	**Desires:** very spicy meat, cold, sour Aversions: bland meats	**Desires:** indigestibles such as dirt or paper, salt, things that are bad for them
Taste: all food tastes as if burnt	**Taste:** everything has a fishy taste	**Taste:** metallic taste, coppery	**Taste:** of pus & blood, sweetish/salty,

COMPARISON OF MIASMIC TRAITS

Polio	Cancer (Psora/Syph/Sycosis)	AIDS
Mental: restlessness, desire to move alternating with despair, forgetfulness, short term memory difficulties, wild optimism followed by deep despair, intolerant and short with people, irritable, whining, often feels aloof or detached from family members and people around them	**Mental:** High-strung, over-achiever, perfectionist, guilt at perception of not having done enough, conflict between what is right and what is socially acceptable, dislike of being contradicted or corrected, yielding to others' opinions (this is a learned, defensive trait), over-extending	**Mental:** lack of boundaries produces vulnerability, openness to the energies of others, builds walls to protect from other's pain that are seen by others as selfishness, feeling isolated and apart but needs to separate self even further, excess & extravagance, confusion
Fear: foreboding, particularly about health matters; deep dread of pain and dying in pain	**Fear:** prolonged fear for own safety, afraid to speak up	**Fear:** being vulnerable, emotions flowing in and out, no boundaries, changes happening too fast to respond to
Physical: stiffness, muscle contractions, paralysis, trembling, clumsy, digestive disturbances with stomach aches, headache, constipation/diarrhea, sinus congestion, weak lungs, tendency to weight gain	**Physical:** insomnia, diabetes, multiple allergies, inflammatory conditions, arthritis, colitis, enlarged glands, varicose veins, mononucleosis	**Physical:** breakdown of immune system, subsequent allergies and auto-immune disorders, flu and non-specific infections, swollen tonsils and lymphatic issues with no specific illness to account for them
Skin: cracks, ulcers, sores develop in folds of skin, itching, old sores open up and weep again and again	**Skin:** eczema, psoriasis, itching without eruption, liver spots, moles, birthmarks, tendency to boils, wounds heal slowly	**Skin:** very dry, especially forehead and cheeks, dry itchy lips, as though water in body has slipped away because there were no boundaries to hold it
Pains: muscle contractions and cramping, constant dull pain in lower back	**Pains:** pains in joints and lower extremities, sciatica	**Pains:** lower body, back, headaches, non-specific
Made Better By: cool applications relieve the paralysis, rainy but not cold weather, cold drinks	**Made Better by:** physical exertion if persistent (exercise feels worse at first), taking a nap	**Made Better by:** music no matter how low the mood (sound floats on the air and knows no boundaries), long sleep, massage, warmth
Made Worse By: approach of night, worse for thinking of ailments, allowing himself to feel dread	**Made Worse By:** result of some type of abuse—made worse by any hint of being controlled or abused in a relationship	**Made Worse By:** music occasionally, worse on first waking in the morning, worse extremes of heat or cold
Desires: little appetite for anything but not experiencing any special digestive distress	**Desires:** craves chocolate and cold drinks; likes music, dancing, and travel	**Desires:** likes to be extravagant, enjoys chocolate, appetite is often voracious but feels just as hungry after eating as before
Taste: putrid, reminiscent of a dental infection	**Taste:** medicinal aftertaste with everything ingested	**Taste:** dislikes food that is lukewarm

Section Three

Comparison of Miasmic Traits

Alzheimer's/Dementia	Vaccinosis (includes drugs, vaccines, and chemical pollutants)	
Mental: weakening and eventual loss of short-term memory, perception of reality is impaired, judgement (what is safe and what is not) is impaired, searches for words, unable to think coherently and complete a sentence, moaning, excessive worrying, fretting, loss of personal identity, inability to recognize family and friends, apprehension, sensation as if they are about to fall forward	**Mental:** variations according to the disease entity and the stabilizers used in that particular vaccine ADHD and behavioral disorders, fear of not measuring up to other people's expectations, lack of trust in others and fear that others do not trust them, unable to feel compassion and connection to others, feelings of worthlessness, feelings that they are deserving of more than they have	The characteristics of this miasm are many and varied. It would be unreasonable to expect each different vaccine, drug, fertilizer, or chemical to produce the same set of symptoms. Because the symptom picture is so varied, the only way to effectively treat for the damage done is to treat by symptom picture just as one would do for anything else. Nosodes used intercurrently should always be considered because of the depth of displacement in the energy. Often treatment is not begun until years after the vaccine was given and nosodes are often needed to reach deeply into the energy and into the past. One researcher (his research is with cats, dogs, and other animals) says that *"vaccinations create a statistical probability of an increased predisposition to the development of the disease vaccinated for without having been physically exposed to the disease except by the vaccine."* ## What? Please read the above quote over again to yourself and then put it in your own words, applying it to your children. It comes out something like, "To protect my infant in case of possible exposure to diphtheria, pertussis, & whooping cough, I will inject something into his system that may develop into one of those dreaded diseases without him even having to be exposed to them."
Fear: there are a lot of fears with dementia such a lost and alone state of being feel they may have committed a crime, fear that spouse is unfaithful	**Fear:** always a fear of inadequacy, many other fears which vary with vaccine type being reacted to. These symptoms include fear of people, fear of crowds, fear of heights and just about any fear imaginable	
Physical: pain and numbness in legs, staggers on walking, excessive perspiration, drinking water in some persons causes nausea, vertigo, great fatigue after even a short walk	**Physical:** convulsions, seizures of non-explainable cause, chronic ill health, recurrent infections all over the body, nervous system damage, headaches, paralysis, encephalitis, neuralgias, fibromyalgia	
Skin: chapped and dry, itching overlying pain, veins under skin distended	**Skin:** eczema, warts, eruptions, acne, areas of extremely dry or rough skin	
Pains: pain in shoulders, upper arms, back, fingers, heels and soles of the feet, pain feels like a hot iron	**Pains:** anywhere on the body, made worse by the pressure created by sitting, lying, or standing	
Made Better By: very short list but seem to be better in the evenings	**Made Better By:** a common keynote is that nothing tried seemed to help significantly	
Made Worse By: from warmth of room or bed, on waking in the morning	**Made Worse By:** pressure to achieve or the imposing of any kind of deadline	
Desires: indigestibles like chalk and sand, a great desire for chocolate	**Desires:** common to all types seems to be the desire for "thrills, spills, and excitement"	
Taste: persistent sour taste with mouth filling with sour tasting water	**Taste:** no particular commonality found	
Both Alzheimer's and vaccinosis patterns have a multiplicity of not well understood causes and neither Dementia or the multitude of drugs and vaccines have been around long enough for us to have enough really good provings of nosodes for their treatment. It will take at least another generation or two for us to really understand what is going on here and what is the best way to cope with it homeopathically.		

Chapter Fourteen - Nosodes and Miasm Descriptions

The Greek word noso is a prefix which is used to communicate the idea of a diseased state. The word is also connected with the Latin word noxa, the root of words denoting noxious or damaged. In ancient days nosocomium was the name for a hospital. Nosodes are remedies prepared from diseased tissues, secretions, or the organisms (bacteria, viruses, etc.) associated with a particular disease.

Hahnemann's theory of miasms was published in a book called <u>The Chronic Diseases</u>. This work was published quite late in his life and career. Shortly after this publication was made available, Hahnemann and other homeopathic physicians—notably Constantine Herring—began provings of remedies meant to be specific for the treatment of miasms and chronic diseases.

Nosodes do not **exactly** follow homeopathic theory because they are made from the tissues affected by the disease, or the disease-causing organisms themselves, rather than being made from something that exists in nature and produces a **similar** response from a healthy body. The law of similars (like cures like) is the basis of homeopathic theory. Nosodes (made from disease entities) and sarcodes (made from healthy tissue) many times are used more on a same curing same basis—rather than like curing like which is a basic homeopathic tenet. It is well known to experienced homeopaths that treatment of this sort often moves the case forward in phenomenal ways but rarely results in a complete cure. A second, intercurrent remedy is needed.

NOSODES AND INTERCURRENT REMEDIES

After seven years of rigorous clinical trials, Constantine Herring stated that "he had never succeeded in curing, but only ameliorating, diseases with their own morbid products"—in other words, by using a nosode. He then gave a classic example of the use of a nosode in a case of suppressed syphilis which was not responding to the clearly indicated remedy, Mercurius. He used Syphilinum, which brought out the eruptions of the syphilitic state. With the disease fully manifested, the case was then completely cleared by another round of Mercurius, followed by Lachesis. Herring reported many similar cases.

For a long time this information was a bit confusing to me. Mercurius, which was not working by itself in this case description, is **NOT** the nosode of syphilis. Syphilinum, which brought out the eruptions, is. I believe that these cases illustrate the homeopathic theory that a nosode—in this case the Syphilinum—would not have worked by itself any better than the Mercurius was working. It takes both the nosode—the "morbid product"—of the disease and an intercurrent remedy, the Mercurius in this case, to accomplish a cure.

The use of nosodes in this way is referred to as treatment with intercurrent remedies. The nosode, a remedy based not on similars but on sameness and referred to as an isopathic remedy, is used along with the remedy that most closely matches the patient's overall symptom picture. Used in this way, the nosode removes obstacles to cure and brings the disease pattern to the attention of the vital force, allowing it to be accessed and cleared by the matching remedy. The nosode and the symptomatic remedy deepen each other's action and make the cure more permanent. An isopathic remedy alone, just as Herring postulated so long ago, seldom produces such as result.

NOSODES AS SYMPTOMATIC REMEDIES

The basic rule of homeopathy is that a remedy is selected based on the totality of a person's symptoms. When a nosode is administered in this way, it is acting as a similinum just like any other remedy.

NOSODES AND MODERN HOMEOPATHIC PRACTICE

Nosode remedies have become extremely important in modern homeopathic practice. They reach deep into the energy system, unraveling complicated damages and alterations. They are, many times, essential to the cure of the really nasty ailments that are a part of our modern world. Nosodes of commonly administered drugs, given with an intercurrent remedy of some kind that matches the specifics of the person's individual reaction to the drug, are proving to be very effective treatments for prescription drug side effects.

It is important that we discover what remedies work against the newer miasms whether they are inherited or acquired because, unfortunately, they are all too common in today's world. Remember, we are talking about the energetic picture here, trying to identify and treat it before it becomes the actual disease. The disrupted energy of a miasm creates emotional and energetic patterns that eventually manifest themselves in our physical bodies as physical and mental illnesses. Nosode remedies seem to be particularly useful for the specific emotional states of miasms.

FLOWER ESSENCES AS INTERCURRENT REMEDIES

As we come to understand the miasms not as evil influences to be stamped out but as weaknesses that may be transformed into strengths, we are able to see ourselves and others, not as broken, but as children of the divine on a course toward perfection and salvation. A person presenting the negative characteristics of a miasm becomes simply a person struggling with a challenge in some area of their lives.

The entire focus of a flower essence is to transform struggle and negativity into strengths and positive characteristics. This makes them absolutely wonderful as an adjunctive treatment to both the nosode of a miasm or a remedy chosen because it is a point-by-point match for the person's unique response to his challenges. When a shift in perspective is needed a flower essence could be the perfect catalyst for change. What was previously a weakness creating havoc in a person's life becomes a strength!

At the end of each miasm/nosode description is a basic list of flower essences and the possible transformations their addition to the treatment might assist in bringing about. There is also a short description of traits that seem to match each particular miasm.

USING NOSODE REMEDIES

The following is a brief summary of nine common scenarios in which a nosode might be used:

1) As a symptomatic or constitutional remedy when the nosode picture matches the totality of symptoms being presented. In this case the underlying miasm has so dramatically deranged the vital force as to produce many of the symptoms of the miasm and leave little room for anything else.

2) When a well chosen remedy which clearly matches the presenting symptoms does not produce adequate results. There may be no improvement at all, or the improvement is of very short duration. This scenario almost always indicates the presence of one of the basic miasms. The nosode will cause more pronounced symptoms to surface so that the appropriate remedy can be given intercurrently with the nosode.

Example A: The use of Psorinum which has the keynotes of lack of reaction; well chosen remedies fail to act, especially in those who are extremely sensitive to cold but suffer from profuse sweating; tend to be pessimistic about recovery; have an unkempt look even when well dressed.

Example B: Tuberculinum bovinum given when the symptoms are constantly changing and well selected remedies fail to bring improvement, especially in persons with narrow chests, low recuperative powers, and compromised immune systems. Other keynotes of Tuberculinum are fear of animals, a deep discontented state with a desire to travel, and a tendency to give in to a desire to break things.

3) When a person presents too few guiding symptoms to make a clear choice from regular mineral, plant, or animal based remedies. Giving a nosode will cause additional symptoms to surface, making the choice of an appropriate remedy easier. Occasionally, if the picture of the nosode matched to any degree the symptoms of the person, the nosode of itself may bring the person nearer to a state of health. This would be operating under rule number one, above, without knowing it because of the scarcity of symptoms.

4) When the symptoms presenting are confusing, disorganized, and cannot be made to fit into any specific miasm or remedy family grouping. Since the symptoms do not point clearly to any particular miasm, unless you muscle test, your choice of a remedy will probably be done by either guesswork or intuition in this case. A flower essence which matches the person's general mood and demeanor may bring things into clearer focus and aid them in moving toward a better pattern.

5) When a person is reporting a "never the same since" syndrome—called NSS in homeopathy. NSS scenarios may have originated due to an accident or trauma, severe illness, drug treatment, surgery, great grief or loss, or any traumatic event. Some examples of NSS situations and homeopathic suggestions are listed below. The nosode remedies are listed in italics with the most commonly helpful remedy in bold italics.

- Vaccination (Thuja occidentalis, Variolinum, ***Vaccininum***)
- Chronic Fatigue/Epstein Barr (Natrum muriaticum, ***Psorinum, Carcinosin***)
- Influenza (Gelsemium sempervirens, *Psorinum*)
- Puberty (Pulsatilla nigricans)
- Miscarriage, birth, or abortion (Sepia succus)
- Grief (Natrum muriaticum, Causticum, Phosphoricum acidum—indicated by emotional flatness, no longer caring about anything at all)
- Head injury—physical or emotional injury (Arnica montana, Natrum sulphuricum, Opium—sleep apnea is the keynote for Opium)
- Hepatitis (Lycopodium clavatum, Phosphorus, ***Psorinum***)
- Mononucleosis (***Carcinosin***)
- Tuberculosis (Thuja occidentalis, ***Medorrhinum***, Nitricum acidum)
- Measles or whooping cough (Carcinosin, Tuberculinum bovinum)

6) When clear progress was being made with the use of a particular nosode but then the improvement not only stops but the re-emergence of old symptoms is experienced. This can be caused by giving the remedy in too deep a potency and/or for too long a time, causing the miasm to display cleared symptoms.

Example A: The giving of the nosode moves the case forward with the removal of the active symptoms. If the improvement is of short duration, a repeat of the nosode may be required. When improvement no longer occurs following the administration of the nosode, it is time to return to the former remedy.

Example B: No improvement is shown following the giving of the nosode. When a sufficient time has elapsed and no improvement has happened, administer the original remedy. The first remedy often acts as dramatically as it did in the beginning and the case moves forward.

7) When the nosode remedy is closely related to the disease, or the problem is the result of a vaccination related to the substance from which the nosode was made.

Example A: The use of Pertussinum (a nosode) against a case of whooping cough. The nosode, in this case, should be used as an intercurrent remedy along with a symptomatic remedy.

Example B: A nosode of the offending vaccination (for example Variolinum—smallpox nosode) to remove the side effects of a vaccination for smallpox. The nosode is almost always best when used as an intercurrent remedy. When dealing with a vaccine, there may not be any need for the nosode at all; the symptomatic remedy is sufficient by itself. The use of the nosode is most appropriate when there is a very stubborn allergic reaction to the organism which was introduced by the vaccine, rather than a reaction to some other substance also found in the vaccine.

8) Nosode remedies are sometimes used to prevent specific infectious diseases. An example of this is the historic successful use of Variolinum in smallpox epidemics. This method of use will be discussed further in the section on the use of homeopathic remedies in epidemics.

9) Autonosodes are made from the person's own disease substances. These homeopathic remedies are prepared from saliva, pus, the weeping material from skin eruptions, other bodily secretions of the sick person, or microbes from the patient grown in cultures. This method has sometimes proven helpful when nothing else has been effective. Autonosodes should be used with another remedy, intercurrently.

It is easily seen that an understanding of the various miasms and the various nosodes is often essential in working out a case. The understanding of miasms is an important part of understanding homeopathy.

Basic Nosode and Miasm Descriptions

The description of the nosode produced with the specific bacteria of the core disease, or diseased tissue containing the bacteria, is the description of the miasm. This is true because the miasm is an energetic reproduction of the symptoms the bacteria creates in the body. This section is a further description of the miasms discussed on the previous pages; these descriptions are also a description of the symptom pictures of the nosodes created from that bacteria.

Psora Miasm/Psorinum Nosode
Struggles to Survive

It is believed by every branch of homeopathy that the psora miasm has been inherited to a degree by every member of the human family. Some, of the Christian faith, even go so far as to link the psora miasm to the changes and challenges that occurred when Adam and Eve left the Garden of Eden for existence as mortal beings.

In our lives, the negative traits of this miasm surface when we are under stress. The depth of the pathology is different from person to person and according to the perceived depth of the stress. The positive traits—once they are discovered by the person, cultivated, and developed—are equally as deep as were the pathologies.

As I have come to view the miasms as the double-sided, negative and positive, attributes of humanity responding to life and learning and growing from it, I can no longer look at the negative traits of psora as something to be "gotten rid of." The struggles with feelings of abandonment can be developed into compassion and connection with others. I see the skin issues as a cry for help in coping with some aspect of their lives that is manifesting at this time with this psoric symptom.

DIFFICULT TO TREAT

Psora characteristics are unique in their difficulty to treat. I believe that this difficulty is directly tied to our mortality. Although we strive for perfection on this earth, the maintaining of it is a continual struggle at this stage of our existence. Nothing given or done for psora symptoms seems to work for more than a few days or weeks. Psorinum, or another antipsoric remedy, given to a deep level is the only treatment that works.

The 'difficult to treat' or 'can't clean up aspect' of Psorinum pathology is found in the psychological issue of chronic depression. In cases where sadness, dejection or anxiety persists long after the source of the unhappiness has been removed, and other remedies have failed to fix the problem, Psorinum should be strongly considered. Continued, inconsolable mourning over anything to do with family (children, home, lost traditions), or a continual looking to the past are keynote indicators.

THE STRUGGLE TO SURVIVE ON EARTH

The immediate needs of survival—a warm and secure place to live, adequate water and nutrition, concern with the weather, and safety from attack, accident, or injuries—are keynotes of the psoric miasm. Survival in a less-than-friendly environment almost always requires the ability to adapt to new, even extreme, situations. Failure to adapt to such things as changes in weather or in the seasons are central to the psora pattern. We fail to adapt—we adapt in inappropriate ways—until we are out of alignment with natural cycles.

The struggle to survive is indicated by poverty struggles—people seem to have one financial reversal after another or who work and work and never seem to get ahead. The administration of Psorinum or one of the other antipsorics that matches the symptoms more closely, changes the mental and emotional attitude toward money in dramatic ways. This is described in some remedy guides as recharging the vital poverty.

VITAL POVERTY

Vital poverty refers to more than money. Psorinum individuals often display a lack of vital heat, an inability to assimilate foods properly, and a deficiency of vital reaction during treatment. This deficiency of vital reaction to a well-selected remedy, is the chief keynote of the remedy and illustrates the basic characteristic of difficult to treat that is so much a part of the psora miasm. The tuberculosis miasm also has this tendency, which supports the contention that the tuberculosis miasm is a composite of psora and sycosis.

APPETITE AND METABOLISM

The psora miasm includes both problems with appetite, too little or too much, and having to eat when not hungry to prevent a headache (hypoglycemia). The underlying theme of appetite issues lies in the *background* of all psora characteristics and remedies while fast or slow metabolism are specifics and give us *foreground* symptoms to choose a remedy by. Some cases of extreme nausea during pregnancy, especially if the nausea did not abate with the use of other remedies, is often an indication of psora being active.

Major psoric remedies such as *Lycopodium, Sulphur,* and *Psorinum* are examples of remedies with fast metabolism in their pictures. They are among the 'hungriest' of homeopathic remedies.

The *Calcarea* remedies and *Graphites* are among the slow metabolizers. No matter how rigidly people needing these remedies follow a diet, they still seem to gain weight.

A third group of psoric remedies are useful for people whose metabolism is so off kilter that they are unable to uptake sufficient nutrients from the foods they eat to maintain health. *Silica* and *Magnesium carbonicum* are two examples of remedies with assimilation issues in their remedy pictures.

APPEARANCE

Another characteristic of psora is a tendency to look unkempt or rumpled. A well-groomed appearance may require enormous effort for a person in which the psora miasm is dominant. Perspiration can be especially offensive and hot showers only make the problem worse by opening the pores. Cold showers and deodorants provide only temporary relief. Psorinum 200C is often used to lessen the offensive odors emanating from terminally ill people and from menstrual blood.

ALLERGIES

Another manifestation of psora's presence is multiple allergies and extreme sensitivity to the environment. Psorinum, given in a constitutional program of 200C, 1M and 10M at appropriate treatment intervals with the right intercurrent remedy, has often had a dramatic effect on even severe allergies. Psorinum, in low potency, is sometimes used as a preventative for seasonal allergies and asthma. Psorinum, if the symptom picture matches, builds up a low constitution by eliminating as much of the psora miasm as is ever possible.

MENTAL/EMOTIONAL

Children in whom psora is dominant are fretful, day and night. The mental/emotional patterns of psora for any age include peevish, irritable, easily startled, and severe ailments from even the slightest emotional upset. Dullness of mind and difficulty concentrating and thinking are also keynotes. Psorinum is a suggested remedy for many kinds of learning disabilities.

ABANDONED/FORSAKEN

Key among the emotional symptoms of psora is the sense, even from earliest childhood, of being abandoned or forsaken. This is not the abandonment issues that occur with the loss of a parent or sibling. It seems that each individual born into mortality feels on a deep, but not quite conscious level, his or her separation from our Heavenly parents. This unconscious feeling of separation drives the deep-seated desire of man to come to know God and learn to serve Him well.

CAUSES

The emergence of the psora miasm and its list of traits and illnesses, when not just the general lot of mortals, can often be traced to an infectious illness from which the person is displaying "never the same since" symptoms. Other causes might include living in a damp or moldy environment, unsanitary or overcrowded living conditions, ingesting toxins and poisons (drugs?), and living on junk food. Just as these may be causative factors, their elimination from our lives may aid us in keeping psora "tamped down."

MODALITIES

The modalities of Psorinum include better for eating with the sad reaction of worse immediately afterward. Symptoms usually improve from rest and pressure applied to the painful part. Symptoms are worsened by cold and changes in weather, particularly the approach of storms, and as evening approaches.

COMPLIMENTARY REMEDIES

The homeopathic remedy Sulphur is a common remedy used in place of Psorinum. Sulphur has many of the same symptoms in its picture as does Psorinum. If one of these remedies has produced results but is no longer doing so, the other may often be given with good results. One major difference between these two remedies is a tendency to coldness with Psorinum and being overly warm most of the time with Sulphur.

HEALING AGGRAVATION

The giving of homeopathic remedies, particularly deep level ones, brings on a reaction to indicate that it is working. This kind of reaction is sometimes referred to as an aggravation of symptoms. The reactions of most remedies—remember these reactions are usually mild and nothing to be concerned about—occur in three to five days. Psorinum is unusual in that the aggravation usually appears a full *nine days* after taking the remedy. This is just another aspect of psora's difficult to treat and slow to respond symptom picture. When giving or taking Psorinum, don't mistake this aggravation for something that needs to be treated for. It is an indication that things are progressing nicely! Mark your calendar and wait it out.

MERIDIAN/REALM RELATIONSHIP

Psora's primary relationship is with the realm of earth, with the earth meridians of stomach and spleen, and with the base chakra.

FLOWER ESSENCES REMEDIES FOR PSORA MIASM

Below is a list of flower essences with a short description, both positive and negative, of traits that have similarities to the descriptions of psora.

BLACKBERRY *Rubus armeniacus (white-pink) North American*

Positive qualities: Decisive action; clear vision of the path ahead; the ability to translate goals into action; the ability to take positive and appropriate action in any situation; radiant enthusiasm for the next step in life or for coming changes.

Patterns of imbalance: Procrastination; inability to put goals and intentions into action; indecisive; sluggish blood; lowered metabolism.

BLACK-EYED SUSAN *Rudbeckia hirta (yellow/black center) North American*

Positive qualities: Penetrating insight into one's own emotional health; self-aware; able to learn and grow from past experiences and traumas.

Patterns of imbalance: Self-destructive tendencies, mental or physical illness as a result of repressing traumatic memories; extreme fatigue, apathy, or depression.

This remedy can be helpful in confronting traumatic episodes from the past that have been repressed.

CALENDULA

Positive qualities: Ability to use the spoken word to create and inspire others; warmth and receptivity that build lasting relationships through positive dialogue.

Patterns of imbalance: Using a talent for the spoken word to argue, badger, belittle, or manipulate.

Calendula is especially indicated for the aspects of psora where lack of communication is damaging relationships or where good communication skills are needed for a teaching assignment or profession. Calendula is also a perfect herbal and homeopathic match for the skin issues of psora.

CALIFORNIA PITCHER PLANT *Darlingtonia californica (green/purple) North American*

Positive qualities: Balance between the desires and foibles of the physical body and the yearnings and aspirations of the Spirit; tremendous physical and emotional vitality; superb instincts, the kind that can only be the result of Heaven's guidance.

Patterns of imbalance: Denial of the emotions and needs of the lower chakras; fears, including fears and issues with sex; physical weakness and lack of the ability to assimilate and metabolize nutrients.

California pitcher plant is a carnivorous plant. Its capacities are closely linked to digestion and especially to the digestion of meats.

CHAPPARAL *Larrea tridentata (yellow) North American*

Positive qualities: Feeling loved, protected and watched over; able to take responsibility for oneself and one's actions; feelings of gratitude and contentment.

Patterns of imbalance: Disturbed dreams; physical and emotional toxicity due to drugs, prescription or otherwise; behaviors as the result of experiencing violence or when suffering from post-traumatic stress disorder; feeling and behaving like a victim; feeling that there is nothing that can be done to make things better; victimizing others as one perceives themselves having been victimized.

CLEMATIS *Clematis vitalba (white) English*

Positive qualities: Ability to both plan for the future and carry out those plans; able to tell the inspiration of the Spirit from wishful thinking and personal desires; inspired ideas but with practical application.

Patterns of imbalance: Not sufficiently present in the here and now; constantly living in the past or talking of the future; drowsy and light headed; prone to daydreaming

Dr. Bach's category: Not Sufficient Interest in Present Circumstances.

GOLDEN YARROW *Achillea filipendulina (yellow) North American*

Positive qualities: Remaining open to others without being overly sensitive to negative energies or reacting inappropriately to the negative actions of others; active social involvement which enriches and energizes others; ability to express themselves gently, but succinctly, when with others.

Patterns of imbalance: Drug addiction, sometimes as the result of over-sensitivity to negative influences; avoiding contact with others because they find it difficult to cope with their own sensitivity

Golden Yarrow helps to create boundaries for energy workers. The herb, yarrow, promotes closing and healing of physical wounds, without scarring. Golden yarrow behaves in a similar fashion emotionally

GREEN CROSS GENTIAN *Frasera speciosa/Swerta radiate (pale green-dark flecks) Range of Light*

Positive qualities: Healing and balance despite challenges and setbacks; able to feel total forgiveness, unconditional love and peace; a desire to serve, help, and heal others; concern for the physical welfare of the earth.

Patterns of imbalance: Deep despair—to the point of depression and inability to function normally—because of man's inhumanity to man; discouragement at the depletion or misuse of the earth's resources.

HORNBEAM *Carpinus betulus (yellow/green) English*

Positive qualities: Unbounded steady state of energy; contagious enthusiasm; connection and joyful involvement in the tasks and events of daily life and work; ability to conceive and carry out new and exciting approaches to old tasks; sufficient strength to carry out life's tasks.

Patterns of imbalance: Fatigue, usually brought on by boredom and lack of connection and attention to the routines of daily life; weariness completely out of proportion to the health of the physical body; living beneath one's potential; lethargy of mind and body; mild depression.

Dr. Bach's category: For Those Who Suffer Uncertainty.

This remedy is especially useful if there has been a head injury; developmental or learning disabilities.

LAVENDER *Lavandula officinalis (violet) North American*

Positive qualities: Spiritual sensitivity; stable physical health; mentally active; ability to relax; overall harmony of body and spirit.

Patterns of imbalance: Lack of focus; distracted, restless; overwhelmed by responsibilities; nervous; agitated; high-strung; physically depleted following agitated states; insomnia; vision problems; neck and shoulder tension.

Lavender is said to teach the soul to temper, moderate, and regulate the previously uncontrolled bursts of energy.

MALLOW *Sidalcea glaucescens (pink-violet) North American*

Positive qualities: Warm, open-hearted sharing; trust and openness in social situations.

Patterns of imbalance: Inability to trust one's self or others; the heart feels frozen and unable to receive or give love; insecure in personal relationships. Mallow is all about the heart and the heart chakra

OLIVE *Olea europaea (white) English*

Positive qualities: Restores a connection to Heaven and inspiration; feeling renewed energy by tapping into the strength of the Spirit; having a strong desire to live life according to the will and inspiration of Heaven.

Patterns of imbalance: Extreme physical symptoms of exhaustion and weariness where the individual needs to reach a higher spiritual plane to gain or regain balance; depression; discouragement; absent-mindedness.

Dr. Bach's category: Lack of Interest in Present Circumstances.

Olive helps bring awareness that the physical self is profoundly connected with the realms of the Spirit

WILD ROSE *Rosa canina (pink or white) English*

Positive qualities: Feeling motivated; being interested and energized by daily activities; a dynamic will to live; feeling great joy.

Patterns of imbalance: Resignation to our current state that deprives us of motivation and vitality; life seems difficult with a continual need to struggle (classic psora) but life no longer seems worth the struggle (unique foreground pattern, not classic psora at all, making this a key note of Wild Rose). Illnesses tend to linger; apathy so deep that it obstructs healing; feelings of helplessness and powerlessness.

Dr. Bach's category: Lack of Interest in Present Circumstances

Wild Rose aids the soul in regaining interest in life after a long or debilitating illness. Returns the emotional and physical bodies to a state of vibrant health and determination to fight on.

UNDERSTANDING THE PSORIC PERSONALITY

If I felt like I was seeing issues belonging to psora in myself or someone I was working with, I would ask myself some questions like the following ones suggested by Ian Watson to help bring things into focus. Journaling these types of questions can be very helpful.

Where is this person struggling with a psoric challenge? Where do they feel that their basic survival needs are most threatened or are not being met? Where in their lives do they feel that they don't have enough or that there is not enough for them and other people too? What are the things that they most fear will be taken away? Where is the basic abandonment insecurity manifesting and how is it affecting their close personal relationships? How can they grow closer to their Heavenly origins and find peace?

Sycosis Miasm/Medorrhinum Nosode
Growth and Reproduction

Medorrhinum was believed by Hahnemann to be the only remedy needed for the removal of the sycosis miasm. Other remedies have been developed and are often used today, sometimes intercurrently with the Medorrhinum nosode. Flower essences are being used effectively as intercurrent remedies with both nosodes and the other remedies used in the treatment of miasms.

EXCESS/EXPANSION

The behavior patterns of Medorrhinum (and the sycosis miasm) tend to excesses. The person has strong desires and passions and is continually looking for an outlet for all this emotion and energy. They want to experience everything—sometimes even the forbidden, immoral, or unlawful. In many areas of life the patient swings from one extreme to another. Whatever they do, they do to excess. They are either A students or F students. They are either very up and energetic, or very low and fatigued. Medorrhinum is a leading remedy in the treatment of bi-polar behavior problems.

Mentally, individuals needing Medorrhinum often have something build up inside them until they must let it out in some expansive and exuberant manner such as yelling or shouting—often while jumping or running. If you have a child like this you are saying to yourself right now, "I know just what you mean!"

The behavior of sycosis/Medorrhinum is often turbulent, and there is a parallel in the overproduction of bodily secretions. Profuse sweat and catarrh are indications. Overgrowth of tissues (warts, moles and polyps) is closely tied to the sycotic miasm and frequently responds to treatment by Medorrhinum.

ATTRACTION

The control of our appetites, desires, and passions—sexual or any other kind— falls under the influence of this miasm. The energy that attracts certain things, good or bad, into our lives and the ability to manifest, materialize and create the things we want in our lives is evidence of strength and positive energy here. The sycotic miasm governs our choices and our ability to distinguish between the things that we want and the things that we really need. One of the positive aspects of sycosis is the ability to really enjoy pleasurable things and appreciate the beauty of the world around us.

HASTINESS/SENSE OF TIME

Individuals in whom sycosis is dominant tend to act in haste without complete knowledge. They often have a distorted or nonexistent sense of time and dates. They may be great procrastinators (they feel that there is plenty of time) who then rush to accomplish things at the last possible moment. Medorrhinum is often considered for hyperactive children whose running and jumping lead them to constantly touch and break things. Medorrhinum people also have a tendency to an overabundance of energy late at night and difficulty with cyclical things like menstruation or sleeping.

SYMPTOM PICTURE

This turbulence and overproduction of secretions does not include an overproduction of symptoms, however. Psorinum has an overproduction of symptoms, while Medorrhinum is often used for people who appear to have strong constitutions and have few or no symptoms at any one time. The sycosis miasm includes people who, while having few symptoms, are the ones who suddenly go down hard with a serious disease or complaint. ("Psoric patients have many uncomfortable sensations in the heart region and think that they are about to die. . . but there is little danger; it is the sycosis heart patients who die suddenly and without warning."—quoted from Roberts repertory.) This is true of more than heart ailments with sycosis people and the symptom picture of the Medorrhinum homeopathic remedy.

THE MIND

Physically, the sycosis miasm impacts generative organs such as kidneys, liver, lungs, and sinuses, but it also has a dramatic effect on the mind. The going to extremes aspect of this miasm produces both a strong memory and the polar opposite of forms of mental retardation such as mongoloidism and autism. Less severe learning disabilities have also been helped with anti-sycotic remedies.

Medorrhinum is known for treating memory problems such as forgetting names and words, and what has just been read. (Syphilinum is tied to forgetting events and occurrences.) With the clearing of the sycosis miasm there is often an improvement, even a reversal, of symptoms connected to the memory.

HEART/EMOTIONAL

An interesting symptom of the Medorrhinum remedy and the sycosis miasm is the sensation that there is a great cavern where the heart should be. This physical symptom seems to be linked to the mental/emotional symptom of things seeming strange, everything in life seeming to be unreal but, at the same time, apprehension that something is about to go terribly wrong. It may also be linked to the sycosis pattern of lack of symptoms—something is wrong but there are no symptoms, only emptiness.

BOUNDARIES

The sycosis miasm and the remedies that treat it have an underlying theme of problems with boundaries. This may manifest as an inability to say "no" when necessary, an over-identification with other people's problems and emotions, panic attacks, the shunning of responsibility because the load feels too heavy to bear, fear of the dark or fear of being followed or attacked.

SENSITIVITY

Often there is the capacity to feel or see energy and be able to observe how it interacts with other energy fields. Any remedy with *clairvoyance* listed should probably be considered a sycotic remedy. This sensitivity can become so overwhelming and painful that the person shuts down to protect themselves. Unfortunately, this shutdown affects the heart chakra contributing to the hollowed-out feeling mentioned above. Too many people, caught in this sycotic cycle, use food to fill the empty spaces. Food cravings and over-eating are problems that are often connected with excesses or shutdowns in these hyper states of sensitivity.

This sensitivity tells us that we are never really very separate. We are part of the whole and brothers and sisters in a very real sense. Sensing another person's presence without being able to see, hear, or touch them with the physical senses creates a very real connection between us. The sycosis miasm, balanced or disturbed, demonstrates how interconnected we are with the rest of creation and presents us with the paradox of finding ourselves and establishing our own boundaries and sense of self. *This is who I am, this is what I think and feel, this is what I wish to become* are central issues in the growth and balance of a positive sycosis personality.

CAUSES

The sycosis miasm is one of extreme sensitivity. The worsening of symptoms often follows verbal or sexual abuse. Because of the extreme sensitivity of out-of-balance states, this abuse may be more perceived than real. Symptoms often become worse from anticipation or just before the need to teach or perform. Bad news, and difficulties or quarrels with another person also often trigger distress and the worsening of symptoms.

MODALITIES

Modalities include better for lying on the stomach, better for bending and stretching backward, and better for fresh air. Worse from three to four a.m. is a keynote of Medorrhinum and all sycosis remedies.

Suppression of an inherited tendency to the sycosis miasm by drug therapies can lead to this miasm's re-emergence as sciatica, arthritis, erosion of cartilage, cramps in the calves and feet, sensations of burning in the legs and feet, pain in the heels or balls of the feet, and other connective tissue disorders. Suppression can also manifest as feelings of being overwhelmed, hurried, anxious, and irritable with a very deep aversion to being touched!

MERIDIAN/REALM/CHAKRA RELATIONSHIPS

The sycosis miasm has a close relationship to all things that are water or of the watery element. For a person struggling with this miasm the kidney and bladder are often troublesome when they are under any type of stress. Whenever bodily fluids become stagnant, negative sycosis symptoms appear. Many bodily functions involve the movement of fluids—urine, bile, blood, mucus, sexual fluids, hormones, or perspiration. These areas can present difficulties as our bodies strive to have the right amount of the right kind of fluids in the right place at the right time.

In health, a person with sycotic tendencies does not retain water or become dehydrated. The capacity to create, absorb, utilize, and eliminate fluids properly is a sign of balance within sycotic tendencies. The sycosis close ties to water make it part of the realm of the sea and a function of the sacral (2nd) chakra.

FLOWER ESSENCES REMEDIES FOR THE SYCOSIS

Below is a list of flower essences with a short description, both positive and negative, of traits that have similarities in the descriptions of psora.

ASPEN *Populus tremula (Green/grey) English*

Positive qualities: Confidence and trust when meeting new experiences and challenges; able to draw inner strength from one's faith; able to receive energetic impressions from others—even, on occasion from the 'other side of the veil'.

Patterns of imbalance: Fear of the unknown and of one's abilities; vague anxiety and apprehension; nightmares; inability to rely on or even remember the spiritual strengths and experiences of the past as a way to cope with the present trial.

Dr. Bach's category: For Those Who Have Fear

BLEEDING HEART *Dicentra formosa (pink) North American*

Positive qualities: Open-hearted ability to love others unconditionally; emotional freedom; ability to fill one's own needs from within or through communication with the divine; intense desire for connection.

Patterns of imbalance: Tendency to form relationships based on fear or possessiveness, emotional co-dependence; loss of boundaries

an amazing remedy for grief or loss of a loved one.

FILAREE *Erodium cicutarium (violet) North American*

Positive qualities: Proper perspective; an ability to see an overview that brings the events of ordinary life into perspective; tremendous inner strength and spiritual reserves.

Patterns of imbalance: Disproportionate, obsessive worry over trifles and unimportant details; failure to see the bigger picture; unable to receive spiritual inspiration and counsel.

IMPATIENS *Impatiens glandulifera (pink/mauve) English*

Positive qualities: Patience, acceptance; flowing with the pace of life; adaptable to others' energies; efficient but patient with self and with the work pace of others.

Patterns of imbalance: Impatience; irritation; hypertension; muscle tension; nervous tension; intolerance; cardiovascular strain and problems; high blood pressure; sudden explosions of temper.

Dr. Bach's category: Loneliness.

LOVE-LIES-BLEEDING *Amaranthus caudatus* *(red)* *North American*

Positive qualities: The ability to move beyond personal pain, suffering, or mental anguish by finding larger meaning, answers, and growth in such suffering; compassionate awareness of and attention to the meaning of pain or suffering;) able to feel and respond to the pain of others.

Patterns of imbalance: Tendency to isolate oneself from others rather than to accept sympathy and assistance (this isolation greatly intensifies the pain and suffering; deep melancholia which focuses entirely on one's personal pain; despair; feeling that nothing will ever change for the better.

PEDICULARIS *Pedicularis groenlandica* *(violet)* *Range of Light*

Positive qualities: Emotional insight and wisdom based on connection as a Child of God; confidence and faith; inner stability and calm; ability to learn from the lessons of history and from the lessons of one's own past

Patterns of imbalance: Hypochondria or hyper-sensitivity to the environment; refusal to participate in things due to possible triggering of sensitivities; fits of crying; water imbalances in the kidneys and cells of the body; excessive emotional responses to small situations.

QUEEN ANNE'S LACE *Daucus carota* *(white)* *North American*

Positive qualities: Spiritual insight; harmony between the higher and lower chakra energies; ability to see both the physical and the energetic, emotional, and spiritual patterns of things; grounded in the physical world while able to access, feel, and see the spiritual.

Patterns of imbalance: Lack of objectivity in viewing other people's motives and intentions—seeing others emotions as just like their own; physical eyesight affected by the ability to perceive reality.

SIERRA PRIMROSE *Primula suffrutescens* *(Pink)* *Range of Light*

Positive qualities: Gratitude for the gift of life regardless of the circumstances of health; strength of character and of the soul; physical vitality; enthusiasm; energy

Patterns of imbalance: Lack of gratitude; little appreciation for the gift of life or for one's circumstances; fatigue; boredom; depression; joyless living; habitually responding dully and with no enthusiasm

SHOOTING STAR *Dodecatheon hendersonii* *(violet/pink)* *North American*

Positive qualities: Open-hearted; generous; caring for all people; deep connection with all creation

Patterns of imbalance: Feeling of complete alienation; not feeling a part of the community or even the human family; holding back from participation in events that involve other people

The imbalances of the shooting star remedy are sometimes created by birth trauma and have been with the person throughout entire life.

VIOLET *Viola odorata* *(violet-blue)* *North American*

Positive qualities: Warmth a perception that is both fragile and beautiful; spiritual perspective; sharing with others while remaining true to oneself; ability to heal and move through loneliness or grief.

Patterns of imbalance: Profound shyness, reserve, aloofness, fear of being lost and overshadowed in groups.

Useful for anyone who is experiencing the isolation and loneliness of grief, suffering or pain.

WALNUT *Juglans regia* *(green)* *English*

Positive qualities: Freedom from the opinions of others which might tell you that you can't succeed at something important to you; making healthy transitions in life; courage to follow one's own path

Patterns of imbalance: Too much influenced by the beliefs and values of family or community, or by one's own past experiences; gastric and duodenal ulcers; allergies; stuck in unproductive habits

Dr. Bach's category: Over-sensitivity to influences and ideas.

WILLOW *Salix vitellina* *(green)* *English*

Positive qualities: Acceptance of others imperfections and acceptance of life as it is; taking responsibility for self and for the life one has made; patience in suffering and with life.

Patterns of imbalance: Feeling resentful, inflexible or bitter; physical rigidity as a result of bitterness and resentment; feeling that life is unfair or that one is a victim of others or of circumstance.

Dr. Bach's category: Despondency and Despair.

UNDERSTANDING THE SYCOTIC PERSONALITY

Asking ourselves (and clients) a questions such as where in our lives and relationships are our tendencies to lose our personal boundaries or cross over the line into either criticism of others or in letting them have too great an influence on us? Am I experiencing hyperactivity, inability to focus and concentrate, manic/depression or bi-polar tendencies? Am I experiencing either the excessive, out-of-control behaviors and emotions or the physical manifestation of excess and over-production of bodily fluids such as perspiration, mucus, or fluid build-up in the tissues?

Syphilis Miasm/Syphilinum Nosode
Destruction and Rebirth

The syphilitic miasm is often called the great imitator because of its ability to mimic other diseases and chronic conditions. Because of this keynote, many other polycrest remedies are mistakenly given where Syphilinum may have been the remedy needed. If Syphilinum seems to be indicated, consider Mercurius as the best constitutional or intercurrent remedy, but never rule out any of the syphilitic remedies. Also, remember the many positive aspects of flower essence treatment with miasms.

FIRE MERIDIAN/BOTH DESTRUCTIVE AND TRANSFORMATIVE

The syphilis miasm's strongest affinity (or, at least, the area that is most frequently out of balance) is in the fire meridian. Like fire, the traits and behaviors of the syphilis miasm can be both destructive and transformative. Fire can destroy but fire is also necessary for transformation to take place. Earthen pots (like earth meridian people) and metals (like metal meridian people) require the refiner's fire to become all that they can be. Trials and suffering can bring refinement and spiritual gifts we would not attain to otherwise. It seems to me that this is true of all of us, whatever our primary miasm might be. More than any other meridian, fire people can display the positive aspects of all of the meridians—but only after their own personal 'trial by fire'. This is a very destructive miasm but also the most amazing if balance is ever achieved.

BREAKING DOWN/LETTING GO

Part of the destructive tendencies of syphilis seem to be connected to the idea that the only way to "fix this mess" is to completely destroy it and start over. This is especially true of relationship issues and plays a part in any self-destruction and self-mutilation. The positive side of this "breaking down" is the getting rid of old ideas and habits that are not serving us well or helping us to be happy and well-balanced.

VIOLENCE

Syphilinum and the syphilis miasm are noted for varying degrees of violence. This can be a confusing symptom because this violence may show up as anything from a tendency to tickle, poke, or pretend to punch, through vindictiveness, inability to let go of hurt and insults, gossip, acts of terrorism, the desire to destroy things, violent jealousy, the desire to kill, and other very destructive mental states. Syphilinum needs to be looked at whenever there are destructive tendencies.

Self-destruction or self-mutilation is a keynote of this miasm. The desire to punch or destroy that is a keynote of the syphilinum miasm has turned inward. Instead of being cruel or destructive to others, the person is cruel and destructive to themselves. This turning on the self can be an indication of self-loathing if the destructive tendencies have led to relationship problems or trouble with the law. The self-loathing may also cover feelings created by abuse of some kind that has occurred or is occurring in the person's life. A 10M remedy is given and repeated if necessary. Hyoscyamus niger is sometimes used here, as an intercurrent or as a follow-up remedy, if the symptoms indicate it.

FEAR

The destructive tendencies of the syphilis miasm are often linked to fear or anxiety, with the anxiety focused on health or relationship issues. One reaction to fear is to hang on tightly to what is already familiar, sometimes resulting in obsessive or ritualistic behaviors. The syphilitic miasm often includes feelings of losing control over their inner selves, needing to exert more and more will power to keep themselves together. They will try to exert control over their environment and their relationships, thinking others feel the same.

There is often a deep aversion to dirt and dirty things and the need to wash the hands repeatedly and clean anything that must be touched. This is a deep level, late to be seen symptom, so don't wait to see it before treating for the syphilis miasm. It is a definite keynote for syphilis when things have reached that state.

INNER DARKNESS

There is a "dark night of the soul" that often occurs with any healing transformation that moves us forward and upward. For people of a syphilitic nature, this "dark night" takes on a special dimension. The scary things out there are seen as a reflection of the really scary dark places they are recognizing within themselves. Syphilis is in so many ways associated with darkness, night, destruction, and loss of control. Remedies with the deepest, darkest pits of despair in their descriptions are among the common syphilitic remedies. These include, of course, the snake remedies.

BONES AND TEETH

Syphilinum people frequently have bone pains, especially in the long bones of the legs and arms and in the cranial bones. These pains are aggravated at night and often show up as growing pains in children.

Structural birth defects such as the deformity of organs, teeth, and bones, or missing organs or teeth, cleft palate, or distortions of symmetry in the skull are all indications of the syphilis miasm.

CHRONIC DISEASES/ADDICTIONS

This nosode is used frequently as an intercurrent remedy in the course of treatment in many chronic diseases, including ones with paralysis. Syphilinum should also be considered whenever there is a hereditary tendency to alcoholism or other addictions.

Pain that becomes more severe or only manifests during the night, and great fatigue, headache and debility in the morning are indications of this remedy. Sleeplessness and mental/physical exhaustion on waking, excruciating headaches (often in the morning on waking) are definite indicators for this remedy and of the syphilis miasm.

MODALITIES

An unusual and I think, terrifyingly sad modality of the Syphilinum remedy and of this miasm is that things—including the mental and emotional depression—are worse from 3 a.m. to 4 a.m. and worse still from sunrise to sunset. This doesn't leave much time for happiness and creates a particular propensity for insomnia. The person develops a real hatred for lying in bed, caught up in depressed thoughts but unable to go to sleep.

SUPPRESSION

Occasionally, treatment with Syphilinum for a headache or other symptom will bring rapid and miraculous improvement and then be followed by an outbreak of sickly, yellow eczema with a red, angry, oozing base. This outbreak will be hard to cure and a continued program of Syphilinum itself has proven to be the best cure. This is rare and is almost always found only in people who have treated a venereal disease (personally and not generational/inherited) with current allopathic medications.

FLOWER ESSENCE REMEDIES FOR SYPHILIS MIASM

BLACK COHOSH *Cimicifuga racemosa (white)   North American*

Positive qualities: Ability to act from a place of courage and clarity in threatening situations or abusive relationships; confronting situations properly rather than retreating or behaving destructively; magnetic and charismatic personality; spiritual life is intense and beautiful

Patterns of imbalance: Caught in relationships and lifestyles which are abusive; addictive tendencies; violent; brooding; giving in to dark emotions; gloom; inability to find clarity and make choices; repeating patterns of seeking relationships with destructive or violent people.

CHERRY PLUM *Prunus cerasifera (white)   English*

Positive qualities: The ability to trust the guidance of the Spirit; feeling both guided and protected by God and unseen beings of light; balance and peace even when under extreme stress.

Patterns of imbalance: Fear of losing control of emotions/mental state; mental and emotional breakdown; destructive impulses based on desperation; fear of becoming erratic, destructive, suicidal or insane.

Dr. Bach's category: For Those Who Have Fear.

CRAB APPLE *Malus sylvestris (white, tinged with pink) English*

Positive qualities: Learning from suffering and imperfection; patience with self and others; balance and clear choices between physical passions and spiritual quests.

Patterns of imbalance: Feeling unclean or unworthy; obsessed with imperfection; unwilling to accept that things in this world are less than perfect; disgust or shame for the physical body; guilt at small or even just perceived imperfections

Dr. Bach's category: For Despondency and Despair.

FIREWEED *Epilobium angustifolium (pink) Range of Light*

Positive qualities: This remedy is useful for restoring balance to the fire (#5 and #6) meridians; ability to recover energy and health rapidly after illness or stress; natural fire and energy; ability to envision the future, see projects in the mind, then carry them to completion.

Patterns of imbalance: Emotional pain and physical depletion following adversity or events that have disrupted one's normal lifestyle; emotional wounding; erratic behavior, and irrationality—often due to events related to fire, heat, light, and technology; severe depression.

GLOSSY HYACINTH *Triteleia lilacina (white) Range of Light*

Positive qualities: The ability to transform darkness into light, negative to positive, confusion into understanding; a remedy to assist as one is moving into understanding and peace following a stressful event or relationship meltdown; recovery and emergence into the light following a "dark night of the soul"; finding the necessary strength and courage to "hang in there" and not give in to despair.

Patterns of imbalance: Profoundly upset by trauma, sorrow, and emotional pain; trauma as the result of coming face-to-face with evil or betrayal; inability to gain perspective or move on from emotional pain or deep emotional wounding

GORSE *Ulex europaeus (golden yellow) English*

Positive qualities: Deep and abiding faith; hope for a better day; joyful acceptance of life as it is; contagious optimism spreading light and joy to others; composure; evenness of temper; inner light; spiritual insight.

Patterns of imbalance: Pessimism; discouragement; darkness; hopelessness; resignation; unable to even imagine or have faith in a happy and positive outcome for the future of current events and circumstances; physical ailments as a result of the persistent feelings of despair.

Dr. Bach's category: For Those Who Suffer Uncertainty.

GREEN ROSE *Rosa chinensis viridiflora (white, tinged with green) Range of Light*

Positive Qualities: Compassion and connection to all living beings; ability to love in such a way that your love engenders trust and feels like a warm embrace to those around you.

Patterns of Imbalance: Fear, mistrust, and defensiveness; fear of being attacked or harmed or even completely destroyed; putting up barriers and heart walls between yourself and others; an uncanny ability to bring those around you into a belief in your fearful perceptions.

JOSHUA TREE *Yucca brevifolia (white) Range of Light*

Positive Qualities: Insight and compassion for family, culture, and country of one's birth; conscious striving for the betterment and unity of the family; ability to change negative family patterns and grow away from cultural conditioning (while remaining compassionate and peaceful)

Patterns of Imbalance: Inability to break free of family or cultural patterns of dysfunction, such as alcoholism, addiction, depression, violence, or hereditary illnesses; loss of individual identity and freedom; lack of insight and understanding of family patterns and cultural influences that are contributing to physical illness and emotional pain.

MUSTARD *Sinapis arvensis (yellow) English*

Positive qualities: Ability to claim darkness and trauma as a transformative, growing experience; light in the soul and in the countenance; able to find joy in life as it is in the here and now; able to find peace, understanding, and acceptance of negative incidences from the past; simple and gentle joyfulness.

Patterns of imbalance: Melancholy; deep gloom; despair; depression tied to deeply repressed, unseen, misunderstood parts of the past; manic-depressive mood swings.

Dr. Bach's category: Not Sufficient Interest in Present Circumstances.

POISON OAK *Toxicodendron diversiloba* (greenish white) North American

Positive qualities: Emotional openness and vulnerability; ability to be close emotionally with others; understanding that sensitive and gentle aspects of one's personality are wonderful strengths.

Patterns of imbalance: Fear of any intimate contact; over-protective of personal boundaries; fear of being violated; hostile or distant towards others; need to "get them before they get you."

ROCK ROSE *Helianthemum nummularium* (yellow) English

Positive qualities: Courage, inner peace and tranquility when facing great challenges; able to take control.

Patterns of imbalance: deep fear, terror, panic; fear of death; use for any extreme of fear, pain, grief or loneliness (Rock Rose is a vital ingredient in the "Five Flower Formula"—Rescue Remedy.)

Dr. Bach's category: For Those Who Have Fear.

SWEET CHESTNUT *Castanea sativa* (green with yellow) English

Positive qualities: Deep courage and faith which comes from knowing and trusting the spiritual world and one's ability to communicate with it.

Patterns of imbalance: Strong despair and anguish; experiencing the "dark night of the soul"; seemingly unable to summon sufficient inner strength to survive.

Dr. Bach's category: For Despondency and Despair.

YERBA SANTA *Eriodictyon californicum* (violet) North American

Positive qualities: Emotions that flow freely from one set of circumstances to another; breathing unrestricted by emotions; able to express a full range of human emotion, especially pain and sadness

Patterns of imbalance: Constriction of feelings and emotions, held particularly in the chest; internalized grief; repressed emotions contributing to physical illnesses.

UNDERSTANDING THE SYPHILITIC PERSONALITY

Asking ourselves (and our clients) questions such as how deep is the depression? Where in our lives or relationships is the tendency to destroy rather than to repair showing itself? Is there violence underlying my behavior and how is it manifesting itself? Am I showing any of the same self-destructive or relationship-destructive patterns that I saw in my parents or grandparents or their siblings? Where in my life has the refining fire of trials and adversity brought about positive changes in me?

Tuberculosis Miasm/Tuberculinum Bovinum Nosode
Dissatisfaction and Aspiration

PHYSICAL IDENTIFICATION

Of all the miasms, the tuberculosis one is the easiest to identify physically, at least. When the tubercular miasm *is an inherited pattern,* the person is usually thin with a narrow chest. They are often extremely thin in spite of eating quite heavily. They often say that they feel totally empty inside they are so hungry. An assortment of food allergies is also common. An allergy to milk is often seen. The face usually has small regular features and the hair is soft and the eyelashes long. The skin is usually fine, clear, and sometimes nearly translucent in appearance.

The above description does not seem to hold true if the miasm was first seen later in life and *was the result of repeated TB patch tests.* In that case, the characteristic thin build and narrow chest, as well as the other physical characteristics may be missing altogether. The person with an acquired tubercular miasm may be of any physical type.

POSITIVE ATTRIBUTES

Literature contains many positive descriptions of the tubercular state. I believe this is because, more than any other miasm, the tubercular energy is one of aspiration and change. This emphasis on improvement has led to a recording of what and where the improvements have taken place—a list of the positive characteristics of this miasm. I wish that we could find (or come to understand on our own) more of the positive attributes of the other miasms.

THE BREATH AND ENERGY MODALITIES

Many spiritual and energy healing traditions emphasize the importance of the breath. They believe that life energy is carried through the breath and that we breathe in new ideas and release negative patterns as we breathe out again.

RESPIRATORY

Since tuberculosis has many symptoms in the respiratory tract, Tuberculinum is outstanding among the respiratory remedies. This remedy should be used when there is a tendency for recurring head colds, constant nasal dripping, recurring bronchitis or pneumonia, or any acute respiratory infection where there is a history of tuberculosis or asthma in the family. Colds from the slightest draft, colds that lodge in the chest, and a persistent, hacking cough that lasts all winter with thick, yellow mucus might be treated effectively with Tuberculinum bovinum.

Any type of problem with restricted breathing or constriction of the throat may reflect a struggle with self-expression or suppressed creativity. Thyroid problems, both hypo- and hyper-activity are often seen.

As with all nosodes, Tuberculinum can be used as a preventative for many types of respiratory infections. Anyone with a tendency to pleurisy, pneumonia, bronchitis, winter asthma, or other chest infections may take Tuberculinum—usually in a low potency—as a preventative in the late fall. Clark writes, "I have found Tuberculinum 30C, 200C, and 1M (given in close succession) the best general antidote for influenza."

LONGING/DISSATISFACTION/RESTLESSNESS

Tuberculinum energy includes a sense that things could be improved, that something essential is missing, or that there must be something more to life than what is being experienced. There is a part of the tubercular miasm person that is never satisfied with things as they are or with being where they are. They are dissatisfied with who they are and what they are doing. This can be a negative trait or it can be the catalyst for growth.

There is a feeling of longing for something that is never quite satisfied because the person is looking outside themselves for solutions and happiness rather than building or relying on strength from within.

There seems to be a deep longing for home, homesickness—not just for their earthly home and family but for the heavenly home they left behind to come here and participate in this mortal experience. This longing for something lost or something better often manifests as a great internal restlessness. This is seen in the person not wanting to be tied down to a job, a place, or any confining situation. Tubercular types often feel a need to travel and travel and travel. If they can't travel about in person they must mentally travel by studying new things and reading about new places almost constantly.

I have seen the exact opposite of this reaction in a tubercular case, believed to have been triggered by continual TB screenings. An interesting note in this case was that the person had been moved frequently as a child and as an adolescent. Throughout his life he often indicated that he had put his roots down deep and never intended to move again. Traveling was sometimes undertaken, but only to visit his siblings or his children—yet another way of returning home or bringing home (his children) closer to him. The inherited characteristics of slender build with a hollow chest did not apply with this man. The symptoms listed above fit easily into Rajan Sankaran's sensation/reaction theory which will be discussed in a later chapter.

ROMANCE/IDEALISM

This longing for home and the seeking for perfection has manifested in the western world as an unhealthy version of romantic love. Falling in love with an ideal rather than the "real" person and then being dissatisfied with your choice or the life you are building together is a recipe for disappointment and disaster in relationships. *Ignatia amara*, *Natrum muriaticum*, and *Luna* are remedies suggested for this type of disappointment.

FREEDOM FROM RESTRICTION

The tubercular miasm always sows a drive for freedom with resistance to any restrictions. An infant with tubercular tendencies, when snuggled close to your chest, will inevitably arch his back away from you. If you wrap your arms tightly around these children, they will do their very best to break free.

Tubercular people feel like they are suffocating if their clothes are tight or restrictive in any way. As they get older they will feel like more and more things are restricting them. First it is being in school, and then it might be religious restrictions, then following house rules and, finally, living with parents or at home at all. Breaking through barriers and restrictions is a driving force of tubercular energy.

CHILDREN/BEHAVIORAL DISORDERS

Children caught in a tuberculosis miasm pattern often display behavioral disorders of very specific types. When confined to a room or situation such as exists at school or church, these children behave in ways that usually get them labeled as hyperactive. They often break other children's toys and do so in a malicious manner. Tuberculinum children can be obstinate or disobedient and may express compulsive or angry head banging. Adults may become fond of ritual and following the same pattern or way of doing things to the point of obsession.

GENERAL SYMPTOMS

Probably the most common symptom of the tuberculosis miasm is exhaustion. The exhaustion can be so total that it is difficult even to get out of bed in the morning. There is also a great sleepiness during the day, with a constant urge to catnap. However, at night the energy awakens, springing to life, and the person finds it difficult to go to bed at a reasonable hour or to obtain restful sleep when they do go to bed. Night is marked by nervousness, restlessness, and nightmares if they do try to sleep.

Tuberculosis is a very changeable miasm. One minute a person feels tired or even angry, and the next minute restless and ready to go somewhere, anywhere. This miasm is also marked by creativity, but the restlessness often leads to an inability to follow through with projects until they are completed.

If there are other symptoms of this miasm present, Tuberculinum is often helpful in cases of bedwetting, diarrhea in children, aching in the bones of the jaw, insomnia, nightmares, and night sweats.

COMBINED PSORA AND SYCOSIS

The tuberculosis miasm is generally recognized as a combination of psora and sycosis. It is helpful to think of its symptoms, modalities, and remedies in this way in order to prevent mistaking it for one or the other by looking at only a few symptoms. The whole picture, both sides of the coin, is needed for diagnosis. The nosode remedy, Phosphorus, is also considered a key remedy for the tubercular miasm.

When a person has been deeply troubled, depressed, violent, or suicidal, I love seeing any of the traits of tuberculosis. I consider it a stop, a way-station, on the way out of the destructiveness of deep syphilis. Many old-style, classical homeopaths consider syphilis almost untreatable. I disagree. But whenever I have seen improvement from really destructive tendencies and traits, the tubercular traits described above came into play for at least a time.

MERIDIAN/REALM/CHAKRA RELATIONSHIPS

The tubercular miasm is very much associated with the air element and with the central and governing meridians—those that run up the center of the body, front and back. The central meridian involves the throat chakra and the ability to express emotions and ideas freely. Sometimes this expression is not done with the voice, but through creative pursuits such as art, dancing, or music. The air element also has to do with travel, communication, and appreciation of nature and of beauty.

There is a symbiotic relationship between the creativity of the sacral chakra and the throat chakra. There are several homeopathic remedies that address suppressed creativity, particularly where the hormones or the genitalia are involved. Among these are Folliculinum, Lac caninum, and Lachesis.

VACCINATIONS

The Tuberculinum nosode remedy does not seem to work well for the person whose symptoms can be traced to repeated screenings for tuberculosis. Thuja or Syphilinum have been recommended by homeopathic physicians for many years in the removal of this block. Once these remedies have been applied, Tuberculinum or another tubercular remedy often moves the case forward to an improved condition.

MODALITIES

The tuberculosis miasm has a strong affinity for the lungs and the air element. This is reflected in the fact that the lung symptoms, and many other symptoms, are better for high mountain air and made much worse when in a confined space or a closed room. Many tubercular symptoms are also worse on first waking.

I have used the words *tubercular* and *Tuberculinum* here; neither is referring to the actual disease.

FLOWER ESSENCES REMEDIES FOT THE SYPHILIS MIASM

BEECH *Fagus sylvatica (red) English*

Positive qualities: A high degree of tolerance with an ability to accept others as they are; ability to understand other people, seeing the good and nurturing them with patience, praise, and kindness.

Patterns of imbalance: Intolerance; judgmental attitudes; critical of others; over-reactive to perceived insults that causes them to react with violent or destructive behaviors.

Dr. Edward Bach placed honeysuckle in the category of Over-Care for the Welfare of Others. It is, of course, possible for care for others to have the negative connotations of manipulation, control, and abuse.

Dr. Bach's category: Over-Care For the Welfare of Others.

BLEEDING HEART *Dicentra formosa (pink) North American*

Positive qualities: Ability to love others with an open heart; understanding that sometimes relationships complete and that loss is a part of life; emotional health and stability

Patterns of imbalance: Tend to become involved in abusive relationships and then stay in them based on feelings of fear; possessiveness or neediness because of one's own emotional co-dependency; pain and a broken heart because of the loss of a treasured loved one or the conflicts existing in a primary relationship.

HONEYSUCKLE *Lonicera caprifolium (red/white) English*

Positive qualities: Living fully in the present; able to acknowledge a longing for one's previous heavenly home and long for a return there, but able to build for the future right where one stands on this earth.

Patterns of imbalance: Nostalgia; homesickness; longing for life to return to how it used to be; unable to enjoy the present because all energy and conversation is concentrated on the past.

Dr. Bach's category: Not Sufficient Interest in Present Circumstances.

LEMON *Citrus limonum (white) Range of Light*

Positive qualities: Clarity of thought; ability to express oneself creatively while remaining aware of the need to live in the here and now; mental clarity coupled with imagination and artistic abilities.

Patterns of imbalance: Mental fatigue; inability to focus or to enjoy life as it is; dreaminess; learning disorders, including attention deficit; nervousness; dissatisfaction.

MADIA *Madia elegans (yellow with red spots) North American*

Positive qualities: Ability to focus on the project of the moment; precise thinking; intense productivity; living up to one's potential

Patterns of imbalance: Easily distracted; inability to concentrate; splintered focus that causes one to be unproductive and ineffective; learning disabilities

MOUNTIAN FORGET-ME-NOT *Hackelia micrantha (blue) Range of Light*

Positive qualities: A soul-deep remembrance of a Heavenly Home and the love of Heavenly Parents; deep spirituality and trust; clarity about the purpose of life and one's place in it; creative, joyful living.

Patterns of imbalance: Dissatisfaction with life and present circumstances; yearning constantly for something better—or, at the very least, something different; grief for the loss of "paradise."

SWEET PEA *Lathyrus latifolius (red-purple) North American*

Positive qualities: A deep commitment to family and community; a firm sense of one's place and role in family and community; ability to form mutually satisfying social and family roots.

Patterns of imbalance: A soul like that of a pilgrim—searching the world over for their place on earth; unable to form caring and committed social bonds; feeling dislocated; prone to frequent travel and moving himself and his family from place to place; feeling that they don't fit in—are "outsiders."

WILD OAT *Bromus ramosus* (green) *English*

Positive qualities: A clear sense of purpose and progression from the pre-existence through this life and on to the next; ability to find purposeful work that matches one's goals and direction in life; responding and living up to what one perceives as their true calling in life.

Patterns of imbalance: Confusion and indecision, especially about a job; trying many activities but chronically dissatisfied and unable to commit to a true vocation; lacking a sense of purpose and direction; working only for monetary gain at a job that lacks satisfaction to the soul.

Dr. Bach's category: For Those Who Suffer Uncertainty.

UNDERSTANDING THE TUBERCULAR PERSONALITY

Questions that we can ask of ourselves or others might include: Is the restlessness I feel and the need I have for perfection damaging my relationships or impeding my forward progress in life? Does my child's (or any child's) behavioral disorders have tubercular roots? Do these persistent lung and respiratory issues have tubercular roots?

Cancer Miasm/Carcinosin
Dissatisfaction and Loss of Self

Cancer has become very prevalent in our society. Statistics show an alarming rise in most types of cancers. The statistics are especially gruesome in the more industrialized nations. In spite of the billions of dollars spent on research each year and cancer centers springing up everywhere, survival statistics for cancer patients have not improved as dramatically as expected over the last 50 years.

COMBINATION PSORA-SYCOSIS-SYPHILIS

It has long been recognized in the healing professions that there are certain common personality and lifestyle traits among people who get cancer, especially among those who suffer repeated cancers. These commonalities are noted here.

The cancer miasm is a very contradictory picture, and that is the main support for the theory that the cancer miasm is a combination of the original three miasms—psora, sycosis, and syphilis. Psora traits are found in the cancer miasm picture, but in much less prominent display than the traits of the sycosis and syphilis miasms unless the cancer is one of the varieties that affect the skin.

It is quite easy to see in the symptom picture of cancer, bits and pieces of the descriptions of all of the original three miasms. That the cancer miasm is a combination of the other three seems obvious. What is not so obvious is why these miasms combine so readily in our day, although the speculation that vaccines, drugs, and chemical pollution of our environment and ourselves enable this combining makes a great deal of sense to me.

INTERNALIZATION

When Woody Allen said, "One of my problems is that I internalize everything. I can't express anger; I just grow a tumor instead," he was describing one important aspect of the cancer miasm's emotional patterns.

The remedy, Conium maculatum, is a key remedy for cancerous conditions and represents the process of internalization and suppression of feelings which can result in an emotional hardness that leads to the growth of hard masses of cancerous tissue.

INDIVIDUAL IDENTITY

People who fit the general description of the cancer miasm, and match the picture of Carcinosin, typically have a poor sense of self. They are dependent on the opinions of others, changing their minds about simple things each time someone else expresses an opinion. They sometimes, when under pressure, display the opposite pole of this trait, becoming for a short time very sure of themselves and of their stand on an issue. It will do no good to argue with them at these times; they are absolutely clear. There is usually no need to argue with them because in this state of mind they have very clear perceptions and very good judgment.

Besides opinions, the cancer miasm personality has a tendency to closely identify with the crowd in which they are living at the moment, taking on the issues and identity of the group until there is little of themselves left. "What will the neighbors think?" is very important to them but because different neighbors think very differently, their own personalities can become a hodge-podge of symptoms that seems to match many different remedies at the same time.

The homeopathic remedy, Carcinosin, at first glance, looks like many other remedies all mixed together, too, making it useful for the symptoms discussed in the previous paragraph. Carcinosin is often indicated when two or three or four polycrest remedies all seem equally well-indicated. This can be considered a keynote of this remedy and when a dose of Carcinosin has been given, the person will often begin to show a clear picture of only one remedy.

Usually, in this case, Carcinosin should be given intercurrently with the now clearly indicated remedy. This is a very positive sign of progress. The new personality may not be pleasant to live with at this point, however. There may be anger or resentment surfacing, but at least the emotions are genuine and they are being expressed openly. One practitioner claims that he takes it as a positive sign when his client complains to him that they are simply unable to keep up the appearance of being nice to everyone.

SUPPRESSION/CONFORMITY
Emotional suppression, mentioned earlier, is not the only kind of suppression displayed by the cancer miasm. While only expressing opinions and emotions that you think others will find acceptable is a big part of the picture, the suppression seems to extend into every aspect of individuality. It is a matter of spending one's life trying very hard to be something one is not.

Far too many cancer patients have very definite ideas about what is the best mode of treatment for themselves but, when it comes down to committing to a treatment pattern, they will say, "I will be doing chemotherapy and surgery. My husband or wife would worry too much if I didn't." Then they will follow through with the treatment that they think will worry their spouse the least. When fighting cancer, a person cannot afford to conform and comply rather than listen to the whisperings of the Spirit. Whatever the choice of treatment, statistics indicate that the survival rate goes way up for those who have confidence in the treatment they are receiving.

SELF-ESTEEM
Somehow, in some way, some people pick up the idea from statements in scripture that to be humble means to put yourself down, almost to the point of abuse. This "false humility," besides damaging our own psyche, invites others to treat us as though we are of little value. If we learn to love/respect ourselves in the same way that we love/respect others, we are much more balanced and, in my opinion, closer to living the scriptures. A healthy respect for oneself "fills your own well" and gives you energy to then share with others.

The self-esteem issues of the cancer miasm are deeply connected to relationships with others, even more so than to job performance, intelligence, or good looks, for example. When a person is battling cancer they are often forced to break a lifelong habit of putting everyone else's needs before their own. They may, for the first time in their lives, need to allow others to take care of them, at least for a time. Perhaps, how well they learn this life lesson has an impact on the final outcome and on future bouts with cancer.

SAYING NO
One trait of cancer personalities that the remedy, Carcinosin, or some other cancer remedy usually changes is the inability of the person to say "no" to requests that are made of them. The typical cancer miasm personality usually tries to do everything for everybody, taking little or no thought or time for themselves.

SELF-ESTEEM/RELATIONSHIPS
Emotionally, when the cancer miasm is present, there is an almost pathological need to take care of everyone and everything except themselves. A cancer personality person is often compulsive about projects and housework. Everything must be finished on time and to the absolute best of their ability. Often, there is a dark side of hopelessness, with anxiety growing into fear, about one's health. This miasm often manifests as the result of abuse, or prolonged stress and fear. Insomnia and interrupted sleep patterns are common.

TAKING RESPONSIBILITY

Successfully working our way through the cancer miasm usually involves learning to take responsibility for our own lives and leave others to take responsibility for their lives. Part of this miasm's picture is a tendency to blame other people—usually the ones we are taking care of—instead of dealing with our own problems. The cancer miasm is a classic example of the victim or martyr mentality. Unfortunately, victims and martyrs tend to pick one or more of their children to pass this pattern of 'serving others at the expense of themselves' on to. Cancer—the disease itself—and the miasm tend to run in families and follow the person who adopts the cancer miasm attitude of their cancer prone parent.

I am not talking about giving up serving others. Service is essential both to the society and to the soul. But service must be done joyfully from a heart full of gratitude and compassion, not grudgingly out of duty or obligation or a need to feel worthy and accepted by others.

INDICATIONS/KEYNOTES

The cancer miasm symptom picture has a special craving for ice cream and chocolate, but both upset the digestive tract producing stomach, bowel, or kidney problems. The cancer miasm is also indicated by poverty consciousness. The feeling is that there is never enough money to meet their needs no matter how much money they have and there is certainly not any extra money to share. The removal of this miasm brings about the most remarkable change in this particular attitude.

Some other interesting keynote symptoms of this remedy are the person's love of dancing, enjoyment and excitement from thunderstorms, and marked improvement from taking short naps.

The confusion of words, or a struggle to remember a word, is another keynote of this miasm. Repeated small strokes and mental confusion are also seen. Cancer miasm people tend to swollen lymph glands, pneumonia, severe acute diseases, diabetes, pernicious anemia, cysts and tumors, panic attacks, and mononucleosis. If any of this seems familiar to you (as it does to me and many members of my family too much of the time) treatment, whenever the symptoms present themselves, would be well advised. Used in this way, the nosode is acting as a preventative remedy, a prophylactic, which is discussed below.

Carcinosin is often indicated when there is a strong family history of diabetes, hypo- or hyperglycemia, tuberculosis, or where there was a severe case of pneumonia or whooping cough early in life. Chronic insomnia, chronic fatigue, mononucleosis, anemia, brittle bones, and inflammation or arthritis are symptoms that would lead to the consideration of Carcinocinum.

Multiple allergies are also associated with the cancer miasm. Allergies that change, with something one used to be allergic to presenting no problem this season but other allergies coming into being with a vengeance, is a keynote of this miasm.

MERIDIAN/REALM/CHAKRA RELATIONSHIPS

The most outstanding affinity of the cancer miasm lies with the blood and the immune system. The function of the immune system is to create a semi-permeable barrier between oneself and others, to distinguish between what is really you and what is an outside invasion, and to detect friends from foes. With the cancer miasm, this ability to distinguish self from others has broken down.

The triple warmer and spleen meridians also play a great role in the cancer miasm and they are usually out of balance in the months or years before cancer or other diseases of this miasm strike. When these meridians are out of balance in childhood—and the cancer miasm just beginning to show itself—there is often a history of especially severe or even repeated bouts with childhood diseases such as chicken pox. The child will have a history of sudden, recurring, high fevers of unknown origin, usually with swollen lymph glands.

In adults, wounds that are slow to heal and slow recovery and slow convalescence from disease are an indication of this miasm. There are almost always deep emotional wounds as well; wounds from which the person has not been able to recover or put behind them. Deep grief, sadness, guilt, or anger are always found somewhere in the remedy picture of cancer miasm remedies.

CAUSES/LINKS
Sexual and physical abuse, prolonged time spent in an abusive relationship, prolonged fear, and prolonged unhappiness are considered to be precursors to the emergence of the cancer miasm in many cases.

Carcinosin, along with Psorinum, should be considered whenever a well selected remedy fails to act or the improvement being experienced does not hold for as long as should be expected. These two remedies should also be considered whenever the symptom picture is constantly changing. The need to chase ever-changing symptoms using different remedies is an indication of weak constitutional vitality and that the presence of the psora miasm is underlying everything else that is going on. The intercession of a major nosode can correct the generationally inherited flaw and allow the indicated constitutional remedy to work more effectively.

PROPHYLAXIS
Carcinosin is also used to prevent the return of cancer in a person who is in remission from a previous bout with some form of cancer. When Carcinosin is used in this way, or is used in an attempt to combat cancer, it is always recommended that it be used alternately (intercurrently) with a remedy specific to the organ, or organs, involved with the cancer. This is also true of the other nosodes and the diseases they are used to treat. This method was pioneered by Dr. A.U. Ramakrishnan and proved so successful that it has become a standard treatment modality around the world.

If there is a history of cancer on one or both sides of a person's family tree—and who of us can say that there is not?—there may exist a predisposition to the emergence of the cancer *miasm* when we are under a lot of stress. This does not necessarily mean that there is a predisposition to cancer or that we will get cancer just because our life is particularly stressful. This miasm manifests in many ways, with most of them being unpleasant even though they are not cancer itself. Carcinosin is a polycrest remedy for a great many debilitating chronic diseases.

VACCINOSIS
Carcinosin is one of the leading remedies in the treatment of unpleasant reactions to vaccination, and while not the leading polycrest remedy, has often been useful in the treatment of some aspects of a vaccinosis miasm. Carcinosin, more than any other remedy, encompasses the symptoms of many other remedies at the same time.

CANCER—THE DISEASE
The lack of boundaries between what is self and what is rogue is the definition of cancer as a disease and the cancer miasm as a whole. When cells become "cancerous" they either begin to replicate uncontrollably (doing too much for those around them) and/or they start to invade neighboring tissues (taking undue responsibility for others around them). They may even metastasize to a different location altogether (taking care of the whole world at the expense of self).

The common theme is an aggressive self-assertion of an individual group of cells. Perhaps this is a correlation with cancer miasm emotions such as trying to do too much for others without being able to determine their own needs and what is really in their own best interest.

HEALERS AND VULNERABILITY
People working in the healing professions are at particular risk for the development of this miasm. We must learn to be open and compassionate with our clients while maintaining boundaries We must not identify too closely with their problems and, certainly, not take them on as our own! We must always recognize when we have, ourselves, become the wounded healers who are struggling on a deep level with many of the same issues as our clients. "Physician, heal thyself" is good advice for anyone working in a healers capacity.

CANCER TO ALZHEIMERS
Arsenicum album and Nitric acidum more nearly correspond to the morbid anxiety that eats away at a person which is one aspect of the cancer miasm. The appearance of repeated cancers during the course of a lifetime is statistically connected to Alzheimer's at a later date. The confusion of the cancer miasm seems to slide into the Alzheimer's miasm all too often.

FLOWER ESSENCE REMEDIES FOR THE CANCER MIASM

CENTAURY *Centaurium erythraea (pink) English*

Positive qualities: Having sufficient inner strength and stability to serve others but with a healthy recognition of one's own needs; strength and purpose but able to say "No" when no is appropriate.

Patterns of imbalance: Life lived in response to the requests of others; servile; acting to please; difficulty saying "No," when no would be best for everybody; neglecting one's own needs to take care of others.

Dr. Bach's category: Over-Sensitive to Influences and Ideas.

CERATO *Ceratostigma willmottiana (blue) English*

Positive qualities: Able to trust what one knows by the Spirit; intuition; self-confidence; certainty; healthy respect for the opinions of others while keeping sight of their own principles and desires.

Patterns of imbalance: Uncertainty or doubt of one's own principles, desires, and like and dislikes; invalidating and apologizing for what one knows; over-dependent on the advice and opinions of others.

CHICORY *Cichorium intybus (blue) English*

Positive qualities: Love given freely and selflessly, but always respecting the freedom and individuality of their loved ones

Patterns of imbalance: Expressing 'love' by being possessive, demanding, and needy; getting attention through negative behavior; selfishness and self-centeredness.

Dr. Bach's category: Over-Care for the Welfare of Others.

GOLDENROD *Solidago californica (yellow) North American*

Positive qualities: Strong and secure sense of self; respect for own individuality and individuality of others.

Patterns of imbalance: Inability to be true to oneself and one's own values and opinions; easily susceptible to peer pressure or the demands, however unreasonable, of the group to which they long to belong.

JOSHUA TREE *Yucca brevifolia (white, tinged with a bit of pink) Range of Light*

Positive qualities: Ability to transform past unhealthy family patterns into patterns of selfless service while honoring each person's individuality and uniqueness; compassion for family members; insight

Patterns of imbalance: Inability to break free of family patterns of addiction, depression, violence, or hereditary illnesses; loss of individual identity and freedom due to lack of insight into the dysfunctional family patterns of the past.

MONKSHOOD *Aconitum columbianum (purple) Range of Light*

Positive qualities: Positive, courageous, and spiritually based leadership skills; ability to understand others.

Patterns of imbalance: Paralysis or denial of spiritual guidance due to prior traumas or satanic cult abuse.

PINE *Pinus sylvestris (reddish brown with yellow) English*

Positive qualities: Self-acceptance; self-forgiveness; freedom from inappropriate guilt and blame; ability to move forward, building on the lessons learned from past mistakes.

Patterns of imbalance: Guilt, self-blame; self-criticism; inability to accept one's value and contributions; paralyzed by fear of making the same mistakes as in the past.

RED CHESTNUT *Aesculus carnea (red) English*

Positive qualities: Caring for others with gentleness and calm; inner peace; trust in the future and the unfolding events of life

Patterns of imbalance: Obsessive fear and worry for the well-being of others; worry in anticipation of problems that may be coming for other people, especially loved ones.

Dr. Bach's category: For Those Who Have Fear.

ROCK WATER *Solarized spring water (clear and sparkling) English*

Positive qualities: Inner personal lives full of rich currents; spontaneous; in touch with their feelings.

Patterns of imbalance: An inability to enjoy life; adhering to hardened and rigid doctrines; setting standards that are too rigid for oneself; self-denial; too bound by every rule or regulation.

Rock Water is the only Bach flower remedy that is not made from a flower. It is made from the essence of an underground spring that is considered sacred. Natural forces of nature seem to be concentrated and consecrated for healing there.

Rock Water is sometimes useful for those beginning flower essence therapy but are unable to feel the energy and change being stimulated by the remedies. Rock Water opens the body and soul to experience the flowing, flowering qualities of life and of these remedies.

Dr. Bach's category: Over Care for the Welfare of Others.

SIERRA PRIMROSE *Primula suffrutescens* (pink) Range of Light

Positive qualities: Joyful service from the depths of the soul; physical vitality and enthusiasm; profound gratitude for life

Patterns of imbalance: Lack of gratitude or reverence for life; joyless service done while pushing through one's own depression and fatigue.

VERVAIN *Verbena officinalis* (pink/mauve) English

Positive qualities: Ability to inspire and lead others; strong, passionate idealism while respecting the thoughts and ideals of others; possessing the fiery light of testimony and spirituality which radiates from their person and from the eyes of their soul; ability to moderate these tendencies when necessary.

Patterns of imbalance: Incredible intensity which may over-ride and overwhelm the wishes and autonomy of others; pushing one's own body beyond its natural capacity; inner tension and intensity that sometimes results in nervous and digestive problems and even a nervous breakdown.

Dr. Bach's category: Over-Care for the Welfare of Others.

VINE *Vitis vinifera* (green) English

Positive qualities: Selfless service; tolerance for the individuality of others; a strong will with organizational and leadership abilities; selfless instead of selfish.

Patterns of imbalance: A tendency to be domineering and tyrannical; forcing one's will on others; compulsive need to be in control; a king who rules rather than a shepherd who guides.

Dr. Bach's category: Over-Care for the Welfare of Others.

UNDERSTANDING THE CANCER MIASM PERSONALITY

Questions that we can ask of ourselves or others might include: Am I too willing to do for others what they could, and probably should, do for themselves at the expense of my own health and well-being? Am I a perfectionist, even about little things that don't really matter in the eternal scheme of things? Do I internalize emotional pain, rather than risk looking less than perfect to someone by expressing my emotions and needs? Is there a family inheritance of more than a few of the symptoms mentioned for this miasm?

Polio Miasm/Poliomyelitis Nosode
Emotional Fluctuations

PHYSICAL MANIFESTATIONS

The early physical symptoms of polio as a disease are reported to be trembling, clumsiness, fever with headache, and muscle pain, upper back and shoulder pain with stiffness in the neck and hands, stomach aches and pains, and constipation alternating with diarrhea. As the disease (and the miasm) worsen there is stiffness in the muscles so severe that it leads both to paralysis and painful contraction of muscles. In severe cases, muscular atrophy is seen.

OTHER SYMPTOMS

Other physical symptoms include sinus congestion, weakness in the lungs and respiratory tract, frequent ear infections in children, shortness of breath, itching, eruptions on the skin, and a tendency to weight gain.

EMOTIONAL/MENTAL PATTERNS

This miasm includes short term memory loss, restlessness, and forgetfulness. Being intolerant of other people or feeling detached from them, feeling remote or aloof and unwilling to be in the company of others, anxiety, and irritability are also parts of the polio miasm picture. There is also little desire for food because of a putrid taste in the mouth.

EMOTIONAL FLUCTUATIONS

Emotionally, this miasm is one of wide fluctuations. The person feels fantastic one moment and then depressed and hopeless the next. This depression often centers around the perception that there is little chance for complete recovery and a return to normal living.

The emotional pattern of wild optimism followed by deep despair, when severe, becomes a form of manic depression. Both the manic phase and the depressive phase of the cycle include being accident prone, although the types of accidents experienced change within the motion patterns of each cycle. The manic-depressive cycles may play out every few hours or have a cycle pattern that is several days long. During the manic phase the person usually becomes very excited about future plans and projects, talking about them incessantly. As they slide into the depressive cycle, all enthusiasm, desire to work on the projects, and faith in themselves disappears entirely.

LINKS/TRIGGERS

The polio miasm has been tentatively linked to Parkinson's disease, Alzheimer's, cerebral palsy, Lou Gehrig's disease, autism, certain types of ADD, and some learning disabilities in which memory loss or inability to memorize are factors. For example, a person may spend hours studying for a test, feel that they have a good grasp of the facts and details only to have, under the stress of exam taking, much of what they had learned disappear from their memory. Other early indications may be forgetting where you put your purse or car keys, difficulty remembering phone numbers that you have always known well, or a newly developed tendency to daydream.

Possible triggers, according to the symptom pictures of the remedies that seem to be useful, are feelings of fear, sudden fright, after receiving bad news. The physical effects of Lymes disease closely mirror many aspects of the polio miasm.

MERIDIAN/REALM/CHAKRA RELATIONSHIPS

This miasm seems to involve the lung meridian and the solar plexus chakra. The digestive tract is always involved but this seems more a product of the paralysis than a problem in the meridians and chakras related to digestion. Paralysis and structural problems in the muscles and bones are usually associated with the realm of earth.

MODALITIES

The muscle contractions and paralysis of this miasm are relieved to an extent by the application of cool cloths and compresses. Symptoms are also made better by rainy weather but if the temperature turns off cold, the stiffness and contractions become worse. Cold drinks seem to decrease the head, throat, sinus, and stomach symptoms.

PROPHYLAXIS

In polio epidemics in the last century on-coming polio was too often mistaken for a summer cold. There are interesting statistics about the prophylactic (preventative) treatment of summer colds with anti-polio remedies such as Lathyrus sativus.

REMEDIES

Gelsemium sempervirens should be considered as an intercurrent remedy, as well as for the final stages of the disease and both the early and 'almost gone' stages of the polio miasm.

Other possible remedies are listed under Ringworm/Polio in the miasmic classification of remedies list.

FLOWER ESSENCES REMEDIES FOR THE POLIO MIASM

CALIFORNIA WILD ROSE Rosa californica (pink) North American

Positive qualities: Seeking to serve others, believing that doing so is one's own personal life calling or vocation; vibrant forces of the heart; enthusiasm for life, for daily tasks, and for human relationships.

Patterns of imbalance: Apathy as the true opposite of once loving feelings; inability to take emotional risks in relationships with others; anesthetizing themselves from the possibilities of pain and suffering; deep-seated social alienation.

California Wild Rose is among the most beautiful and fundamental of all flower remedies because it helps a person to take a firm hold on his own personal responsibilities and tasks on earth; walking one's own spiritual path.

CALIFORNIA VALERIAN *Valeriana capitata* (white) Range of Light

Positive qualities: Confidence for the future because of the soul's understanding of our premortal and post earth lives; tranquility and inner peace of soul and conscience.

Patterns of imbalance: Shallow breathing due to anxiety about the future; lack of faith; nervous agitation alternating with insomnia and disconnection.

CASSIOPE *Cassiope mertensiana* (white) Range of Light

Positive qualities: A warmth of soul that radiates into and out of the body through the solar plexus chakra; joy and appreciation for physical existence; warmth towards others as the source of personal well-being

Patterns of imbalance: Lack of appreciation for the spirituality which exists in the physical world and in each person; aloof or removed from nature, other people, and their own body.

LAVENDER *Lavandula officinalis* (violet) North American

Positive qualities: Spiritual sensitivity and highly refined awareness of others along with stable bodily health; highly receptive of spiritual forces; energy sensitive; awake and mentally active; able to use the highly sensitive spiritual and energetic abilities in sync with the physical body.

Patterns of imbalance: Depletion of physical forces; insomnia; so energy sensitive that they often absorb far more energy than can actually be processed through the body; high strung; wound up; headaches, vision problems, shoulder and neck tension.

MALLOW *Sidalcea glauscens* (pink-violet) North American

Positive qualities: Able to experience the warm glow that comes from loving exchanges with others; learning to trust the feelings of the heart.

Patterns of imbalance: Insecure in relationships; paralysis in reaching out to others, resulting in social barriers; heart walls; lack of trust in others and in one's ability to relate warmly to others.

NICOTIANA *Nicotiana alata* (white) North American

Positive qualities: Inner peace that is centered in the heart and heart chakra and in the lungs and lung chakra; physical and emotional well-being.

Patterns of imbalance: Rigidity of the body; blunted feelings; shallow breathing; numbing of the feelings; coping with pain or risk by numbing normal feelings.

PINK MONKEYFLOWER *Mimulus lewisii* (pink) North American

Positive qualities: The courage to take emotional risks with others; understanding that only by being open and vulnerable can one experience deeply the warmth of human love and affection.

Patterns of imbalance: Fear of exposure and rejection, usually due to prior abuse or trauma; hiding or masking themselves as a form of protection; highly sensitive; bearing deep pain within themselves.

VIOLET *Viola odorata* (violet-blue) NorthAmerican

Positive qualities: Spiritual perception; sensitivity; ability to trust the warmth, love, and acceptance of others

Patterns of imbalance: Feeling fragile in group situations; feeling a great deal of inner warmth, but appears cool and aloof to others—even the body and hands may lack circulation and warmth; great feeling of loneliness

Like the violet flower which only shares its fragrance when the sun shines upon it, people needing this remedy express their own warmth best when they have learned to trust the warmth that is being offered by others.

WATER VIOLET *Hottonia palustris* (pale mauve with a yellow center) North American

Positive qualities: Quiet and self-contained, with an ability to handle difficult situations with calm and gracefulness; soul qualities that set them apart as quiet, competent leaders.

Patterns of imbalance: Aloof; withdrawn; disdainful of others; proud; haughty; arrogant.

It is interesting to note that not one flower essence remedy listed for the polio miasm originates in England. This fact becomes even more worthy of contemplation when it is noted that although England experienced a 10-fold rise in polio cases during the 1940's and 1950's compared to the earlier years of that century, the number of polio cases in the United States (proportioned according to population) dwarfed those of England. The citizens of America, especially our children, were hit hardest by this epidemic. Why was that?

UNDERSTANDING THE POLIO MIASM PERSONALITY

Questions that we can ask of ourselves or others might include: Do I feel intolerant of or detached from the people around me? Am I either anxious or irritable a great deal of the time? Am I on an emotional "rollercoaster" ride, with wild optimism and enthusiasm followed by deep despair and discontent? Do I often begin projects with great enthusiasm and then slide into a depressive state, leaving the project unfinished?

AIDS Miasm/Aids Nosode
Self in Relationship to the Family and the World

BOUNDARIES

In Peter Fraser's theory of what brings a new miasm into the world, the electronic age is responsible for the sudden surge of the modern-day miasm referred to as the AIDS miasm. Fraser notes that with electronic devices and the World Wide Web, boundaries of time and place are being dissolved. Boundaries play a part in many of the symptoms of this miasm, but differently from the way boundaries play into the cancer miasm. Boundaries, as they play out in this miasm, produce very contradictory symptoms.

First, there is a lack of boundaries as communication is accomplished on a global scale but rarely face to face coupled with a need to knock down remaining boundaries in order to more fully join the cosmopolitan world. There is a need to knock down societal boundaries and norms contradicted by a need to build barriers between themselves and others, especially family members.

FEELING VULNERABLE

The dissolution of boundaries creates a feeling of vulnerability—people, relationships, and emotional attachments flowing into and out of their lives with no restrictions. They feel open and exposed to a violent world. There are often vague and disturbing memories of abuse and mistreatment. The flip side of this vulnerability is a great ability to communicate and connect with people in certain circumstances.

MOTHERING TROUBLED INDIVIDUALS

This is a very left-sided remedy, indicating an ascendancy of the female energies of multitasking and communication. This energy, though feminine, is very strong, even brittle and hard at times. In women, especially, this miasm includes a need to protect and mother those in trouble emotionally. This aspect sometimes leads the woman into danger and abuse and encourages her to stay in bad relationships past any kind of good sense as she tries to mother troubled individuals.

PARANOIA/SECRECY

With boundaries gone, there is a feeling of being continually watched by "big government" and judged by everybody else. There is privacy and secrecy—including the hiding of "dirty little secrets" that is part of the syphilis miasm from which AIDS springs. This secrecy plays against a desire to be known and recognized for who they really are—the feeling that they are separate and not understood by family. Estrangement from family brings feelings of isolation and despair. People caught in this miasm often feel that they have been mistreated and abandoned by those who should have loved them best.

SEPARATION

An early sign of this miasm is the need to be alone (or the desire to be left alone much of the time). This seems like a contradiction in one who feels separate and abandoned. One person, during a proving of *Plutonium* as a possible remedy for the AIDS miasm, explained it this way, "It is when I am in the company of others that the feeling of being separate from them becomes most apparent to me. I feel such a need to be alone with myself." In the early stages, AIDS miasm people crave the re-connection with self that comes from periods of time spent with only themselves for company.

The relationship issues of this miasm seem to center more around having a relationship with or an understanding of all—or at least as many as possible—other cultures around the world. This aspect of need often leads the person to travel widely and make friends from all cultural backgrounds and, in some cases, to learn to speak several languages.

LIMITS

This miasm seems to have a great deal of confusion as to what the physical body can do and can tolerate. There is a tendency to over-work, drug abuse, and radical diets. Positive aspects include an increased respect for the body on an energy level and a respect for cultures different from our own and for individuals who think and act differently from the way we do. There is an understanding (sometimes, finally) that we cannot mistreat our bodies without paying the consequences at some future time, probably very soon.

ENERGY SENSITIVITY

The vanishing of boundaries also leaves the individual open to the bombarding negative energies of others. As this unwanted energy builds up it often creates very severe headaches. Eventually, the person learns to build strong energetic barriers and to avoid those people who make them physically ill.

The establishment of these boundaries may be interpreted by others as the person being hard hearted with a lack of compassion, or it is interpreted as simple selfishness instead of the self-protection that it really is. Sometimes, to their discredit, they use this sensitivity to avoid serving and doing things for others that they probably should do. Whether they serve others or not, most AIDS miasm people have an incredible ability to get others to serve them and take projects and responsibilities off their shoulders.

Energy sensitive people, with their walls and boundaries, are often accused of not caring about the feelings and pains of others, even when they are contributing to that pain. They are often heard to say, as an excuse for hurting someone, that they "didn't feel comfortable" doing whatever it was they should have done.

CONFUSION

Confusion is another keynote of this miasm. This includes confusion about words, names, and about time in general. Communicating over the World Wide Web messes with our sense of time as the person we may be communicating with is experiencing a different time of day (or night) from our own. There is confusion about their place in the family and their position in the world. This confusion is often compensated for by competitiveness and a strong desire to succeed and be recognized by the world.

The confusion of identity with forgetfulness and ideas disappearing from the mind are symptomatic of a move toward the Alzheimer's miasm that is even more deeply destructive of self than is this miasm.

NEEDS VERSUS CONSEQUENCES

The emotional keynotes of the AIDS miasm include a lack of responsibility or a refusal to take responsibility for the consequences of one's own actions. There is an overriding attitude of living for today and not worrying about, or even being able to see, the connection between today's choices with tomorrow's happiness. This lack of responsibility sometimes includes a denial that such things as right and wrong exist. Their attitude is something similar to "Whatever a person does is OK" or "If you can get away with it and no one is seriously hurt by it, why should anyone care that you do it?" They often have a high degree of need to have their own wishes gratified and their desires met—and met right now!

This wanting it right now attitude is part of every phase of their lives. It certainly extends to their health care. Whatever remedy or procedure utilized is supposed to work instantly and with little effort on their part. They want life in the fast lane—faster computers, faster cars, faster food. There is often a craving for sweets and an addiction to sugar. (Is sugar addictive? "If you are addicted to it, then it is an addictive substance!")

The natural result of avoidance of responsibility is denial of reality and a pathological inability to see one's self and one's actions with clarity. Just as it is possible to present any face at all over social media, people caught in this miasm remake themselves and rewrite reality by retelling events in their minds, making themselves look better than their original behavior warranted and, usually, painting someone else as the villain. Usually they believe their own stories and nothing can ever convince them of the truth.

AIR ELEMENT

Music is an art form that floats on the air, knowing no boundaries, heard by and available to all. Music resembles the freedom of cyberspace and the electronic age. AIDS miasm individuals respond to music and usually display great talents and abilities in various areas of musical ability. One prover said, "In a black mood, any sort of music pulls me out of it!" Their high degree of sensitivity may also allow for their symptoms to be aggravated by music.

Of the four elements, air and water are the most free of boundaries. Many of the remedies for this miasm come from animals that live in the air or in the water. Any plant remedies that apply are plants that spread rapidly and prolifically. If you place a few leaves of Rhus toxicodendron (poison oak) in a jar with a tight lid overnight, the *air* in the bottle—there will be no need to touch the leaves—will make your skin rash up.

The air element is, of course, associated with the realm of the sky, especially in the sense of living free in the air, with information being passed through the air. People in this miasm often have a high degree of clairvoyance and psychic gifts and, when they seek for it, display an amazing connection with light and knowledge that is transmitted by the Spirit.

PHYSICAL SMYPTOMS

The physical symptoms of this miasm are many and varied. The keynotes, of course, center around the destruction of the immune system which allows the body to be ravaged by any and all diseases.

Other physical symptoms include flu and other non-specific infections, feelings of suffocation, asthma, feeling of the chest being crushed, glandular swellings which include swollen tonsils, a tendency to constant colds during the childhood years, and lymphatic congestion. The physical symptoms are composed of bits and pieces of both the cancer and tuberculosis miasms being combined in some new and unique ways.

CHILDHOOD PATTERNS

Some practitioners recommend treatment for this miasm early in the life of any child showing addictive behaviors, a need for the thrills and spills associated with speed, either over-concern for or a lack of a sense of responsibility and concern for other people, a high sensitivity to the energy fields of others, or the attitude of never being satisfied with what they have. An 'entitlement attitude' is often seen very early and is too often fostered by our society.

FLOWER ESSENCES REMEDIES FOR THE AIDS MIASM

CALIFORNIA POPPY *Eschschoizia californica (gold) North American*

Positive qualities: Spirituality that is light-filled and heart felt; living a life that aligns with personal values and principles; able to see one's actions and attitudes clearly; taking responsibility for one's actions; a yearning for quiet inner development and spirituality.

Patterns of imbalance: Pulled toward the "false light" of Satan's delusions; drawn to glamour and fame; seeking the limelight; making themselves look better than they deserve at the expense of others; failure to seek for truth and to strengthen their inner spiritual life.

CHRYSANTHEMUM *Chrysanthemum morifolium (red-brown) North American*

Positive qualities: The spiritual part of ourselves is immortal. The balanced state of chrysanthemum desires to be continually growing and moving forward spiritually.

Patterns of imbalance: Fear of aging and death; too much emphasis being placed on achieving fame and fortune; materialism; identity crisis such as a mid-life crisis or a life-threatening illness.

FAIRY LANTERN *Colochortus albus (white) North American*

Positive qualities: Acceptance of adult responsibilities; functioning as a capable adult but with the joy and spontaneity of a child; healthy maturation and aging processes—physically, mentally, and spiritually.

Patterns of imbalance: Clinging to the damaged "inner child"; dependence on parents or peers for a definition of who one is; needy; unconscious living with childlike attitudes throughout their adult lives.

IMPATIENS *Impatiens glandulifera (pink/mauve) English*

Positive qualities: Mentally brilliant; extremely capable; ability to slow down and experience the beauty and flow of life.

Patterns of imbalance: Tendency to rush ahead in life—leave for college early, date young; fiery life forces that flair up suddenly into irritation, impatience, intolerance, and anger; diseases and pre-mature aging due to burn out.

Dr. Bach's category: Loneliness

IRIS *Iris douglasiana (blue-violet) North American*

Positive qualities: Inspiration and inspired vision of the material world; artistic and vibrantly creative; in touch with the Spirit and inspiration; alive and intensely luminous with vitality and strength.

Patterns of imbalance: Lacking soul vitality; lacking inspiration or creativity; feeling weighed down by the drab ordinariness of the world; sitting as a spectator of life rather than a participant.

MUSTARD *Sinapis arvensis (yellow) English*

Positive qualities: Emotionally steady; ability to endure suffering and setbacks with joy, a positive attitude, and the ability to learn from the experiences of life; understanding and experiencing the dark times as a step in the process of growing toward perfection.

Patterns of imbalance: Overwhelmed by gloom and despair, particularly when called upon to endure hardship or pain; bouts of creativity bordering on mania followed by depression (bipolar); triggered into the depths of despair by a word, a look, or even a person casually encountered.

Dr. Bach's category: Not Sufficient Interest in Present Circumstances

PINK YARROW *Achillea millefolium var. rubra (pink-purple) North American*

Positive qualities: Able to discern and respond to others needs with love and compassion while not overly identifying or being affected by other people's energies; the maintaining of appropriate emotional boundaries and responses

Patterns of imbalance: Lack of emotional balance and clarity; dysfunctional empathy for others; taking on or being affected by the energy of others; loose and ill-defined emotional boundaries; one's own energy being exhausting or overwhelming to others.

PUSSY PAWS *Calyptridium umbellatum (pink) Range of Light*

Positive qualities: Openness to touch; touching others, physically and emotionally, with grace and gentleness; understanding that life and death are parts of life's experiences; able to comfort others in their times of grief

Patterns of imbalance: Fear of being touched; unable to allow their softer side to be seen or exposed to others; suffering emotional hardening of boundaries as the result of sexual abuse or violence

QUEEN ANNE'S LACE *Daucus carota (white) North American*

Positive qualities: Spiritual insight, vision, and inspiration; clear-seeing concerning issues and people, especially in relationships that are feeling stress or pain; perceptions of energy fields, either visually or through the other senses of the body and spirit.

Patterns of imbalance: Distortion of energetic perception or physical eyesight due to sexual or emotional imbalances; lack of harmony between the lower chakras and the higher chakras, including the "third eye" by which we see clearly the intentions of others.

SPREADING PHLOX *Phlox diffusa (deep pink) Range of Light*

Positive qualities: Able to accept the help of like-minded souls as they seek to discover their own personal path and calling in this life; ability to recognize and build on relationships that began before this life; moving comfortably into relationships that foster one's life purpose and destiny.

Patterns of imbalance: Caught up in meaningless social activities and social circles; inability to identify opportunities that connect to one's personal mission and life path.

SUNFLOWER *Helianthus annuus (yellow) North American*

Positive qualities: Unique individuality; soul forces and positive energy that radiate like the sun; strong solar plexus chakra; warm and loving compassion; truly able to bless and heal others through the Light that radiates from within themselves.

Patterns of imbalance: Distorted or constantly changing sense of self—simply unable to decide who they are or who they want to be; inflation of one's importance to others or feelings of worthlessness; low self-esteem or arrogance; poor relationship with their father; distortion of motives and actions of the men in their lives; lacking in the qualities of light that should illuminate the soul.

WILLOW *Salix vitellina (green) English*

Positive qualities: Acceptance of the past; forgiveness; taking responsibility for the decisions and actions one has taken (instead of blaming others); able to ride out the storms of life's changing fortunes and circumstances.

Patterns of imbalance: Feeling angry and resentful; inflexible; rigid; sometimes having inaccurate memories (as we all sometimes do) which have turned to anger and then bitterness; blaming others; behaving as though one were a victim and the only one to whom bad things have ever happened.

Dr. Bach's category: For Despondency and Despair.

UNDERSTANDING THE AIDS MIASM

Questions to ask ourselves or things to look for in our children might include: Is there a constant confusion between what I think really happened and what others around me observed? Are there tendencies toward addictive behaviors of any kind? Am I overly sensitive to the energy of others? Do I isolate myself or build walls to avoid the negative energy of others? Do my physical ailments reflect a compromise of my immune system?

Alzheimer's Miasm/Aluminum Oxydata (possibly)
Lost and Gone from the Here and Now

There are some in the homeopathic community who consider Alzheimer's an extension of the AIDS miasm. AIDS, in their view, would be the active, out-going, dynamic expression with Alzheimer's being the more passive, deeply internalized, version rather than being a miasm in its own right. Whichever is the case, a miasm in its own right or an expression of the AIDS miasm, Alzheimer's is so totally destructive of the individual's sense of self and is prevalent enough in our society at this time to warrant its own description here, in my opinion.

NOSODE/DISEASE AGENT

One of the criteria of miasmic status is that there be a clear nosode remedy available that has been made from the "disease agent" that causes the illness of the same name. No such nosode exists for Alzheimer's. If there is an infectious agent responsible for the destruction of the mind and memory, it has not yet been identified but there is a whole list of other possible causes for this malady.

A few of these possible causes include formaldehyde in glues used in new books and carpets, sugar substitutes, exposure to molds, and flukes or parasites in the brain. It is also known that an autopsy on the brains of people with Alzheimer's show higher levels of mercury making dental amalgams and other sources of mercury objects of suspicion.

Aluminum in cookware, foil, utensils, deodorants, and in water and juice packaged in aluminum foil is also suspected as being the cause of at least some cases of Alzheimer's. One thing is certain—the symptom picture of the homeopathic Aluminum oxydata matches very closely the symptoms of Alzheimer's and what we know of the miasm. Aluminum oxydata is a mineral remedy rather than a nosode.

GENETIC INHERITANCE

Another criterion of miasmic classification is having a genetic component, which Alzheimer's seems to have. If a first degree relative (parent or sibling) has Alzheimer's, you have a threefold risk of developing those symptoms yourself.

EARLY TREATMENT

It would be possible to describe Alzheimer's disease here and probably be quite close to the physical and emotional manifestations of the miasm in its later stages. That description would not, however, give us the mental and emotional symptoms that precede this miasm or exist in its earlier stages. It is believed by some homeopaths that the emotional patterns of the cancer miasm deteriorate into the dementia and complete loss of self that is Alzheimer's and the Alzheimer's miasm.

It is at the early emotional stages that miasmic treatment is the most effective at prevention, especially with something as deep and disturbing as the cancer, AIDS and Alzheimer's miasms. We all seem to experience some memory loss when we are under stress and as we age. Using the muscle test to identify remedies for ourselves, as needed, may assist us in treating the early stages of these miasms and diseases and aid us in preventing the manifestation of these conditions in our lives as we age.

The homeopathic remedy, Aluminum oxydata, is a slow-developing remedy; care should be taken not to give up on it too soon by moving on to another remedy without giving the Aluminum oxydata time to get the job done.

MENTAL/EMOTIONAL SYMPTOMS

There is not a lot of information available as yet about the emotional and mental symptoms of the Alzheimer's miasm by itself, although the symptoms of the disease are clearly identifiable. The various aluminum remedies, however, fit the physical and emotional symptoms of Alzheimer's very closely and it is probably a pretty good bet that the composite description of these remedies contains a good description of the mental and emotional patterns of this miasm.

Of particular note among these symptoms is alternating moods, sometimes happy but then followed by moroseness and depression. There is also a great deal of agitation and worry over trifles. These traits may have played only a small part in the person's personality in the years previous to the Alzheimer's diagnosis, but become more pronounced as the person ages or the miasm worsens.

CONNECTIONS TO OTHER MIASMS

There are some symptoms that are common to both this miasm and to the cancer miasm. One such symptom is a struggle to find the right word when speaking. The person hesitates, trying to remember a word that they have known perfectly well for years but is escaping their mind at the moment. Another symptom seen is that when asked a question, a person in the early stages of the Alzheimer's miasm, gives vague or inappropriate responses.

The perfectionism and concern for what others may be thinking of them causes a person in the early stages of the Alzheimer's miasm to go to great lengths to hide their forgetfulness from friends and family, often carrying off the deception (and keeping hope alive in their families) for years.

A strong family history of diabetes, hypo- or hyperglycemia, tuberculosis, or where there were severe cases of pneumonia or whooping cough early in life (just as with the cancer miasm) often precede the Alzheimer's miasm. Chronic insomnia, chronic fatigue, mononucleosis, anemia, brittle bones, and inflammation or arthritis are symptoms that are part of Alzheimer's, AIDS, and the cancer miasm.

CAUSES/LINKS

I am always alarmed at the appearance of these symptoms. These symptoms tell me that there is, quite possibly, a series of small strokes going on in the person's head and that they are possibly at risk for further strokes, yet another cancer (there has usually been one or two scares already), and—eventually—Alzheimer's. Statistically, these three aliments are very closely linked to one another.

MERIDIAN/REALM/CHAKRA RELATIONSHIPS

This miasm has an affinity for the heart meridian and the solar plexus chakra. The connected realm would have to be the realm of the sky. Alzheimer's patients have lost their connection to earthly reality and almost seem to have "gone from this world" already. The realm of the sky may not quite describe it. Perhaps, one should consider an additional realm, the realm of heaven, when considering Alzheimer's patients and the effects of this miasm.

FLOWER ESSENCES REMEDES FOR THE ALZHEIMER'S MIASM

QUAKING GRASS *Briza maxima* (green) *North American*

Positive qualities: Able to see one's place in the group, whether in the family, in the work place, in the community, or in a social contexts.

Patterns of imbalance: Dysfunctional and uncomfortable in group settings and social situations; inability to compromise when working with others.

REDBUD *Cercis occidentalis* (deep pink) *Range of Light*

Positive qualities: Acceptance of the natural cycles of life; aging gracefully; vitality as the result of making the best of each of the cycles of life.

Patterns of imbalance: Going to extreme lengths to preserve the physical youth and outward appearance of the face and body.

SHOOTING STAR *Dodecatheon hendersonii* *(violet/pink) North American*

Positive qualities: Feeling a connection with and a love for all of humanity and for the privilege of life on this earth; qualities of love, compassion, and understanding; a healthy and sharing heart.

Patterns of imbalance: Profound feelings of alienation; lack of participation with others and with life; may even have suffered birth trauma as they held back from experiencing the challenges that would come with life on this earth.

STAR OF BETHLEHEM *Ornithogalum umbellatum* *(white) English*

Positive qualities: Sense of one's place as a child of the Divine; exceptional recovery from deep shock or trauma; the ability to move beyond trauma, either current or from the past.

Patterns of imbalance: Lack of recovery from shock or trauma, either recent or from the past; a need for healing and comfort from the spiritual world but unfortunately linked to an inability to receive or accept the comfort of the Spirit

Dr. Bach's category: For Despondency or Despair.

UNDERSTANDING THE ALZHEIMER'S MIASM PERSONALITY

Understanding this miasm is not so much a matter of questions as of observing the person's life. Have they displayed symptoms of both the cancer miasm and the AIDS miasm? Do they tend to become agitated and overly concerned over trifles? Do they have a tendency to perfectionism? Do they believe themselves to be the victim of childhood abuse? Is there a tendency to forget common words when speaking?

Vaccinosis and Toxic Substances Miasm/Toxic Substances Nosodes
A Variety of Possible Nosodes Depending on the Cause

It is believed by some homeopaths (and certainly by me) that chemicals, drugs, environmental pollutants and other toxic substances not only have a very strong causative connection to cancer, AIDS, Alzheimer's, and polio-like patterns but that the presence of these toxic substances has allowed the original three miasms to combine in new ways, creating ever more destructive patterns.

CATEGORIZING TOXIC SUBSTANCE MIASMS

Some homeopathic practitioners place all *drugs, pollutants,* and *vaccination* related patterns under the category of what they refer to as the vaccinosis miasm. Others place only patterns that have been shown to be directly related to a *vaccination* under the title of vaccinosis. I tend to think of the vaccinosis miasm as any pattern created by a toxic or poisonous substance. In addition, a part of many vaccine reactions seems to be related to toxins in the vaccine rather than the original disease agent. It is hard to tell whether any miasmic pattern that develops as the result of a vaccination was brought about by the disease agent in the vaccine or by the other toxins that the vaccine contained.

There are simply too many toxic substances on this earth to start listing them as separate miasms—although I have seen some internet sites that are trying to do so. Theses sites are also trying hard to provide a nosode remedy for as many of the vaccines and toxic substances as possible. I salute them and their efforts!

Vaccinosis and toxic substance miasms are a very broad group of problems and the remedies that would match them would be an equally long list no matter how that list would be arranged. If we consider all the damage done to our bodies by chemicals of any sort as part of this miasm, we have a miasm that we cannot possibly ever completely categorize or understand. It is probable that the symptom picture is different for every single drug, vaccination, chemical, and toxin in our world.

It may also be impossible, or at least very daunting, to create a homeopathic nosode remedy from each toxic substance or to unravel the mystery of which remedy to apply in which situation. Even among vaccine reactions alone, there could only exist similarities in symptoms if the toxin causing the destruction is something common to all vaccines. It would not be reasonable to expect the same side effects from the smallpox vaccine as from the tuberculosis vaccine—unless the side effect is being caused by an additive or one of the immune suppressants that is common to more than one vaccine.

"Never the same since a particular vaccine or drug treatment" is a phrase which practitioners in all fields of alternative medicine hear too frequently and it may, when all the facts are in, turn out to be caused by a toxin or toxins common to many vaccines.

MATCHING SYMPTOMS TO A REMEDY PICTURE (HOMEOPATHY)

Bringing about improvement with homeopathy is **always** done by matching as many of the presenting symptoms as possible with the symptom picture of a particular remedy. When the chosen remedy has cleared all of the symptoms that it can, the situation is re-evaluated and another remedy is applied. If we had the proper nosode for every chemical and vaccine and could use it with the appropriate companion remedy, we could probably work through our symptoms quite efficiently. But all the while, in our modern environment, we will be coming across new poisons every day, resulting in the constant need for more treatment.

Even without a nosode for each toxic substance, patterns should be able to be cleared by matching the presenting symptoms to the picture of a remedy. It may be necessary to use two remedies—one being the best symptom match and the other being a flower essence—to completely remove the negative energetic patterns that have developed.

GENETIC ALTERATIONS

The burning question all over the world is, "Do drugs, vaccines, food additives, fertilizers, genetically altered foods, and poisoning by chemical and technological toxins create damage to the genome of the human body which is then passed down to future generations?" Alterations to the genetic code or to the inherited mental and emotional pattern is the definition of a miasm. I am afraid that the answer to the question is a resounding "yes." New miasms are being created with every new toxin that is developed.

The presence of these new—or combined—miasms certainly complicates things and has brought us to the state where we see new diseases with very severe symptoms that are extremely resistant to conventional treatment protocols. We also see a worsening of overall health. Cancer, arthritis, allergies, and asthma, to name just a few, are much more common and debilitating than they have ever been before.

IS THERE HOPE FOR A CURE?

Can we cure ourselves of our environmental, drug, and vaccine related diseases? I believe so. Since homeopathy is a method of treatment based on symptoms and the clearing of those symptoms to a deep, genetic level, I believe that it is possible. To some extent, maybe, the origin of the problem can be set aside. Herbal remedies, essential oils, and working directly with the energy systems of the body will also be essential.

I don't know if drug side effects can be totally eradicated by either herbal or homeopathic remedies, but the only course I see as maybe having even a chance of success would be to treat homeopathically according to the totality of the symptoms. Perhaps the gentle nudging of the immune system by continually treating homeopathically would eventually stimulate the vital force to throw off these poisons and their energetic effects. Liver cleansing herbs and clay foot soaks will also be helpful.

SUSCEPTIBILITY

It must be remembered that not everyone is affected equally by any destructive force. Susceptibility plays a large role in human illness and suffering. Building strong, healthy, resistant systems is even more crucial to good health in our day than it has been in the past. Perhaps susceptibility is also governed by the presence or absence of one of the original three miasms—psora, sycosis, and syphilis—just as Hahnemann and the early homeopathic pioneers believed.

VACCINES

Perhaps, with more research and understanding, it will be made clear exactly what effects vaccinations are having on us as a civilization and how they fit into the miasmic picture. Hahnemann actually supported the smallpox vaccine in his day. Of course, it was the only vaccine at the time and very little follow-up research had been done. Within a few years of his death, homeopaths everywhere were deploring the side effects of this and the other vaccines being introduced. Even Dr. Salk, creator of the polio vaccine, eventually turned against it.

Dr. Dorothy Shepherd, an orthodox physician in England who became a homeopathic physician, had some strong beliefs about the negative impact of vaccines.

MULTIPLE VACCINATIONS IN THE SAME SHOT

It was Dr. Shepherd's belief, based on her vast experience and observation, that when travelers or soldiers were forced to have multiple vaccinations against several diseases at or near the same time, the effect on the body and on the cells was much more devastating physically and mentally and much more confusing from a homeopathic viewpoint.

She found that when soldiers who had these multiple inoculations later developed influenza, it was generally a particularly virulent type and did not respond either to the usual conventional or homeopathic treatments. Interestingly, according to her reports, their flu responded to Pyrogenium (in high potency). Pyrogenium is recognized as a major remedy for the ill effects of vaccines and the vaccinosis miasm.

It was not common in Dr. Shepherd's day for anyone other than travelers or soldiers to be given multiple vaccinations at the same time. Today, babies are begun on a regimen of vaccinations, often including shots with multiple components, when only a few hours old. Worse yet, the immune systems of newborns are just developing. They do not have macrophage protection yet. Such immature immune systems are often just not ready to take on the injection into the body of possible disease entities with toxic stabilizers and immune suppressants included.

SCIENTIFIC RESEARCH

I would like to include here part of an article by Richard Moskovitz, an American homeopathic physician, who has researched the efficacy and impact of vaccinations. Moskovitz says,

"Vaccines have become sacraments of our faith in biotechnology in the sense that:

1) Their efficacy and safety are widely seen as self-evident and needing no further proof.
2) They are given automatically to everyone, even by force if necessary, in the name of the public good.
3) They ritually initiate our loyal participation in the medical enterprise as a whole.
4) They celebrate our right and power as a civilization to manipulate biological processes ad libitum (at one's pleasure) and for profit, without undue concern for or even any explicit concept of the total health of the populations about to be subjected to them."

NOSODES

Moskovitz recommends a nosode approach to dealing with vaccine reactions. A homeopathic preparation, made from the specific batch of the vaccine which triggered the reaction, is used along with an intercurrent remedy specific to the patient. This is sound advice from a homeopathic standpoint. The problem is in obtaining any of the vaccine to make your homeopathic remedy from if you are not a medical doctor. Parents trying to obtain the syringe used to inject their child are usually flatly turned down and sometimes questioned intensely about their motivation for such a request.

Moskovitz's advice is only for extreme reactions to the vaccination itself which occurs within a few hours of administration. An extreme reaction might justify heroic measure sto obtain some of the serum but by the time you work your way through the legal hassles, the exact offending serum might not be available. He does not address the long term health concerns nor any miasmatic connections that may still exist even without a severe and immediate reaction.

Remember, nosode remedies may be used by themselves if the entire symptom picture matches. The remedy would be used in the same way as a basic constitutional or acute remedy. When a nosode is used to combat a miasmic pattern, it must be matched and used intercurrently with an appropriate organ or ailment specific remedy.

IMMEDIATE VACCINE REACTIONS/NEVER THE SAME SINCE REACTIONS

Dealing with vaccines using the symptomatic approach of classical homeopathy has two categories that need our consideration. The first thing to treat for is the immediate reaction to the vaccine over the first day or two following the administration of the vaccine. There are some homeopathic remedies whose symptom picture is very similar to the more common reactions that children and adults have to vaccines.

The second concern is the ***never the same since*** the vaccination symptoms. These effects may be as many and as varied as there are batches of vaccine and people who get vaccinated. The answers to these problems lie in symptomatic, constitutional treatment over however long a period of time it takes to return to wellness.

One famous homeopath has this suggestion on his website. He recommends following constitutional treatment protocols to strengthen the body against the vaccines before submitting to them. This advice will be hard to follow before they vaccinate your baby in the hospital on the day it is born! The mother being in the best possible health, mentally and physically, will help but there may still be inherited predispositions unique to the new little individual.

BECOMING BULLET PROOF
For adults, working through your issues homeopathically is very good advice, but I would go one step further. Strengthen the body against everything (I call this becoming bullet proof) using homeopathy and *every other natural thing you can think of* every day of your life. In every epidemic there are people who work among the afflicted and never catch the disease themselves.

TO VACCINATE OR NOT TO VACCINATE—PERSONAL CHOICE
My personal belief is that a well person has more to fear from the vaccine than from a disease such as polio or smallpox which he has very little chance of exposure to (except through vaccination). A newborn baby has very little to fear from many, if not most, of the things it will be recommended that he be vaccinated for. He cannot make this choice for himself. The parents have an obligation to have done the research, and the praying, as they make this important choice for their children.

Remember, all vaccines come with built-in immune suppressant drugs.
Something as serious as deliberately suppressing your immune system needs thoughtful consideration.

VACCINOSIS REMEDIES
Below is a list of some of the more common vaccinosis remedies and brief, very general descriptions of their remedy pictures.

THUJA OCCIDENTALIS
Antibacterial action against the disease agent in the vaccination. Never well since an innoculation. Neuralgia, skin problems, abscesses, collapse and weakness, convulsions, lung congestion after vaccination. Thuja has been the #1 vaccination remedy for many years, but vaccines have changed and other remedies are often better for the newer vaccines.

MALANDRINUM
Modifies many of the side effects of vaccinations, especially the small pox vaccine. May prevent reactions if given immediately after vaccination.

Some symptoms include dry rough skin, beginning shortly after the vaccination and possibly remaining with the person for years. Other symptoms include headache, dizziness, confusion, lassitude following a vaccination.

MEZERUM
Eczema and itching eruptions appearing shortly after a vaccination. Mezerum affects skin, bones, nerves and mucus membranes of the mouth and stomach. The mind symptoms of Mezerum include forgetfulness and the vanishing of thoughts while speaking. The out-of-balance Mezerum personality is often quarrelsome and censorious, reproaching those around them and picking fights and quarrels.

SILICA TERRA - THJA OCCIDENTALIS - VACCININUM
Abscesses form and/or convulsions are experienced following a vaccination. Each remedy has its own unique symptoms other than the common ones listed above.

VACCININUM
Growth of scar tissue after vaccination. This scar tissue, over time, becomes keloids or ulcerated sores. Emotionally, there is restlessness and feelings of being tired all over. Mentally, the mind sometimes becomes confused, not remembering words or other things when the memory is needed.

APIS MELLIFICA
Sudden puffing up of the whole body after vaccination; burning, stinging sensations. These symptoms are usually accompanied by great anxiousness, restlessness, and fidgeting.

BELLADONNA
Fever with localized inflammation at the site of the vaccination. Glands may also become swollen, tender, inflamed, and bright red.

ANTIMONIUM TARTARICUM
Drowsiness and abdominal pain following a vaccination

SARSAPARILLA
Itchy eruptions on the skin, especially the face, following vaccinations. Despondent and gloomy without any apparent cause unrelated to the vaccination just experienced. Kidney disorders, including kidney stones. Sarsaparilla purifies the blood.

VARIOLINUM
Used as a preventative to side effects from the smallpox vaccine. Variolinum is also used to treat infections that sometimes occur at the site of a recent vaccination. Variolinum is also an excellent remedy for shingles.

Vaccinations - Statistics and Opinions

You have probably ascertained by now that I am very anti-vaccination. I have spent many years following the research on this controversy. I could write an entire book on vaccines and drug therapies, but an excellent job has already been done by many people. There are some books, articles, and facebook posts out there that are little more than rhetoric and opinion, but there are some excellently referenced and researched books also. Always check the facts and statistics presented to you—from both sides of this issue—and form your own opinions. Some people do not mind misrepresenting facts or fitting them to their prejudices.

STATISTICS AND THE PERTUSSIS VACCINE

I came across some interesting statistics about the pertussis vaccine recently. As is my custom, I confirmed those facts. I found confirmation in a couple of places, the most interesting being in the New England Journal of Medicine. (I love quoting the medical establishment when proving an herbal or homeopathic point of view!)

I will sum up this article, briefly, here. In 1993 there was an outbreak of pertussis in Cincinnati, Ohio, which had a population of 1.7 million people.

Statistics relevant to this outbreak: From 1979 to 1992, a period of 13 years, there had been a cumulative total of 542 cases of pertussis in Cincinnati. In 1993 (in just that one year) there were 352 cases.

Interesting facts: A vaccination campaign had commenced in the city, beginning in the fall of 1992. At the time of the outbreak, Cincinnati boasted an average of 69% of children 12 years old and younger that had been vaccinated—some of them 3 and 4 times. The national average at this time for vaccinated children was estimated at just under 30%. The vaccines came from 2 major manufacturers. When the investigations were over, it was determined that the vaccines were up to standard and made by acceptable methods.

The *New England Journal of Medicine* stated (This is copied from their report, verbatim):

> Conclusions: Since the 1993 pertussis epidemic in Cincinnati occurred primarily among children who had been appropriately immunized, it is clear that the whole-cell pertussis vaccine failed to give full protection against the disease.

There are many more studies and statistics and many good books written about nearly every vaccine ever produced. Later, in Section Four, we will talk about polio epidemics around the world and the efficacy and safety of polio vaccines.

SOME THINGS TO THINK ABOUT

There are many questions that come to mind when reading about this epidemic and other similar ones.

Some of them are:

Do vaccines really provide immunity? (Maybe, but the science supporting immunity is iffy, at best. In fact there are many studies and statistics that indicate that some cases of epidemic disease, including among them and leading statistically polio, got worse after immunization programs were put in place.)

Do vaccines, with their built-in immune suppressants, damage the immune response? (Absolutely. The research is clear. Statistically, getting a flu shot often increases your risk for getting a different type of flue within a couple of weeks.)

Do vaccines create any short-term or long-term health risks? (According to research and statistics, this is a resounding YES!)

Are children at more risk from the vaccine or from the disease for which they are being vaccinated, should they actually encounter it and then actually contract it? (Statistically, in the United States at this time, the vaccine presents both more risks and more side effects than the disease.)

What day-old baby needs protection in the form of a statistically dangerous vaccine for a disease he has a very low likelihood of encountering? (None)

Many diseases have been eradicated almost completely in America. Were vaccinations responsible for this? (Cases of polio had fallen off dramatically 2 full years before the Salk vaccine was marketable. This is only one example.)

Even if the vaccines did accomplish the eradication of the disease (which statistics do not support), are we paying too high a price in long-term poor health and side effects? (From what I have researched and seen, this gets a resounding YES vote from me.)

Most importantly—Is there a better way? (I have devoted a good portion of my life to finding answers to health questions and the answer to this one is, in my opinion, YES.)

Samuel Hahnemann's Concept of Drug Therapies

Samuel Hahneman, gave his opinion of drugs as healing agents in his book, <u>The Organon of Medicine and Chronic Diseases</u>. Much of this section is a summation of Dr. Hahnemann's theories. The rest is based upon my own research and the opinions I have formed because of what I have learned. It is interesting that with very little scientific research available to him, Hahnemann had a clear understanding of the side effects of drug treatments. I have placed Dr. Hahnemann's statements within quotation marks to eliminate confusion about who said what, but much of the rest of this section is a summation of what he believed and wrote.

DRUG SIDE EFFECTS OF DISEASES STATES

Hahnemann described drug side effects (remember he died in 1835) as *"the most tragic and most incurable of all the chronic diseases."* He said that *"when these diseases have gone beyond a certain point it is probably impossible ever to discover or imagine any means of curing them. In homeopathy benevolent providence has given us relief only for natural diseases."*

Because of the prevalence of allopathic drugs in our modern world, much of what we are treating for, and what has been given names as diseases, is nothing more than the negative side effects and energy disturbances created by the drugs the person has taken in their lifetime. Many drugs, especially the ones that treat mood disorders and learning disabilities, leave much of their original dosages intact in the body for many years. These drugs may re-enter the bloodstream under the right circumstances.

Dr. Hahnemann: *"No human means can ever repair those innumerable abnormalities so often produced by pernicious allopathic treatment. Their prolonged use always adds new disease conditions to old ones. "*

DRUGS AS A CURE

When a person takes a drug allopathically they often believe that the drug is meant to eradicate the disease entity. (Allopathically means the giving of a contrary or opposite rather than a similar as is done in classical homeopathic treatment.) Eradicating the disease in this way is impossible, according to Dr. Hahnemann, because the drug temporarily hides the symptoms from the vital force by presenting the opposite picture. This contradictory picture results in neither the disease state nor the foreign medicine being recognized by the vital force.

When the vital force acts it is often by means that produce discomfort—fever, diarrhea, vomiting, etc. In the presence of the drug, the body for a time, no longer recognizes that it has a problem. The result is that the vital force—the immune system—does not act against it and manifests no pain or discomfort. Let me re-emphasize. With no visible disease signal to act upon, the vital force does not activate against the disease.

The symptoms usually produced by the drugs are also hidden because they are in direct opposition to the disease itself. Energetically, the symptoms of the drug and the symptoms of the disease cancel each other out. This effectively hides the symptoms and the disease from the immune and energetic responses that should kick in to eradicate them both if they were occurring separately.

The medical world, and the patient, view this lack of discomfort as a cure but when you remove the medication you find you have left the original disease unchanged. It may even have worsened considerably because it has been left unchecked by the body's own defense mechanisms during the time in which the drug was confusing the immune system and the energy defenses of the body.

DRUG SIDE EFFECTS

Since the allopathic medication given is usually toxic and must be given in fairly large doses, a counter reaction from the vital force is initiated when the initial period of time has elapsed. The liver scoops up these poisons that were used as medications and takes them out of circulation in the body. This can only be done by linking these poisonous substances to harmless nutrients in order to pass them through the kidneys and intestines without damaging those vital organs. Drug side effects are often the symptoms of a deficiency of whatever vitamin or mineral was used up in the excretion of the drugs. It should always be remembered that there are no drugs without side effects.

NOXIOUS SUBSTANCES AND UNHEALTHY LIFESTYLES

According to Hahnemann, diseases brought about by prolonged, deliberate exposure to avoidable noxious substances should not be called chronic diseases. He included ailments brought about by:

- the habitual indulgence in harmful food or drink
- all kinds of excesses that undermine health
- prolonged deprivation of things necessary to life
- dwelling in unhealthy places such as cellars, damp workplaces, or closed quarters
- lack of exercise or fresh air
- physical or mental overexertion
- continuing emotional stress

These self-inflicted disturbances go away on their own with improved living conditions if no chronic miasm is present, and they should not and cannot be properly named *chronic diseases*. I am sure that many an alternative practitioner would be out of a job if these ailments were eliminated by improvement in lifestyle by the people they work with.

ALL DISEASES AFFECT THE ENTIRE ORGANISM

Hahnemann believed that if there were symptoms visible on the outside of a person they were inwardly sick as well. In his book <u>Chronic Diseases</u>, Hahnemann illustrated this principle with a story about rabies. He said,

"Among many persons bitten by a mad dog, only a few are infected; often . . . only one out of twenty or thirty persons bitten. The others even if ever so badly mangled by the mad dog usually all recover, even if they are not treated by a physician. But with whomsoever the poison acts, it has taken effect in the moment when the person was bitten and the poison has then communicated itself to the nearest nerves and therefore, without contradiction, to the whole system of the nerves, and as soon as the malady has developed in the whole organism (which requires several days if not weeks), the madness breaks out as an acute quickly fatal disease. Immediate amputation or excision of the infected part does not protect from the progression of the disease within. . . ."

The same is true of any acute disease. It is certainly true of contagious diseases such as measles and chicken pox. Hahnemann referred to them as "fixed or acute miasms." He believed that the person was ill from the time of exposure, not just from the time that the symptoms became manifest. This makes sense, of course, since many time and with many contagious diseases a person may expose others before they are displaying any symptoms themselves.

Chapter Fifteen - Miasms and Plant Remedies

Based on the Work of Rajan Sankaran

Rajan Sankaran, a homeopathic practitioner with vast experience in India, has written several works and commentaries based on his personal research and observations of many years. My favorite is a two-volume work titled *An Insight Into Plants*. In these volumes he explains some interesting concepts and ways of looking at the human psyche and homeopathic miasms.

Sankaran has a concise, but deeper, approach to the emotions underlying miasm categories than I have seen elsewhere. In order to understand Sankaran's classifications and categories, it is necessary to understand at least a little about the basic concepts and philosophies that he follows. It is also necessary to have a basic understanding of how he categorizes the miasms. His category lists are a little different from other researchers—just as theirs are different from each other.

I tend to use Sankaran's lists more often than any other because his lists are categorized by depth of the energy displacement, the degree of desperation displayed by that miasm, and the severity of the resulting ailments. I find the ordering of the lists by degree and depth of the problem very helpful. For the most part, I agree with the order in which he places the miasms. Since he has far more experience than I have, I acknowledge that time and patience will probably bring these minor disagreements into greater clarity and focus.

Sankaran's work has been helpful to me many times in understanding how my mind works, and how my perception of my environment is affecting my health and happiness. It has been helpful to me in identifying a homeopathic remedy that I am in need of, and then understanding why and how it can help me make changes for the better.

Basic Concepts of Sensations, Actions, and Sensitivities

THE VITAL SENSATION

Sankaran observes his clients closely in an attempt to ascertain what he calls the vital sensation that they are experiencing at the present time. Sensation is much deeper than just a state of mind or a passing emotion. Sensations are the beliefs, real or only perceived and imagined, by which the person is living their life. This sensation is the basic perception of self, of others, of the way life works, and of how people interact with each other. From this basic perception spring all of the behaviors, emotions, actions, and reactions that are displayed by that person from day to day. These emotions and behaviors eventually manifest in the body as pain, illness, and disease.

As I look for this vital sensation in myself and others, so much about the symptoms being presented in the present moment becomes clear and understandable. The vital sensation becomes the marked puzzle board onto which all the pieces of the symptom picture fit together. This is true whether you are considering a person and their ailments, or trying to understand the mental/emotional picture of a particular remedy. Always looking for the core perception that drives all of the other emotions, and lies beneath the physical manifestations of their ailments, is a very perceptive and effective way to analyze and understand a case. It is also a good way to understand yourself and how you relate to the people in your world.

When I do not know what direction to go in a situation, looking at the person in the light of the original vital sensation brings clarity. The vital sensation that a person is feeling is sometimes so core that it often remains with them in one form or another for their entire lifetime. At other times, this vital sensation is the result of major trauma to either the emotions or the physical body, and has drastically changed from what was perceived and thought before the traumatic event.

SENSATIONS, ACTIONS, AND SENSITIVITIES

The behaviors that a person displays, based on their core perception of themselves and life in general, are referred to as actions. Sensitivities are those things that we have difficulty doing or very much dislike doing. These struggles are based on our perceptions and our fears, usually having to do with our value as a person and our safety in particular situations. It must be remembered that we are talking about perception here, not necessarily reality and fact.

Actions, reactions = the behaviors that are displayed
Sensitivities = things that are difficult for us to do but at which we may learn to excel

Through observation of hundreds of clients, Sankaran developed some basic rules for interpreting these actions, reactions, sensitivities, and the basic sensations that drive them. His work has been done mostly with plant remedies because he considers the mineral and animal kingdoms to be well-documented already. His later lists however, include some mineral and animal remedies with which he is familiar.

Concepts of Interpreting Sensations, Actions, and Sensitivities

ACTIONS AND SENSATION ARE EQUAL AND OPPOSITE

The actions displayed by a person will be in direct opposition to the sensation he feels, and the intensity of his reaction will be in proportion to the intensity of the sensation as he feels it.

If a person states that he sometimes feels like killing someone (this is the sensation he is feeling) it can be assumed that there exists for him also the fear of being killed (this is the opposing reaction). The fear of being killed has created the need to get people before they get you. Alternatively, the desire to harm others has triggered the notion that others probably feel the same way about you.

These sensations and reactions are often expressed in dreams, interests, and hobbies (such as an interest and participation in martial arts). You will also find the core sensation expressed in the things they say every day. The person might use phrases such as "my shoulder is *killing* me."

Example A: Feeling indignant and insulted by others who he thinks consider themselves better than him. On reflection, he feels that these people are only better looking (but shallow) while he is himself great and good and wise (This basic thought pattern of his is, of course, very insulting to others.)

Example B: Feels contemptuous or mocking of his relatives but also experiences the opposing feeling that his relatives are continually mocking and feeling contemptuous of him.

SENSITIVITIES INCLUDE BOTH WEAKNESS AND A POTENTIAL STRENGTH

This brings to mind the scriptural assurance that weak things can become a strength to us.

Fear of public speaking shows a sensitivity to public speaking in general that is manifesting as a weakness in that area. This weakness indicates a potential to be a very good public speaker. It is the sensitivity that causes the fear. Fear & courage/faith are two sides of the same coin. This sensitivity might have manifested in other ways, such as seeking the limelight or speaking out of turn in classes, and displayed different opposite states.

Example C: Person emphasizing peace and harmony holds within himself the potential for violence. The person claiming he is afraid of nothing probably harbors fears and lack of confidence in himself. *If the opposite sensitivity is not true for a person, the sensitivity is not a keynote for them.*

THERE IS NOTHING OUT THERE OTHER THAN MYSELF

All of us tend to see in others what is most amiss in ourselves. All too often these are the only things that we do see about them and, sometimes, we see other people this way whether or not it is really true of them. We usually perceive in others what we are struggling with (or sensitive to) ourselves. This viewpoint is what we understand best and are most capable of perceiving and knowing.

The remedy that is correct for a person may not match what they tell you (or perceive) about themselves; rather it will match what they see in the people around them. A person's description of their spouse or coworkers will often be a description of where their sensitivities and struggles in life are. Having a client describe their mother, father, or siblings is often a very good way to discover clues to the homeopathic remedy that they need.

Example D: Two daughters describing their mother so differently that a stranger would have a hard time believing that it was the some woman. Each daughter is revealing her own sensitivities and should be prescribed for, or matched to, a remedy as though she were describing herself (for that is what she is doing).

You Will Do to Yourself What You Perceive Others Are Doing to You
and/or
You Will Do to Others (or to Things) What You Would Like to Do to Yourself

If you look up a remedy for suicidal tendencies, you will find that the remedy suggested also has indications for homicidal tendencies, and if it doesn't it should, because the tendency is there. There is a corollary between the desire to hurt others and the desire to hurt one's self. So it is with injury and everything else. If a person has a desire to hit his head against a wall, there is also a desire to do an injury to other people or things. Victims and aggressors are two sides of the same sensation.

If a remedy lists the sensation of mocking, it can be assumed that the remedy (and the person) also has the perception of being mocked. This is true even if the repertory and remedy guide does not list this symptom. When I began applying this concept I found the descriptions in the remedy guide fit myself and others much more closely. I should have realized it, without Sankaran pointing it out, because people frequently said, "That doesn't fit me. In fact, I am exactly the opposite," when I would read to them the description of a remedy I had muscle tested for them. It was frustrating! Knowing what I now know about sensations and their opposites, studying a muscle tested remedy is very educational!

So many experiences that I have had with people and homeopathic remedies make sense when looked at according to these concepts. Fear of being hurt and fear of hurting someone else are opposite sides of the same picture. If you cannot find the symptom you have observed listed in the remedy you have chosen, consider carefully as you look for this opposite. Conversely, when you cannot find a remedy listed under your symptom in the repertory, try looking at the remedies listed for the opposite feeling. "Kill, desire to" and "kill, fear of being" are results of the same sensation and belong to the same miasm.

EXPRESSION OF SENSATION

The sensation that is being felt can be expressed in four different ways:

1) as the sensation itself (sensation is feeling hurt or injured)

2) as a passive reaction (passive reaction is to just sit there feeling dazed and unable to cope)

3) as an active action/reaction (active action/reaction is to strike right back)

4) or as compensation. Example: The compensation is to become the tough one that no one can hurt or the tough one that hurts before being hurt. A person will often have one preferred way of reacting to situations. On the other hand, they may react differently according to the situation or the people involved. (This makes analysis tricky, but interesting.)

Depth of Pathology (order)

Sankaran identifies 10 miasms in his work. These miasms are listed below. The order in which they are listed has been determined by the depth of the pathology and the desperation of the action/reaction to the perception. In other words, the syphilis miasm is much deeper and more disruptive to the person's life than is the acute miasm. It will take more patience, more time, and more remedies to effectively clear the deeper miasms.

The Sensations and Actions of the Miasms

This following list is the miasms as they are seen by Rajan Sankaran, with the addition of a section for a vaccinosis miasm. They are arranged in order, from the least severe to the deepest and most desperate.

Sankaran has listed an age with each of his miasms. It is recognized in energy work that in each stage of our lives a different type of energy opens and becomes active. Here, briefly, are some examples: age two—I can do it myself; 4-5 years—growing away from mother, independence; 8 years of age—age of accountability in many cultures; at 12 years—emotions and hormones, the beginning of adulthood; 18-21 years—energy to the intellect and analytical aspects of the mind; and on through life.

When a person is manifesting one of the first three miasms—acute, typhoid, or psora—which represent infancy, childhood, and the teen years, perhaps they are displaying a psyche that is stuck somewhere in a trauma or pattern from those early years. One of the results of a failure to mature emotionally on all levels is a misunderstanding of what adult roles and behaviors should be. Being stuck displaying childlike reactions to situations results in behaviors that are inappropriate or destructive to the person himself, and often, to those who are close to him and care about him. Understanding the miasmic patterns and struggles of the human family can help us be more compassionate and, perhaps, of more assistance to them.

For each miasm, I have listed a few key words, the age pattern of the displacement, and the sensation and subsequent action that results from the sensation that is perceived. KEY WORDS are simple descriptions of what the person might be feeling, or the words you might hear him say in describing himself or his situation.

Acute Miasm
(The Least Deep of the Miasms)

SENSATION Feeling of an acute threat or danger of some kind. Threat is too big and too sudden.
ACTION Strong and instinctive reaction to that threat. An attempt to escape.
KEY WORDS acute, sudden, instinctive (reaction), panic, violent, escape, helpless, terror, fright, immobilized by fright
AGE PATTERN infancy

Typhoid Miasm

SENSATION Feeling that a critical situation, if properly handled for this critical period of time, will end in total recovery or resolution (example or trigger: sudden business loss or other crisis that needs attention right now).
ACTION An intense struggle against the situation. Taking over or taking chances.
KEY WORDS crisis, intense, recover lost ground, emergency, homesick, critical period, collapse, impatience, demanding
AGE PATTERN childhood (1-12 years)

Psora Miasm

SENSATION Feeling of a difficult situation where one has to struggle in order to succeed. Comes with a lot of anxiety and with doubts about his ability to cope. A Psoric person is usually hopeful and does not consider situations as unsolvable or failure to be the end of the world.
ACTION Struggling on to recover or maintain his position in the world. Getting the job done as best he can.
KEY WORDS optimism, effort, struggle, anxiety, doubts, hope, effort, giving up, lack of self-confidence, inattentive
AGE PATTERN teen years

Psora is a miasm that seems to be universal in scope. No plant remedies were identified by Sankaran. He feels that the plant remedies usually associated with this miasm fit better in the typhoid, ringworm, and malaria miasms. I believe that plant remedies, because they are of the earth, are often a necessary part of working with psora.

Malaria Miasm

SENSATION Underlying feeling of being lacking or deficient. There are intermittent periods where there is a feeling of acute threat.

ACTION Sudden and acute, from time to time, with lengthy quiet periods in between. The mild despair of accepting his real or perceived limitations.

KEY WORDS limited, stuck, intermittent attack, persecution, misfortune, harassed, hindered, obstructed,

AGE PATTERN childhood to middle age

Ringworm (Polio) Miasm

SENSATION Alternating periods of anxiety about success, followed by periods of despair and giving up. Often feels that a difficult situation is beyond an easy solution and/or may never be fixed.

ACTION Extreme effort and success and then the alternate pattern of no action taken. Sunk into despair.

KEY WORDS trying, doing the best I can, giving up, accepting, irritation, discomfort, impatient, inattentive, depressed, manic depression, poor memory

AGE PATTERN 25-35 years

Sycosis Miasm

SENSATION Feeling of unfixable weakness within himself.

ACTION An attempt to hide his unfixable weaknesses from others with secretiveness, egotism, compulsive acts, being defiant, or any other action that keeps other people out of his business and personal space.

KEY WORDS cover up, hide, guilt, secretive, avoidance, accepting, remorse, self-reproach, self disgust, neurotic, resentment, lack of perspective

AGE PATTERN 35-50 years

Cancer Miasm

SENSATION The need to perform exceedingly well and live up to very high expectations, but with an underlying feeling of weakness and incapacity. Life feels like a prolonged struggle with no end in sight.

ACTION Superhuman effort, stretching himself beyond the limits of possible. Failure is simply unacceptable. Failure would mean death with eternal damnation and destruction.

KEY WORDS perfection, fastidious, control, expectations, order from chaos, loss of control, self control, beyond my ability

AGE PATTERN 60-70 years

Tuberculosis Miasm

SENSATION Feeling of intense oppression and a desire for change. Feels caught in a situation which is suffocating. Feels that there is not enough time to do what is needed.

ACTION Intense, hectic activity in order to break free from this oppression or to get the work done which he thinks needs to be accomplished.

KEY WORDS caught, suffocated, compressed, narrow, trapped, closed in, change, activity, freedom, defiant, oppressed, intensity, desire to change

AGE PATTERN 60-70 years

Leprosy Miasm

SENSATION Feeling of intense oppression and isolation accompanied by intense hopelessness and disgust with himself. Feels an intense desire for change.

ACTION Will be to isolate himself even further. The possibility exists that contemplations of homicide or suicide will be acted upon. These people need help and they probably need it right now!

KEY WORDS isolation, loneliness, despair, hopelessness, oppressed, outcast, secluded, confined, disgusted, dirty, sadistic

AGE PATTERN 60-70 years

Syphilitic Miasm

The deepest of the miasmic energy displacements that were identified by Dr. Hahnemann. Difficult, but NOT impossible, to treat.

SENSATION Feeling of being faced with a situation that is not salvageable. This leads to complete hopelessness and despair.

ACTION A desperate effort to change the perceived situation in inappropriate ways that usually result in disaster or destruction.

KEY WORDS destruction, destructiveness, impossible, despair, psychosis, devastation

AGE PATTERN Beyond 80 years in the sense of approaching death and destruction. This pattern can, of course, be seen at any time of life.

AIDS Miasm

Not discussed by Sankaran, but I have added it here to provide continuity and completeness to the information presented.

The AIDS miasm is very real. People all around us can be seen to be suffering from it. The sensations and reaction common to this miasm can be seen everywhere we look. They are having an impact, often destructive, within families and on the political scene and are beginning to define us as a nation and as a global community.

SENSATION Feelings of isolation created by the dissolution of boundaries. Fear, anxiety and paranoia are often experienced.

ACTION Contradictory. A need to establish personal boundaries opposed by a need to destroy the things they see as restrictive—the traditional family or national boundaries, for example.

KEY WORDS vulnerable, energy sensitive, secretive, angry, isolation, depression, despair, mistreated, abandoned, confusion, irresponsible, free, entitled

AGE PATTERN Can be any age at all but our children and young adults (quickly growing into the adult generation), accustomed as they are to the use of electronics and allowed to spend hours disconnected from reality by their use, are particularly at risk from the negative effects of this miasm.

Alzheimer's Miasm

Once again, not discussed by Sankaran but added here. We are seeing more and more heart-breaking cases of dementia and Alzheimer's every day. A family that has not experienced this with a senior family member is becoming very rare.

SENSATION Lost in both time and space. Not knowing who they are, where they are, and not recognizing who they are with, or why they are wherever they are. It is frightening to even contemplate that amount of fear that must accompany this most lost of states.

ACTION In the early stages, there is usually a great need to pretend that the loss of memory and the loss of self is not happening. The need to cover it up and pretend to be normal is very great, especially if there were any of the cancer miasm issues of perfection and never having done things good enough seen in their younger years.

KEY WORDS lost, anxious, vague, disconnected, unhappy, angry, sad, out of time and place, confused, discontented

AGE PATTERN Beyond 80 years and into the next life in the sense that the person seems to have already left this world with all of themselves except their physical body. This pattern can, of course, start to develop much earlier in life.

Vaccinosis Miasm

The vaccinosis miasm is not part of Sankaran's list. I consider it a major contributor to the ill health of everyone that I know, so I have included it here with my interpretation of its sensation, actions, etc.

Because of the number of toxins, pollutants and vaccines in our world, it is difficult to list only one (or even two or three) basic sensations or actions for this miasm. Even so, there do seem to be some commonalities among all of the possible reactions to the chemical exposures that we are all subjected to.

SENSATION 1) Great pressure to achieve, with a tremendous and persistent fear of not being good enough. This fear remains constant in the mind no matter what is accomplished in life to prove otherwise.

2) Has a need for speed, thrills, and excitement that often leads to accidents and injuries.

ACTION 1) A frantic race for accomplishments and accolades to prove one's self. The joy of life is forgotten in the race for more recognition and more credentials. The opposition state of this frantic race is depression and despair when failure is experienced or even contemplated.

2) Daredevil tendencies; running faster than one has strength; taking risks in business and personal life.

KEY WORDS burned out, running too fast, irritability, angry, short attention span, pressured, inadequate, fearful, anxious, skeptical, worthless, deserving, entitled, deadline, excitement, boring, confused, restless

AGE PATTERN Any time in our lives. Since we are all exposed to about a zillion chemicals everyday and immunizations have become the "sacraments" of our faith in the medical model, this miasm is affecting all age groups. Worse, like all miasms, it has the potential to be passed on to subsequent generations.

VACCINOSIS AND POLIO

The vaccinosis miasm is an acquired miasm, meaning that it is the result of things we have taken into our bodies rather than inherited as Hahnemann believed, or the result of changes in the structure of society. These patterns can be and are labeled as miasms because they seem to affect our bodies in such a way that they can be passed on to the next generation. This spin on genetic inheritance makes these patterns miasms in every definition and sense of the word.

From the statistics and information that I have gathered, it seems that at least parts of the polio miasm are also acquired patterns that have developed inheritable characteristics. Whatever Sankaran's reasons for omitting vaccinosis from his list, it is a certain thing that in the United States we deal with the result of chemical poisoning every day and in nearly every person we work with. It is a very rare person, who never in their life suffers from some aspect of this miasm. I placed vaccinosis last on the above list because I could not ascertain the depth or the desperation of the pathology as these aspects vary so widely from person to person.

THE POLIO/RINGWORM MIASM

Also note that the polio miasm as discussed previously seems to be similar in mental/emotional symptoms (sensations) to Sankaran's description of the ringworm miasm. The ringworm miasm has, of course, a lot more skin symptoms than does the polio miasm. Muscle contractions, paralysis, and lung symptoms are the primary physical symptoms of the polio miasm. I cannot account for this except to think that, perhaps, in the warmer/moister climate of India the skin symptoms predominate, while in climates like ours the predomant symptoms are those seen in the polio miasm. It is interesting to note that, statistically, when psoriasis or eczema (skin symptoms) in children is treated with cortisone there is a higher than normal risk of asthma and arthritis within a few years. I believe that this statistical connection demonstrates a connection between the descriptions of the two miasms.

PLANT FAMILIES

Sankaran's earliest published work (a 2-volume set) linked the miasms only to plant remedies. Each plant family has a main theme and then passive, active, and compensation actions which describe it are identified. Plant families do not correspond to particular miasms. Each plant/remedy within the family perceives the sensation to a different depth and degree of desperation and reacts to the perception in a unique way, making it specific to a miasm of matching dept and desperation. At first, I was disappointed by this seemingly random arrangement made by the creator of heaven and earth; on further reflection, it can only be described as brilliant, phenomenal, intelligent, and amazing!

Instead of each plant family corresponding to a miasm, there seems to be at least one remedy in each family which corresponds to each miasm. We don't always know what these remedies are, because they are not among common polycrest remedies at this time (probably for lack of understanding), but there are enough correlations to lead to the assumption that there are plants in each family for each miasm.

It appears that each plant family, all over the world, contains remedies for the less extreme miasms (such as the acute or typhoid miasms), for the miasms of the midrange of desperation and intensity, and remedies for the very nasty miasms like leprosy and syphilis.

It would seem that no matter where you live in the world, a loving Heavenly Father has provided a solution to whatever problem you have at the moment in just the plant kingdom alone. I believe that as Sankaran and others finish their research and analysis, we will find that the same holds true for the mineral and animal kingdoms. In fact, Sankaran explains, more clearly than I have found elsewhere, the differences between remedies of the three major kingdoms—plant, animal, and mineral.

If the plants matched up with the miasms *according to plant family*, there would be some miasms for which there would not be a remedy available in each portion of the world since some plant families are not found everywhere. Put simply, if your miasm was best dealt with by a remedy from the cactus family, you had better be living where cactus plants are available. The same would be true for all miasms. What a marvelous plan—having a remedy for everything in each family wherever that family is predominant in the world.

SENSATION, PLANT FAMILIES, AND INDIVIDUAL REMEDIES

In summary, each plant family has a main theme, a sensation, and corresponding actions/reactions. Each plant, and remedy made from that plant, perceives the sensation to a different depth and degree of desperation. Each plant reacts to the basic perception of the miasm in a unique way, unlike the reaction of other plants in the same family. Thus, each plant within the family is specific to a different miasm.

The same holds true for human beings. We all experience the basic emotions of mad, sad, glad, and scared, but our actions and reactions to these emotions are uniquely our own and different in depth and scope. The difference in depth of feeling and the desperation displayed by our reaction account for the differences in symptoms and behavior patterns. These same principles also apply to the remedies of the mineral and animal kingdoms.

For example, the basic sensation of shock may be felt as panic or as helplessness. The person who has reacted with panic may make a sudden, instinctive, but short-lived attempt to fix the problem and then calm down. If helplessness is their reaction, they may do nothing at all because they believe themselves to be helpless victims and will probably just blame the whole thing on someone else. Another person may perceive this same sensation of shock as being the result of a situation that is absolutely critical, probably can't be fixed but that they must make a desperate effort to set right by some dramatic, long-term something only they can—just possibly—accomplish.

These different reactions are characteristic of very different miasms. The first example, panic or helplessness, is simply two sides of the same reaction. The feeling that the situation is critical, while still the basic perception of shock, is more desperate. Each scenario will need a remedy from the same plant family—the compositae/asteraceae family for the feelings of shock—but will each require the remedy specific to the depth of their reaction. In the first case, a reaction of either panic or helplessness, the miasm is probably acute. In the second case the depth of desperation is very nearly, if not completely, that of the syphilis miasm.

FURTHERING OUR UNDERSTANDING

These theories and concepts are in their infant stages. Sankaran says that his works are in a developmental stage—new things are being learned every day. It is exciting work, and the concepts are important in understanding the human psyche and its relationship to physical health. A look at the underlying sensation and the resulting actions/reactions when analyzing a case can be very helpful. To analyze, after the fact, when the remedy has been arrived at by muscle test, is a wonderful way to learn and understand the different remedies, the way our minds and bodies work, and how to identify and treat miasmic patterns.

Chapter Sixteen - Miasms and the Periodic Table of Elements

Based on the Work of Jan Scholten

INTRODUCTION

Jan Scholten, a Dutch homeopath who wrote the forward to Rajan Sankaran's books <u>An Insight Into Plants</u>, has done his work predominantly with the remedies of the mineral kingdom—the elements. He has observed that there is a very basic difference between the remedies which are salts and the remedies which are minerals. Salt remedies always deal with difficulties in relationships, while the emotional picture of the metal remedies has more to do with a person's role in life or level of performance in that role.

THE PERIODIC TABLE AND HOMEOPATHY

Scholten bases his theories on the position of the elements in the periodic table of elements. This table is a universal system of mathematical beauty and symmetry which outlines the material structure and atomic weight of the elements which comprise everything in the whole universe (as far as man understands it).

Scholten observed that the position of an element in the periodic table of elements corresponds directly with the depth of desperation within basic patterns. He does not call these patterns miasms. He refers to "stages" and "series", with the series corresponding to the basic miasm patterns very well. The stages give us another scale by which to judge and understand the uniqueness of each series/miasm.

Scholten's element theory can be a powerful tool in analyzing and prescribing homeopathic remedies. This method is especially fun if you love order and mathematical precision.

In his research, he has many times predicted what symptoms an unknown remedy would display in its upcoming provings. He determined the symptom picture of the new and unproven remedy based on its place, relative to other elements, in the periodic table. When the provings were completed and the data collated, he has been proven absolutely and uncannily correct every time he has done this.

SCHOLTEN'S STAGES

Jan Scholten's stages are theoretically similar to the miasm theory of traditional homeopathic thought. The series and stages of Scholten's categorization are units based on divisions within the periodic table. Scholten claims that since the elements are the building blocks of everything on earth, the stages can be applied to the plant and animal kingdoms as well. I have not spent the money to buy his expensive books on this topic, yet, because I don't have the time right now to study them the way they would need to be studied. (I have added them to the long list of things I want to know before I die.)

The periodic table, as it stands today, contains 18 columns and 7 rows. In Scholten's theory the 7 rows, each named for an element within that row, are patterns similar to basic miasms. The 18 columns each represent what he calls a stage, a depth of desperation.

Hahnemann identified 3 basic miasms. My version of miasmic theory, at the moment, identifies 12 basic ones and adds another one called vaccinosis, which is a catch-all category for the damage done by drugs and pollutants. Some of the mental/emotional/physical characteristics of Scholten's 7 series and 18 stages correspond very nicely to the descriptions in traditional homeopathy and in Sankaran's descriptions of the miasms. As the basic building blocks of life, perhaps the elements and their corresponding stages finally answer the question of how many patterns/miasms there really are.

As I read and try to understand this very complicated material, I feel like I am standing in a science laboratory trying to analyze and understand the mind of God and the methods of creation with my own very finite mind and too few pieces of the puzzle. The grandeur and complexity of this earth is so awesome. Reflecting on it deepens my appreciation and love for my Creator and leaves me in awe at the scope of His infinite intelligence.

SCHOLTEN'S SERIES

In the common versions in use today, the periodic table has seven rows. These rows correspond, in Scholten's theory, to seven layers of development in pathology and symptoms, with the symptoms worsening as they descend down the table. Each series is named after the most prominent element which occupies that row on the periodic table.

There are 18 columns in the periodic table. Each column represent a family of elements. Each series (row) has 18 possible stages (columns/families), each stage corresponding to the 18 columns of the periodic table. The emotions and mental patterns are similar for each of the elements in a particular column. The further to the right an element's location is in the table, the more severe, dissolute and destructive are the issues in the symptom picture of the corresponding homeopathic remedy.

To be understood completely, the stage of each element (column) must be placed in context with the series (row) in which it is also found. I find that even when I am using Hahnemann's or Sankaran's nomenclature, I like to cross-reference it, using the chart below and the following pages, and study the further information provided by the description of the appropriate stage and series.

They are listed in the chart below, cross referenced to Sankaran's miasms, traditional miasms, and linked to possible emotional age characteristics.

Comparison Chart—Series and Miasms

Scholten's Series	Sankaran's Miasms	Emotional Age Designation	Traditional Miasms	Hahnemann's Miasms
Hydrogen	Acute	infancy	*(Pre-Psora)* *(Perhaps Pre-Existance)*	
Carbon	Typhoid	childhood (1-12 years)		
Silicium	Ringworm	teen years	Psora	Psora
		25-35 years		
	Malaria	childhood thru middle age		
Ferrum/Iron	Sycosis	35-50 years	Sycosis	Sycosis
Silver				
Gold	Cancer	60-70 years	Cancer	
	Polio	25-30 years	Polio	
	Tuberculosis	60-70 years	Tuberculosis	
	Leprosy	60-70 years		
Uranium	Syphilis	beyond 80 years and moving toward either destruction or death	Syphilis	Syphilis
	AIDS			
	Alzheimer's			

A VERY BRIEF CHEMISTRY LESSON

The creation of elements begins with hydrogen, which is matter in its simplest, lightest, and most elemental form. From hydrogen the process of adding protons and neutrons continues, step by step. With each step another element is born, each having gained in atomic mass. This process continues until the atoms become so heavy and complex that their inner stability begins to deteriorate into radioactivity.

Movement downward in the columns of the periodic table indicate that a new outer shell of electrons is being formed. Elements in the same vertical columns have the same valence number (look that up in a chemistry book) and are similar in interesting ways. Movement from left to right indicates that more protons and neutrons are filling each outer shell. As the shells are filled, the atomic weight of the element is increased. When the shell of the element in the far right column is full, the series is completed. A new outer shell forms, shown on the table by beginning a new row at the far left and beginning the process of adding protons and neutrons in the new outer shell.

Brief Descriptions of Each Series

SERIES #1 HYDROGEN (PRE HAHNEMANN'S MIASMIC PATTERNS)
THEME: Coming into being; existence; connection or separateness
APPLICABLE TO: Scholten's stage 1 and Sankaran's acute miasm
AGE: Infancy

The hydrogen series at the top of the periodic table consists of only two atoms, hydrogen and helium, both of which are utilized in homeopathy.

The theme of this series is existence in the mortal plane, coming into being, distinction as an individual, and separation from parents. This simple series of only two represents very well the dualistic principle—either or, one or the other, pairs of opposites, yes or no, to be or not to be.

Hydrogen represents action, affirmation, existence, and presence in this world and time. The gaseous helium represents intangibility and a reluctance to connect with mortal existence and experiences.

The symptom picture of helium is almost perfectly that of autism, and it has been used successfully several times in such cases.

SERIES #2 CARBON (PRE HAHNEMANN'S MIASMIC PATTERNS)
THEME: Development of the body; individuality; questioning "who, what am I?"
APPLICABLE TO: Scholten's stage 2 and Sankaran's typhoid miasm
AGE: Childhood, 1-12 years

The second series, or level, of the periodic table is named after the carbon element. There are 8 light, small, and "young" elements at this level.

Lithium, at the far left, is the lightest element in this series. As a stage 1 (column 1) element it has to do with beginnings and starting out or starting over. Lithium affects every system of the body, all membranes, nerve impulse transmissions, hormones, and metabolism. Several lithium salts are used as medicines.

Some of the other elements and homeopathic remedies at this level, going from left to right, are beryllium, boron, carbon, and fluorine (fluoricum).

The remedies on this level all have to do with development of the body and mind, just like a child growing toward adulthood. There are issues of self-confidence, mental ability, memory, and physical growth as well as vitality running through all of these remedies. As we move further to the right on the chart, the remedies become more and more about personal identity, becoming a unique and separate person, breaking those childhood attachments to mother, and individuality.

SERIES #3 SILICIUM (PARALLEL OF HAHNEMANN'S PSORA MIASM)
THEME: "Ripening" of relationships; development of a sense of self and identity as an individual
APPLICABLE TO: Sankaran's ringworm (polio), malaria and psora miasms and Scholten's stage 3
AGE: Early Adolescence through early middle age

There are 8 elements in level 3 also. They include stages 3 through 9. The elements on the left (sodium and magnesium) have about them the identity crisis of the pubescent/adolescent years with its struggles to decide and define who you are and who you will become. Painful sometimes, to be sure, but lacking the desperation, fatigue, despair, disorganization, and feelings of betrayal that characterize the remedies as you move further and further to the right. You can see the moving into adulthood patterns, and if balance and health is not maintained as the person ages, the patterns show increased dissolution and crumbling. From left to right the major remedies are Aluminum, Silicon, Phosphorus, Sulphur, and Chlorine.

SERIES #4 IRON (PARALLEL OF HAHNEMANN'S SYCOSIS MIASM)
THEME: "Growing up"; work; duty; rules; teamwork; taking responsibility.
APPLICABLE TO: Scholten's stage 10, Sankaran's, traditional, and Hahnemann's sycosis miasms
AGE: 35-50 years

This level shows its grown-up status by the fact that it is the first level to have a full span of the 18 stages. The increasing weight of the remedies is easily seen by comparing calcium on the left to iron as you move further right. The calcareas are full of insecurity and fears and are very much concerned about and driven by what the neighbors may be saying. Sensitivity to criticism often rules their world. Moving left, column 7 shows great strength but still needs support and assistance from time to time. Iron, a little further to the right, stands firm, is persistent and persevering, and can become downright irritable if pushed against.

SERIES #5 SILVER (PARALLEL OF DEEPER LAYER OF HAHNEMANN'S SYCOSIS MIASM)
THEME: Creative genius; mediators; maintenance of the status quo
APPLICABLE TO: Between sycosis and cancer on both Sankaran's and traditional lists
AGE: Midlife

The remedies made from the elements of row 5 show a need to explore their world and create something memorable. There is a need to improvise and invent, but also a need to shine and to be appreciated. Here again the patterns of aging, the accumulations of failures and missed opportunities begin to show in degenerative diseases like arthritis, etc. The iodatums, from column 17, crave escape from their problems and sometimes begin to show obsessive or neurotic behaviors. The metal remedies show their fixation with achievement and performance very clearly at this level. Physically, the weight leads to heaviness in the extremities.

SERIES #6 GOLD (PARALLEL TO DEEPER LAYER OF HAHNEMANN'S SYCOSIS MIASM)
THEME: Leadership; responsibility; power
APPLICABLE TO: Scholten's stages 12-16, the cancer, polio, tuberculoisis, and leprosy miasms of Sankaran's and traditional thinking
AGE: All the way from young adulthood to 70 years of age

The miasms included here are an illustration of all the ways that power can be misused and how avoiding responsibility can create havoc in our bodies. The gold series also includes the development of inner strength, integrity, and autonomy if we move into old age in harmony with who we are and who we were meant to be.

SERIES #7 URANIUM (PARALLEL OF HAHNEMANN'S SYPHILIS MIASM)
THEME: Dissolution and death—resurrection and new life
APPLICABLE TO: Scholten's stage 17 and the syphilis miasms of Sankaran, traditional thought, and Hahnemann
AGE: Beyond 80 years

This level is about destruction and destructiveness, physically and emotionally, or it can be about mellowing toward perfection and contentment.

Brief Descriptions of Each Stage

The stages, as described by Jan Scholten, show a definite pattern of youthful insecurity in the early stages which matures into accomplishment and power in the middle stages. Then there is a gradual descent from confidence and power into negative emotions such as boasting, looking to the past, and eventual destruction. Remember, the elements in each column of the periodic table (the stage) share similar characteristics but they are displayed against the overall background of the miasm/series (the row of the periodic table).

This makes an orderly looking pattern on paper, but *if Sankaran is right about a sensitivity indicating both a weakness and a possible strength, perhaps these descriptions should be expanded to cover both the positive and negative traits. I don't believe that old age or the completion of a project has to be a descent into destruction. It is attainable to be well balanced, happy and productive at all stages. Homeopathy is meant to help us, along with faith and inspiration, to achieve this.*

In my mind, the stages are ways of analyzing myself (and others, when they ask) to see if negative aspects of any of the stages are present in my life. The purpose is to recognize my faults and fix them, now!

STAGE #1 The theme of stage 1 seems to be impulsiveness and action taken without thought or reflection. Sometimes the description of this type of behavior might be naive, simplistic, childish, or foolish. Sometimes this impulsiveness, especially in an adult, can become narrow-mindedness which appears rigid and domineering. Often there is loneliness or a sense of being alone.

STAGE #2 This stage is characterized by insecurity and lack of appreciation for one's worth and contribution. Because a person in this stage does not value himself enough, he tends to be passive, sitting back and watching rather than contributing. The opposing action of watching is the feeling of being watched; sometimes these people are good at hiding and being invisible in social situations. Because they feel overwhelmed and bewildered much of the time, they want to be protected and supported by others.

STAGE #3 This stage is also one of insecurity and underestimation of one's own worth, but stage 3 is characterized by a searching for just the right thing to do or become. At this stage, the search is not completed because, lacking confidence, decisions are avoided and commitments are not made.

STAGE #4 Moving on from stage 3, we begin to see conclusions drawn from searching. A decision is made, a direction decided upon. There is still much vacillation, back and forth, about whether or not the decision made was a good one. This stage is one of irresolution and astonishment if plans made begin to show signs of working out.

STAGE #5 The decision and direction have been decided upon. Plans and proposals start to come together, work is begun but the work looks horrendous, much to big to be accomplished. This stage is, to often, one of discouragement, disappointment, and alternating between the decision to go on and the desire to give it all up. There is procrastination out of fear that the goal was unrealistic all along.

STAGE #6 Commitments have been made. There appears to be no way out but forward, proving one's ability. This stage is about finding courage and fortitude. Sometimes, the nagging fear of failure and inadequacy is expressed as risk taking and overenthusiasm. At other times, the fear leads to secretiveness as the person, afraid he may fail, tries to keep others from seeing what he is doing until he has found success.

STAGE #7 Shows signs of maturity. Education, training, and experience have begun to build confidence and a desire to learn more. There is usually an ability to cooperate with others in an attempt to learn from them. There is often a desire to teach others and help them find success without the struggles that he endured.

STAGE #8 Column 8 is a stage of productivity and power, where everything learned and dreamed seems to be coming together. Life is characterized by perseverance, accomplishment, and power. The downside of this stage is feelings of pressure, lack of time, and the stress of deadlines. Often there is impatience and irritation with other people which must be overcome.

STAGE #9 Stage 9 is an interesting stage. It is characterized by the let-down feeling that sometimes follows accomplishment and completion of a project. Sometimes there is also an undercurrent of fear that a mistake will be discovered or that whatever was accomplished will not be appreciated—or maybe, wasn't worthy of appreciation in the first place.

STAGE #10 In this stage, pride can sometimes be seen. Accomplishments seem to all be the result of our own talents and abilities. There can be such a feeling of self-sufficiency that the need for others, even God, is forgotten and unrecognized. An attitude of "my way is the only right way, and I am smarter than you, and almost smarter than God" can enter into the picture.

STAGE #11 There is a mellowing in this stage. It is the need to hold on and maintain the success and position attained. There is a need to relax and enjoy the feeling of a job well done. There is often a feeling of benevolence toward others, but there is also a feeling of the tremendous weight of caring for others and maintaining one's position.

STAGE #12 Unlike stage 11, which a person needing this type of remedy seems to have skipped over (there is little of the mellowing mentioned above), this stage demonstrates abuse of power—tyranny. When one becomes so caught up in the feeling of one's own greatness, it is easy to feel threatened, attacked, envied from all directions. Suspiciousness and tyrannical defense of one's power and position lead to opposition from others, which only underscores the feeling of threat. There are a lot of negatives here. Boasting, overdoing, overstating one's own importance, or the creating of tension and disharmony to keep others off guard and make them less of a threat.

STAGE #13 This stage is one of looking back to the glory days. There is a nostalgia for things past, a feeling that the old days and ways and things were better than anything available today. A need to stay on top, to be admired, renders the clinging to old ways and old things impossible, but there is a great deal of conflict about it. Sometimes, there is a drawing away from things of the present and the future.

STAGE #14 This stage is heavy with the feelings of being pushed aside, past one's prime, dismissed, seen as useless. Often the person will be maintaining the facade of their former life and power, but they feel powerless, drained, and empty. There are often deep feelings of insecurity based on wondering how long they can keep up the pretense or maintain any usefulness to their organizations or families. Depression and the degenerative diseases of old age often enter into this stage.

STAGE #15 This a deeper stage of the disappearance of all that was achieved and an even further descent into a loss of the sense of self. Often felt in the body much the same as a shock from an accident or traumatic experience. There are two responses to these feelings. The first is to fight and resist, insisting on staying in the picture and staying in control. The other is surrender, capitulation, and abdication of roles and responsibilities. If one can achieve balance here there will be forgiveness of self and others and deep satisfaction.

STAGE #16 If stage 15 is allowed to disintegrate further, stage 16 becomes a stage of ashes and decay. Physical symptoms include the odors and problems of very advanced age. Only memories are left and these memories may bring sorrow or they may bring an exaggerated fantasy of former greatness. There can, of course, be a deepening of faith and insight, a greater love for family, and a reconciliation of the coming of death. Lazy or simply content? I suspect it is a choice, most of which was made long ago in other stages.

STAGE #17 Another step toward the final scenes. People either hang on, fighting tooth and nail as they view life as a force that is trying to annihilate them. Holding on sometimes manifests as taking things without asking, acting as though everything belongs to them and their every wish should be someone's command. Sometimes there is a gentle letting go of everything—might be memories or might be things and people in the present (dementia). This letting go can be full of fear or it can sometimes be accomplished with humor.

STAGE #18 This stage is described as the denial of action and connection. It can be nothing more than the taking of a rest, a holiday, or a nap. It also represents meditation, coma, and death. Externally, there seems to be nothing going on, internally there can be transformation—the view of death as the portal to the next level of existence. This stage need not be just about death. It can be a deep manifestation of the water meridian cycle of life—everything frozen, underground, but preparing for the budding stage of spring.

Chapter Seventeen - Mineral Remedies by Element Families

Single Minerals

This group includes nosodes and sarcodes. Reactions are everything or nothing both physically and emotionally. Third party description processes—my head, my foot, my headache—as though they were not a part of the whole of them.

The personality has a disconnected quality—bipolar and manic depression is often seen here. Extremes of mood and covering one emotion by another emotion are also keynotes. Examples: masking fear with anger, or lack of self-esteem with judgmental attitudes towards others.

There is a clear distinction between salts and metals. A person needing a salt remedy has misperceptions and problems in his relationships, while a person needing a metal remedy has problems which center on his role or performance in some way.

In the periodic table used by chemists, the elements are arranged according to atomic weight. The further down in the table the element sits, the heavier is its atomic weight. There is an obvious corollary between the atomic weight of an element and the depth of the miasm it is able to treat. The heavier the element, the deeper it reaches into the vital force. This was explained in a little more detail in chapter 16 when discussing Jan Scholten's theory of elements in homeopathy.

Some minerals and metals occur, of course, by themselves and they are utilized this way in homeopathy. For example, a homeopathic remedy has been made from zinc (Zincum metallicum) and from gold (Aurum metallicum), to name just two. Many of the elements are found combined in nature; others are artificially combined by man in laboratory settings. Combining two family groups makes for some interesting symptom pictures, and makes analysis both more complicated and more fun. Experienced practitioners often find the descriptions created following Scholten's theories more accurate than the descriptions of provings in the Materia Medica.

Carbonicums

> Full of self-pity
> Needs constant care or nurturing
> Always wants mother available
> Needs attention
> Has issues with self-awareness
> Doesn't seem able to see other people's needs

SCHOLTEN: Series 2, individuality with stage 14, feels that he is being pushed aside and seen by others as useless and powerless.

CALCAREA CARBONICA: Protection and withdrawal combine with homesickness and needing mom to come and spoil them a little bit and take over their responsibilities for awhile. Calcareas are often indicated during pregnancy and postpartum.
KALI CARBONICUM: Duty and self-pity combine to make a remedy (and a person) of alternating moods. A keynote is wanting company but, when they come, treating them horribly or waiting for them to go.
MAGNESIA CARBONICA: This combination links magnesia passive/aggressive tendencies (mostly passive) to the self pity and need for attention of the carbon family.
NATRUM CARBONICUM: The combining of natrum grief with carbonicum self-pity creates profound sadness and depression. The person is overwhelmed by grief. Sometimes the person becomes pathologically cheerful (faking it), sacrificing own feelings to make others feel better. Wants more from mother than she is willing or able to give or feels that what mother is doing and giving is not enough.
OTHERS: *Ammonium carbonicum, Baryta carbonica, Lithium carbonicum, Magnesia carbonica.*

Nitricums

Desire for space, expansion, going out
Desire for enjoyment and entertainment
Congestion/explosion
Tension/relaxation
Fighting to stay in control or the abdication of all responsibility

SCHOLTEN: Series 2, and found in column 15, is immediately to the right of carbon so the pathology can be expected to be slightly deeper.

KALI NITRICUM: Has the tension/relaxation of the nitricums but with the kali connection to duty and principle. The closed in personal relationships lead to isolation and deep sadness whenever they are alone. There can be depression when the desire for enjoyment is unfulfilled because of the inability to establish relationships with others.
NITRICUM ACIDUM: Acids are always implicated in fatigue no matter what the other part of the remedy is. When combined with the nitricum theme, the fatigue often manifests as anxiety, fear, and the holding on to grudges for long periods of time.
URANIUM NITRICUM: Uranium is a stage 17 remedy. It is a picture of disorganization, instability, and destructive forces at work. The focus is ill humor, irritability, and ill health with deepening depression.
OTHERS: *Argentum nitricum*

Fluoratas

Superficial relationships and contacts
Glamour, glitter, money, clothes
Part of the "in crowd", looking good
Sex with little emotion
Hard, smooth, fast
Fear of death or loss

SCHOLTEN: Series 2, Stage 17. This is an advanced state of negative pathology with little real connection or feeling for others. Literally fighting tooth and nail to hang onto something, anything to keep old age, death, and annihilation at bay for another day or hour.

CALCAREA FLUORATA: The sensitivity to criticism and the opinions of others characteristic of calcarea combined with the superficiality of relationships of the fluoratas makes this a very difficult pattern to live in. All fluoratas manifest with frightening and uncomfortable symptoms in the body.
FLUORICUM ACIDUM: The negative and desperate patterns of fluorata have taken their toll. The pattern of all acidums is extreme fatigue.
NATRUM FLUORATUM: Most often the hard, fast, smooth aspects of the fluoratas become agitation accompanied by deep depression. A completely closed off state, lack of inclination or ability to speak.
OTHERS: *Cadmium fluorata*

Natrums (Sodiums)

Grief and depression
Pessimistic, gloomy "Eeyore"—things not too bad, but never likely to get much better
Emotionally sensitive; moved by music
Restrictions, denial, closed, alone
Holding onto destructive relationships, horrible jobs, and bad situations

SCHOLTEN: Series 3, Stage 1. This is puberty and adolescence in every sense of the word. There is a seeking to find one's identity and move into adult relationships coupled with impulsive, thoughtless, almost childish behavior. This pattern is sometimes held onto far into adulthood.

NATRUM PHOSPHORICUM: The phosphorus focus on family and friends combined with the gloominess, grief and depression of natrum becomes indifference to loved ones and mental confusion.

NATRUM SULPHURICUM: This is one of the most desperate and scary of the homeopathic remedies. It is often indicated after head injuries. Relationship problems and the absence of joy that are characteristic of sulphur combine with the gloom and depression of natrum to form a very deep pathology. Irritability and estrangement from family decline into suicidal impulses. The Materia Medica description includes having to use self-control to keep from shooting oneself. The childishness and irresponsibility of stage 1 combined with stage 16 negative patterns is alarming! A lot of bi-polar attributes as a result.
OTHERS: *Natrum arsenicum, Natrum carbonicum, Natrum muriaticum*

Calcareas

What will the neighbors (others) say?
Sensitive to criticism
Insecurity
Full of fears
Protection and withdrawal
Tends to be cold or get cold easily
Tends to weight gain
Commonly required during pregnancy—because the symptom picture fits so well

SCHOLTEN: Series 3, Level 2. Trying to establish one's own identity, but struggling with issues of self-worth and confidence. Calcareas often feel like the whole world is watching them and deciding that they are not quite good enough.

CALCAREA IODATA: Attempting to establish one's own identity while experiencing self-confidence issues and insecurity. All of those calcarea insecurities coupled with iodine's compulsiveness, busyness, and need to escape is a volatile mix.

CALCAREA PHOSPHORICA: This is a very sensitive pattern as it combines the calcarea sensitivity to criticism and insecurity with phosphorica's anxiousness and vague bad feelings about something happening to loved ones. Problems manifest in bones, teeth, and with growth issues.

CALCAREA SULPHURICA: There is a lot of "what will the neighbors say about my appearance," or a contrasting thumbing of the nose at the neighbors' opinions appearance, and everything else.
OTHERS: *Calcarea carbonica, Calcarea fluorata*

Magnesiums

Pacifism - unable or unwilling to be in the middle of conflict
Aggression - if pushed hard enough becomes aggressive
Fear of loss, worries about family members and friends
Sensitivity to pain

SCHOLTEN: Series 3, Level 2. Once again the pattern of establishing one's own identity, coupled with insecurity. Magnesium tends to behave passively, sitting back watching, avoiding conflict to the point of hiding or choosing to become completely isolated.

MAGNESIA PHOSPHORICA: Phosphorus brings in a lot of restlessness and anxiety and a great sensitivity to noise and/or excitement. Phosphorus is level 15 on the table so the pathology is very pronounced.
OTHERS: *Magnesia carbonica, Magnesia sulphurica, Magnesia muriatica*

Phosphoricums

Open Communication
Sympathy
Friends, acquaintances, neighbors (all love them dearly when balanced)
Homesickness
Language and learning; curiosity and travel
Restless and anxious; bad feelings about something vague
Feels out of touch with people
Puts everybody's needs before her own

SCHOLTEN: Series 3, Level 15. Being a stage 15 remedy, phosphorus has a lot of issues about loss of power, autonomy, and sense of self.

KALI PHOSPHORICUM: The combination of the phosphorus deep love of people and a tendency to put other people's needs ahead of one's own gets blown way out of proportion by the kali sense of duty. The result is nervous prostration, mental and physical fatigue, and general weakness.

OTHERS: *Calcarea phosphorica, Magnesia phosphorica, Natrum phosphoricum, Ferrum phos.*

Sulphuricums

Clothing and appearance—sometimes manifests as the opposite total lack of concern for appearance
Beauty, grace, harmony
Absence of joy
Love and relationships, jealousy

SCHOLTEN: Series 3, Level 16 The homeopathic remedy, sulphur, is the embodiment of Level 15 symptoms. Murphy's Materia Medica lists "imagines himself to be a great person." Senility and senile dementia are part of the sulphur picture.

KALI SULPHURICUM: Stage 16 decay and disorganization dominate this remedy with weariness, vertigo, absentmindedness, anxiety, and deep sadness. Physically, there is a lot of deep yellow mucus and discharges as well as heart palpitations.

SULPHURICUM ACIDUM: Fatigue is always part of the acid picture. The fatigue of the acids added to the stage 16 deterioration can be an ugly picture, indeed. But keep in mind that the purpose of homeopathic treatment is to return the body to a state of balance. In this case, a deepening of faith, insight, compassion, and sufficient strength for the day are the goals of treatment.

OTHERS: *Cadmium sulph, Calcarea sulphurica, Ferrum sulphuricum, Hepar sulphuris calcareum, Natrum sulphuricum, Zincum sulphuricum.*

Kalis

Duty and principlese—task oriented, "stick to it no matter what"
Closed and reserved in personal relationships
Optimistic, hold on to a situation or person too long—even a bad situation
Family or job, takes responsibility for everything and everyone
Holding on—people, events, the past (usually with accompanying constipation)

SCHOLTEN: Series 4, Level 1. The kali remedies are part of the iron series and show a surprising amount of strength for a far left remedy. The strength of a kali, however, is somewhat fragile—brittle, narrow-minded, rigid, and closed off from others.

KALI BROMATUM: The guilt of the bromatums is combined with the duty to principle of the kalis. This often manifests as guilt about religious duties or guilt about past mistakes or about inability to live totally up to every principle and requirement. Feels like he can never do enough to be good enough.

KALI IODATUM: Kalis are about duty, principle, family, and taking responsibility while iodatums seek freedom and escape. These combine to make a nervousness that must be walked off and an inability to cope with the myriad details of everyday life. Often a headache just above the nose and spreading over the eyes.

OTHERS: *Kali arsenicosum, Kali bichromicum, Kali cyanatum , Kali muriaticum, Kali phosphoricum, Kali sulphuricum.*

Ferrums (Iron)

Perseverance, persistence
Firmness, stands ground
History of abuse
Irritability

SCHOLTEN: Series 4, Level 8. The height of productivity and power with the perseverance to make it all work. Stress and pressure sometimes lead to impatience and irritation with other people who are less gifted.

FERRUM PHOSPHORICUM: This remedy combines the rigidity and perseverance of iron with the phosphorus focus on family. In a balanced state, this would be a good thing. Out of balance it creates a rigidity of thinking and irritation when opposed. Wants both to be left alone and to be a good family member. Often alternates between states of anger and apathy. Anemia usually plays a part in this pattern.
FERRUM SULPHURICUM: Firm stance and perseverance, with rigid thinking and an absence of joy that sometimes becomes anger and jealousy.
OTHERS: *Ferrum metallicum, Ferrum iodatum.*

Bromatums

- Guilt, feelings of failure
- Restlessness, escape
- Passion
- Psychosis from guilt with the guilt usually tied to work
- No acceptance of atonement—must "save" self

SCHOLTEN: Series 4, Level 17. As is often the case, the deepening pathology that occurs the further right you go in the periodic table dominates any remedy in which bromatum is found. With homeopathic treatment, there can be peace, acceptance, and humor at this stage instead of the more negative pathologies.
KALI BROMATUM: The kali tendency to hold on to people, events, jobs and everything else combines with stage 17 pathology and becomes a pattern of hanging on by whatever means it takes. This remedy is also characterized by failing mental faculties and loss of memory.
OTHERS: Ammonium bromatum, Arsenicum bromatum, Cadmium bromatum, Radium bromatum.

Iodatums

- Escape
- Food, issues about
- Working, busy, restless, freedom of movement
- Obsessions
- The right to exist
- These are "endocrine system" remedies and are "hot" remedies

SCHOLTEN: Series 4, Level 17. Series 4 has a need to explore and create, but also a deep need to be admired and appreciated. Combined with the patterns of stage 17, there is a tendency to neurosis.

CALCAREA IODATA: The combination of calcarea's sensitivity with iodatum's business and need for approval too often creates burnout. Emotional picture of this remedy is complete indifference and indolence. I include it here because it is a remedy for enlarged tonsils, thyroid tumors, and cysts.
FERRUM IODATUM: Ferrum's rigidity mixed with iodatum's obsessiveness becomes an overblown attention to trifling matters.
OTHERS: *Ammonium iodatum, Arsenicum iodatum, Baryta iodata, Kali iodatum, Plumbum iodatum.*

Metallicums

- Weakness, mind and body
- Rigid thinking, even in depression
- Rigidly negative
- Always right, very stubborn
- Ferrum (iron) - anemia with weakness

SCHOLTEN: Metallicums are found throughout the periodic table and cover several series and stages.

EXAMPLES: *Argentum metallicum, Arsenicum metallicum, Aurum metallicum, Cadmium metallicum, Cuprum metallicum, Ferrum metallicum, Plumbum metallicum, Zincum metallicum.*

NOTES: Acids are always implicated in fatigue. Consider **Bromatums or Iodatums** whenever dealing with **endocrine system** imbalance.

Polycrest Combination Mineral Remedies

As you compare these combinations and the ones listed in the "other examples" sections of the previous pages, try to determine which symptom listed belongs to which family group. For example, in the first remedy which symptoms belong to the calcarea family and which to the carbonicas?

The mentals are most often combined into partnerships—with the resultant combining of two symptom pictures. Studying the remedies by groups—and coming to understand how one group interacts with another is a fascinating thing to do. Besides which, it is easier to remember what is what when thought of in this way.

THE CALCAREAS

All Calcareas are better for warmth and dryness; worse for cold, dampness, drafts or cold applications.

CALCAREA CARBONICA

MENTALS:
 Overworked, overwhelmed
 Strong sense of duty & responsibility
 Works to complete exhaustion
 Anxiety about health
 Feels mind is weak; everybody must know it—this becomes a self-fulfilling prophecy

GENERAL:
 Obesity, flabbiness, puts on weight easily
 Weakness, fatigue, inner trembling, difficulty climbing stairs
 Perspiration back of neck during sleep
 Uterine fibroids with profuse bleeding
 Craves eggs, sweets—pastries & ice cream
 Back weakness, low back pain
 Arthritis, worse from cold and damp
 Cold feet in bed (wears socks to bed)

CALCAREA FLUORATA

MENTALS:
 Indecision, depression
 Anxiety about state of own health
 Prolonged grief from unexpected, sudden loss
 Unreasonable fear of financial loss, poverty, heights, mice

GENERAL:
 Hot flashes w/palpitations then chilliness
 Teeth crumble and break easily; insufficient enamel on teeth—(family genetic pattern seen in children)
 Large, hard uterine fibroids (also Epihysterinum)
 Arthritis, joint pains (nodes), bone spurs
 Stiff neck with a great deal of pain
 Craves sweets, salt, pickles
 Varicose and enlarged veins
 Acute indigestion when fatigued

CALCAREA PHOSPHORICA

MENTALS:
 Peevish, discontented; constantly complaining
 Slow comprehension
 Can be open, friendly, and sensitive
 Never satisfied and easily bored, sighing
 Prostrated by homesickness but when home, wants to go anywhere else
 (Remedy for mentally & physically handicapped children)

GENERAL:
  Obesity, flabbiness, puts on weight easily
  Enlargement of tonsils
  Soft, thin, brittle bones; osteoporosis; spine curvature
  Chronic stomach aches, slow teething in children
  Craving for bacon, ham, salted or smoked meats
  Tip of nose is icy cold

CALCAREA SULPHURICA
MENTALS:
  Always feels hurried
  Sits and thinks and thinks about imagined misfortunes
  Despises those who do not agree with him
  Complains that his views are not understood
  Grumbles about just about everything
  Extreme jealousy

GENERAL:
  Keynote—suppuration—pus, thick, yellow mucus discharges
  Acne, often quite severe
  Abscess, boils—any location will have thick yellow pus
  Craves green, unripe or sour fruit
  Burning, itching of soles of feet
  ***Worse in a warm room**

THE MAGNESIUMS

Magnesiums are noted mainly for anxiety, sadness, and fear of conflict, quarrels, or contention; the symptom pictures vary greatly according to the other half of the remedy.

MAGNESIUM CARBONICUM
MENTALS:
  Anxiety; sad moods all day; trembling and fear of accident; better in the evening on going to bed
  Peacemakers; intolerant of quarrels, confrontations or disharmony
  Fear of aggression or violence
  Sensitive to noise
  Doesn't like to speak in the morning on waking

GENERAL:
  Persons of lax tissues and sour smells.
  Often used in chronic fatigue syndrome and in failure to thrive in infants
  Sleepless from 3 - 4 AM; wakes un-refreshed—comes alive an hour or so later
  Worse before menses—gets a sore throat every month
  Menses flows only at night—stops during day
  Worse for rest—must get up and walk around; hates to be uncovered

MAGNESIUM MURIATICUM
MENTALS:
  Aversion to quarrels; peacemaker; great passivity
  Cannot cope with life; depression
  Anxiety worse in bed, lying down, eyes closed
  Sensitive to noise
  Convinced looks old and has suddenly aged
  Uneasiness; anxiety; tends to weep easily and often
  Anxiousness is better outside in open air

GENERAL:
  Cannot digest milk—diarrhea and abdominal pain
  Liver enlargement
  Loss of smell and taste
  Craves sweets; hungry but doesn't know for what
  Craves vegetables, fruits, light foods, salads
  Palpitations, heart pain worse sitting—better moving
  Likes lying on left side—worse lying on right side
  Most things better from hard pressure
  Very unrefreshed on waking
  Toxic feeling of dullness

MAGNESIUM PHOSPHORICUM
MENTALS:
  Irritable
  May experience phosphorus type fears
  Learning and thinking clearly are difficult
  Ailments and drowsiness brought on by study
  Discontented, dissatisfied
  Oversensitive to pain, noise, excitement
  Pain brings on anxiety
  Talks to himself constantly (feels like it to others) but also often sits in moody silence

GENERAL:
  Liver less affected than with other magnesiums—irritable, but less so and sour, but less so
  Facial neuralgia, right-sided; pain behind ear
  Bloated full sensation in abdomen
  Menstrual cramps, pain before flow
  Heart—palpitations, constricting pains
  Cramps in calves
  Writer's cramps
  Toothache better for heat and hot liquids
  Pain is better for pressure, bending
  Better from heat, warmth, hard pressure, rubbing
  Worse from cold air, drafts, night
  Worse on right side

THE KALIS

The most important characteristics of the kali salts is the strong sense of duty. Each salt then picks up the basic characteristics of its "other half," making some very interesting mixes. These remedies, especially Kali bromatum, are dramatically effective when the symptoms clearly match.

KALI PHOSPHORICUM
MENTALS:
  Mental/physical exhaustion after stress
  Brain fatiguee—mental exertion aggravates
  Slightest labor feels like a monumental task
  Hypersensitivity to noise, etc.
  Feels unable to cope; nervous dread/anxiety
  Strong emotions such as anger, grief, or fright bring on illnesses
  Gloom sliding into deep depression
  Weak memory; forgetful; loss of memory
  Shyness; dislike of meeting new people and talking with them
  Nervous anxiety with dread

GENERAL:
  Famous remedy for exhaustion/chronic fatigue
  Kali sense of duty combines with the phosphorus need to communicate & to keep friends informed about each other's lives
  Kali duty with phosphorus tendency to be upset at bad news (should have been able to fix or prevent it)
  Humming and buzzing in the ears
  Sleeplessness from worry, too much mental activity, or business troubles
  Temperature—neutral

KALI CARBONICUM

MENTALS:
  Compulsive adherence to rules
  Obstinate, dogmatic
  Full of imagination and fear
  Stoic; uncomplaining
  Reluctant and resistant to any type of change

GENERAL:
  Kali sense of duty with the carbonicum's need for values and rules; this can get out of hand
  Anxiety produces nausea/pain in stomach
  Swollen eyelids
  Asthma, worse during the night (2-4 AM)
  Back pain during the night
  Severe back pain during menses, pregnancy, labor, or following a miscarriage
  Ineffectual labor pains
  Sleeplessness—"can't let go of day's events"
  Worse at night and from cold—even cold drinks

KALI NITRICUM

MENTALS:
  Anxiety about health
  Hold grudges when others fail in their duty
  Feels it is their duty to work hard before they can play (not workaholics—they do play, especially with their children when their work is done)
  Fears confinement and limits

GENERAL:
  Asthma, worse night and must sit up
  Cravings for fats
  Temperature: warm but generally worse for heat

KALI BROMATUM

MENTALS:
  Combine kali rigidness with bromatum guilt—Guilt about duties/responsibilitiese—often religious
  Feels forsaken by God or singled ouT for special punishment because they did not do their duty
  Need to escape "righteous" punishment

GENERAL:
  Nervous system problems
  Convulsions; catatonic states; autism; night terrors
  Wringing of hands
  Temperature: warm

THE NATRUMS

Eeyore attitude—gloomy; great sensitivity but feel they must carry their grief, burdens and sadness inside. Because of their pervading sense of loss, all natrum people tend to hold on to situations, people, memories.

NATRUM CARBONICUM

MENTALS:
  Mild and kind
  Need to find value or reason in life's experiences
  Aversions to certain people
  Profound sadness, depression, and melancholy
  Suffers grief with dignity
  Excessively cheerful—even when sad inside
    "cheerful" is not usually a Natrum characteristic, you must notice "sad inside, faking it" part

GENERAL:
  Indigestion; overall weak digestion; food allergies; sensitive to milk
  Headache from the sun or from exposure to hot weather
  Weak ankles; easily dislocated and sprained
  Worse from milk and starches—creates diarrhea

NATRUM MURIATICUM

Nat mur is a very commonly needed remedy—the emotions (deep grief and sorrow) touch us all

MENTALS:
  Ailments from grief and disappointment in love
  Sad yet unable to weep—finally hysterical weeping
  Aversion to company
  Severe depression and feeling of isolation

GENERAL:
  Headache, migraine—worse from light
  Hay fever; cold sores; cracked lips
  "Bashful kidney"—unable to urinate
  Asthma—in the evening
  Back pain—better for hard bed or pressure
  Insomnia—thinking about past or day's griefs

NATRUM PHOSPHORICUM

MENTALS:
  Extremely refined
  Easily frightened
  Startling from noise
  Fears dark and thunderstorms
  Fears of Phosphorus—tends to the depression of the natrums with the need for communication of the
    phosphorus remedies but, like all natrums, consider it wrong to share certain parts of themselves
  Lonely and depressed after death of close confidant

GENERAL:
  Yellow coating of tongue, base of tongue and throat
  Craves eggs, particularly fried and salted
  Asthma—worse in evenings
  Worse from acids and citrus fruits
  Hives, especially around the ankles

NATRUM SULPHURICUM

MENTALS:
 Confusion after head injuries
 Suicidal longings; won't usually commit suicide because of how it would affect their family
 Serious, overly responsible
 Sensitive to music

GENERAL:
 Asthma—worse early mornings
 Liver and gallbladder disorders
 Headache after head injury
 Craves yogurt, fish, ice, sweets, chocolate
 Eyes are unusually sensitive to light
 Worse for warmth and humidity
 Worse for damp weather

THE FERRUMS

FERRUM METALLICUM (IRON)

MENTALS:
 Firmness; stands ground
 Forceful; determined
 Preoccupied with business matters
 Irritable—especially when contradicted
 Overly sensitive
 Often quite aggressive and domineering
 Great sensitivity to noises such as paper rustling when they are "working"
 Feels that people are compelling them to act "against their wishes"
 Often these people suffered beatings and abuse as a child

GENERAL:
 Anemia
 Flushes of heat with slight exertion but feels worse from resting
 Long, continual headaches—often lasting 3-4 days
 Periodic headaches—every 14 days is common
 Pale face which flushes easily or red flushed face (color in this face is not a sign of health)
 Craves sweets, bread and butter, and tomatoes—Aversion: eggs, tomatoes

FERRUM PHOSPHORICUM

The characteristics of Ferrum and Phosphorus are nearly opposites, making people needing this remedy particularly difficult to identify.

MENTAL:
 Characterized by extremes—very talkative and excited or keeps very quiet. Anger or apathy
 Often averse to company or fears going into crowds

GENERAL:
 Acute: high fever—usually 102 degrees or higher. Fever but no local or individual symptoms
 Paleness of face alternating with redness
 Sensitivity and fear of light. Triggers headache with fever
 Anemia. Blood disorders. Hemorrhages
 Conditions are usually right-sided (pneumonia, shoulder pain, etc.)
 Tonsillitis. Tonsils red and swollen
 Useful for first stages of all inflammatory disorders

Additional Mineral Remedies

CAUSTICUM
Great remedy for chronic diseases. Affects all organ systems with special affinity for the nervous system and connective tissues. Affects all 3 of the basic miasms.

GENERALS:
 Mild paralysis is a keynote
 Manifests in brain as memory loss. Can manifest throughout the body as lack of involuntary muscle
   control (bladder, vocal cords, eyelids, muscle coordination), voluntary muscles (rheumatisms,
   contraction of tendons, trembling, cramps here and there)
 Restlessness at night, particularly the legs which are constantly "on the go"
 Burning sensations, whatever the area or symptom, is a great keynote

MENTALS:
 Great sympathy, great anger over injustices, political activism, rebellion
 Strong sense of duty; takes care of everybody when they are threatened (perceives threats everywhere)
 Symptoms arising from great grief is a prominent keynote
 Short term memory loss; confusion in speech
 2-sided nature: strong, reliable, stable, even tempered, self-respecting, great speech skills, intelligent, quick thinking
  or fierce anger, righteous indignation, distrust of authority, confrontational, rebellion against authority

MODALITIES:
 Better from cold drinks, damp weather, warmth of bed, gentle motion
 Worse from clear weather, dry cold air, winds, extremes of temperature, 3-4 am, evening 6-8 pm
 COMPARISONS: Natrum muriaticum, Phosphorus, Sepia succus, Staphysagria

GRAPHITES NATURALIS
Powerful anti-psoric; effective for wide variety of ailments if mentals and emotionals fit.

GENERALS:
 Strong anti-psoric—particularly useful to close a case
 Sluggish metabolism
 Unhealthy skin; tends to eczema, psoriasis; tends to scabs and fissures everywhere
 Cobweb sensations on the face
 Thickening of skin, glands, nails, old scars
 Edema of legs
 Particular affinity for the digestive system, the skin, mucus membranes and the metabolism

MENTALS:
 Needs creative self-expression
 Lacks self-confidence in their thinking skills
 Has trouble concentrating. Can memorize without understanding
 Anxious, fastidious—control of details lessens anxiety
 (controlling the details means being prepared and that means survival—can relax)
 Music brings tears

MODALITIES:
 Better in dark and all wrapped up, yet better from walking in open air; weeping
 Worse from hot drinks; cold; drafts; suppression of eruptions; fats; warmth, too warm bed at night

COMPARISONS:
 Pulsatilla nigricans, Antimonium crudum, Cina maritima, Calcarea phosphorica, Hepar sulph calcareum

HEPAR SULPHURIS CALCAREUM
Consider whenever there is abscess with suppuration and copious amounts of mucus, whether the abscess is internal or external.

GENERALS:
  Splinter like pains
  Works on skin and gastrointestinal issues
  Very cold remedy
  Vulnerable to infections, sepsis, weather changes, chemicals, excess noise and light
  Every little injury suppurates
  Deep cracks on hands and feet

MENTALS:
  A great sensitivity to pain and any outside stimuli
  Violent impulses, especially when offended
  Attraction to fire
  Hypochondria
  Irritable, impatient, critical, hurried
  Vulnerability; feelings of being threatened; feelings of vulnerability lead to despair and suicidal thoughts
  Impulsive; impulses to commit violent act

MODALITIES:
  Better in damp weather
  Worse from slightest draft; From wrapping head
  COMPARISONS: Nux vomica, Lycopodium clavatum

MERCURIUS SOLUBILIS THIS POLYCREST REMEDY FOR USE WITH SHINGLES
Remember the symptoms by thinking of human thermometers—sensitive to heat and cold. Mercurius should be considered whenever the patient is worse for both hot and cold. #1 anti-syphilitic remedy according to Hahnemann.

GENERALS:
  Inherited weakness in vitality. Over 60 listed factors that aggravate, only 8 that improve
  Affects lymphatic system (all membranes, glands), internal organs, bones, tissues, blood, etc.)
  Affects profoundly the reproductive organs of both sexes
  Indicated for cases of trembling, especially in the hands, Parkinson's disease

MENTALS:
  Intense emotions held in as impulses (to scream, to poke, tickle, jab, injure oneself on seeing knives, etc.
  Irresolution, constantly changing one's mind
  Poor self-confidence
  Loss of will power
  Weak memory, forgetful
  Feeling of being dominated by dictatorial authority
  Need to escape
  Weary of life; indifferent to everything (in extreme cases)
  Overall syphilitic dominance (situation is beyond repair and must be drastically altered or destroyed)

MODALITIES:
  Better from moderate temperature; sensitive to both hot and cold—made worse by both heat and cold
  Better from rest
  Worse at night and from heat and cold. Cloudy, damp weather. Drafts. Wet feet. Touching anything cold. Warmth of bed. Rainy weather. Glare of light

SILICA TERRA (SILICEA)
Helps improve defective nutrition when lack of assimilation is the problem; especially useful for children. Removes splinters, bits of glass and other obstructions from the body

Silica terra is commonly seen in flint and sand; this is reflected in the remedy—certain grittiness, a tendency to form hard lumps, etc. Sand is parent material for glass, thus, the brittleness of this remedy

GENERALS:
Can stimulate the body to reabsorb fibroids, scar tissues and deal with pus formation
Lack of vital heat
Tends to easy exhaustion
Symptoms brought on by ill effects of vaccination
Person has tendency to brittle bones, nails, teeth, hair
Also tendency to growths, cysts, abscesses, deposits and chronic dry nasal obstructions

MENTALS:
Lack of self-confidence, overwhelmed by task
Anxiety from noise
Stage fright

MODALITIES:
Worse in winter (feels cold, chilly, hugs the fire, and wants warm clothing)
Averse to fats, milk
Often adversely affected by vaccination
Better from heat and massage

This is a remedy that I use often; lack of assimilation is so common these days, creating problems with hair, skin and nails. Silica terra will also remove a sliver or embedded piece of glass, etc. Because of its effects on the pus of early infection. Silica is a follow-up (companion remedy) of Pulsatilla nigricans

SULPHUR
Great anti-psoric. Use when carefully selected remedy fails to act in acute diseases, or the person relapses.

GENERALS:
Headaches, often as if a band about the head or burning on the vertex
Particularly bright red lips
Eye infection and irritation with the sensation of sand or grit in eyes
Empty hungry feeling every day at 11 AM
Heartburn, from dietary indiscretions
Weak back, slumps in chair
Insomnia, sleeps only for 3-4 hours, then wakes and dozes for rest of night
Itching. Skin afflictions

MENTALS:
Egotism, bragging
Indifferent to appearance
Disgust at odors, objects, people (slovenly himself but critical of it in others)
Extroverted, boisterous, friendly, bossy as children (sometimes as adults)

MODALITIES:
Better from dry, warm weather, lying on right side, from curling in a ball, from open air, motion, walking
Worse for standing, resting, stooping, reaching high, much warmth in bed, milk, atmospheric changes

COMPARISONS:
Nux vomica, Psorinum, Lycopodium clavatum, Argentum nitricum

Chapter Eighteen - Remedies of the Plant Kingdom

Dr. David Stewart (The Chemistry of Essential Oils Made Easy) claims that plant classification varies quite a bit from country to country around the world. Sometimes a plant is categorized in more than one country in the same year or two, but the discovery and classification did not make it into common texts for some years after that. Other times, the variation in classification is the natural result of the variety and complexity of the plant kingdom. Sometimes also, a name for a class or family has been changed, but old texts and references do not contain that change. Since we are talking about Sankaran's idea of the theme of each family, it only makes sense to use the classification and naming system that he uses.

Many family groups have only one representative among the well-known homeopathic remedies. These remedies are placed in alphabetical order at the end of this chapter. The index provided at the end of this book will provide an alphabetical listing of the remedies with the pages on which they are mentioned.

I will not attempt to write a complete Materia Medica here in this small book. There are great ones on the market already. Hopefully, you have already purchased at least one of these. I will provide you a few keynotes and mental symptoms. I will also give you insights into which plants for which miasm, according to Sankaran and others, wherever possible.

I will also try to point out how one member of a family differs from another. It is these differences that determine which miasm a remedy is best suited to treating. As stated previously, miasms differ in the intensity of the symptoms and the desperation with which the sensations are met and handled. The list of miasms on pages on 100 through 102 are listed from the least severe, acute, to the most severe and desperate and destructive, syphilis.

Anacardiaceae Family (Cashew - Poison Ivy)

MAIN THEME: stuck. Sensations: caught, not allowed to move, tight, stiff, restricted. Passive reactions: paralysed, immobile. Active reactions: wanting to break out and move constantly, aggravated by being still, but pain on beginning to move. Compensation: always on the move.

ANACARDIUM ORIENTALE (MARKING NUT)

This remedy is often used in treatments for cancer; considered an antidote to poison ivy; mental disorders, manic depressive states, hearing voices; very easily offended; forgetfulness; Alzheimer's; eczema with intense itching.
KEYNOTES: Pressing pains as if a plug in any locality. These pains are connected with neuralgia but may occur in the abdomen, eyes, head or anywhere. All symptoms better during a meal.
SANKARAN MENTALS: Leprosy miasm: in a very tight corner, completely controlled, and not allowed to move. The reaction to this perception is cruelty.
MIASM: Cancere—must somehow maintain control even though being held tightly or in a very tight corner; also the leprosy miasm
COMPARISONS: Rhus toxicodendron, Rhus radicans, Apis mellifica, Ferrum metallicum, Lycopodium, Pulsatilla nigricans, Causticum, Thuja occidentalis

RHUS RADICANS (CLIMBING IVY)

There is much dispute about whether there is a substantial difference between Rhus radicans and Rhus toxicodendron. Note the slight differences that Sankaran points out between the mentals of each remedy as they relate to the miasms of malaria and typhoid.
AILMENTS: From straining a single part, muscle or tendon. Backaches and stiffness of back and neck. Eruptions on skin. Neuralgic pains. Intermittent fevers.
KEYNOTES: Inflammation of the joints with wandering pains and stiffness.

SANKARAN MENTALS: according to Sankaran: Caught in a tight spot where there is a feeling of being attacked. These feelings are not constant but occur from time to time, intermittently.
MIASM: Malaria
COMPARISONS: Rhus toxicodendron

RHUS TOXICODENDRON (POISON OAK)
One of the most important polycrests. Often remembered only as an arthritis remedy, Rhus toxicodendron also covers many mental disorders and deep pathologies of the nervous system and spine, the heart and almost all other organ systems!! Low back pain and sciatica, usually worse for stillness, which causes stiffness. It is interesting to note that the people suffering the physical symptoms of arthritis, back pain and sciatica often do not show the typical mental picture of anxiety and restlessness because movement is so painful. They feel it, however. Consider this remedy for shingles, chicken pox, connective tissue disease, eczema, impetigo, Parkinsons's disease; ailments brought on or worsened by financial loss
KEYNOTES: Always considered for injuries and sprains, particularly to joints.
SANKARAN MENTALS: Stuck in a bad situation; must escape immediately before it gets more dangerous.
MIASM: Typhoid
COMPARISONS: Ruta graveolens—Rhus toxicodendron is more general and commonly used than Ruta graveolens

Berberidaceae Family (Barberry)

MAIN THEME: I recover from sudden changes in my life by changing my nature, just as suddenly, to match. The situation is viewed as temporary and, if handled properly by changing themselves *temporarily*, a complete fix is possible. Sensations: of sudden, intense, rapid changing at the mental and physical levels. Passive reactions: confusion, dullness, confusion of identity. Active reaction: the rapid change of character, and sometimes location and job status. Compensations: learns to easily adapt to situations and people

BERBERIS AQUIFOLIUM (OREGON GRAPE)
Syphilis is a deep and difficult miasm to treat. This is one of the most important remedies for these situations, *if a plant remedy rather than an animal one is indicated*. Intense pulsating headaches in the forehead—a two inch band around the head pulling tighter and tighter. Pain in joints of hands and lower back. Slower metabolism with incomplete digestion; all symptoms worse in the evening and at night.
KEYNOTES: Unhappiness and depression coming on suddenly; pimples, skin eruptions and scaly skin.
SANKARAN MENTALS: The combining of the Berberidaceae change and adaptability with the destruction and destructiveness that is characteristic of the deep and difficult syphilis miasm, gives us a person who is destroyed by sudden change. They simply lack any ability to adapt to new types of situations. Thus, marriage, the birth of a child, a job change, or a move to a new city can bring out the characteristics of the syphilis miasm (which is the worst and deepest of the earliest recognized pathologies).
MIASM: Syphilis
COMPARISONS: Sulphur, Psorinum, Arsenicum album, Hydrastis canadensis

BERBERIS VULGARIS (BARBERRY)
Inflammation of kidneys with severe pain; kidney stones; gallstones; tearing, sharp pains in chest; beating or fluttering noises in the ears; dryness and burning of the eyes; headache that is like a tight cap over entire head; eczema; sleepiness during the day; nausea before breakfast, better after.
KEYNOTES: Rapidly changing pattern of symptoms; pains radiate out from one point; pain often described as bubbling.
SANKARAN MENTALS: The malarial feeling of stuck in a situation; the situation is that you have to keep dealing with totally different situations in quick succession, one right after another, forever.
MIASM: Malaria
COMPARISONS: Ipomoea purpurea, Aloe socotrina, Lycopodium, Nux vomica, Sarsaparilla, Thuja occidentalis, Arsenicum album, and many others

CAULOPHYLLUM THALICTROIDES (BLUE COHOSH)

Special sphere of this remedy is women in labor. Acts primarily on the uterus, and to a lesser extent on the muscles. One of the best remedies in labor, especially when labor pains are weak or irregular due to lack of tone in the uterus or exhaustion on the part of the woman; arthritis of the fingers or toes; thrush; headache over left eye, with pressure behind the eye; fretful, irritable, and apprehensive.
KEYNOTES: Habitual miscarriage from uterine debility; weak or irregular labor pains; false labor; arthritis of small joints.
SANKARAN MENTALS: Intense need to hide and cover up a sudden change that has occurred.
MIASM: Sycotic
COMPARISONS: Viola odorata, Cimicifuga racemosa, Sepia succus, Gelsemium sempervirens, Belladonna, Calcarea phosphorica, Lilium tigrinum, Magnesia muriatica.

PODOPHYLLUM PELTATUM (MAY APPLE)

In digestive difficulties Podophyllum peltatum affects mostly the duodenum, small intestines, and liver. Hemorrhoids. Prolapsed uterus. Stools yellow with undigested food. Dislike of change. Mind going quickly from one subject to another.
KEYNOTES: Alternating conditions—headache/diarrhea, diarrhea/constipation, hot/cold; most afflictions will be on the right side of the body.
SANKARAN MENTALS: The typhoid sensation that a critical problem can be fixed if handled properly combines with the Berberidaceae to convince the person that if they change themselves quickly enough to meet the situation, all will be well.
MIASM: Typhoid
COMPARISONS: Mandragora, Aloe socotrina, Chelidonium, Mercurius, Nux vomica, Sulphur.

Cactaceae Family (Cactus)

MAIN THEME: The remedies in this family are used predominantly for the heart, in both homeopathy and herbal medicine. The main theme is tightness and constriction. Sensations are constricted, made smaller, trapped, downtrodden, oppressed, weighed down. The passive reaction is to shrink or feel shrunken. The active reaction is to expand in opposition to the oppression, becoming boundless and released. Compensation—to never allow oneself to be affected by contraction and restriction.

CACTUS GRANDIFLORUS (NIGHT BLOOMING CEREUS)

General weakness and prostration; irregular circulation; sadness; apprehension; fear of death; fluttering and palpitations of the heart, made worse by lying on left side; numbness of left arm; cold sweat on face; coldness of limbs; cries but doesn't know why; is made worse by consolation from others; right-sided facial pain; congestive headaches.
KEYNOTES: Heart and circulation tonic; symptoms of heart attack; spasmodic pains; feels compressed.
SANKARAN MENTALS: Feeling of being stuck in a situation, then suddenly released.
MIASM: Malaria
COMPARISONS: Digitalis purpurea, Spigelia anthelmintica, Lachesis muta, Belladonna.

CEREUS BONPLANDII (A VARIETY OF CACTUS GLANDIFLORUS)

Gloomy and restless, desire to be useful; pain in chest running down toward spleen; pain in left arm and left lower ribs; sighing with breaths, as though chest is being compressed; occipital headaches with pain in the eyes; mental and physical pains alternate with only one or the other present at a time.
KEYNOTES: Antipsoric of great power; itching, eczema.
SANKARAN MENTALS: Feels oppressed and shrunken, almost choked and suffocated. The reaction is the need to perform useful deeds at a hectic pace.
MIASM: Tuberculosis, Psora
COMPARISONS: Cactus grandiflorus, Spigelia anthelmintica, Kalmia latifolia.

Compositae Family (Aster - Daisy - Sunflower)

MAIN THEME: The main theme is injury. Sensations are injured, hurt, insulted, shocked, fear of being touched. Passive reaction is physical and emotional numbness. Active reactions are touchy, cruel, violent, hurts others. Compensates by being the tough guy, protecting others so they avoid being hurt.

ABROTANUM ARTEMISIA (SOUTHERNWOOD)

A very powerful children's remedy. Malnutrition in children, with failure to thrive. Intense indigestion. Ravenous appetite but emaciation, nevertheless. Alternating diarrhea/constipation. Movement of symptoms from place to place—for example, pain first in one joint and then others. Weakness after illness.
KEYNOTES: Great appetite but emaciated anyway, particularly in the lower limbs. Progression of symptoms throughout the body or system. Food passes undigested.
SANKARAN MENTALS: Feeling oppressed and suffocated by an injury, hurt, or insult.
MIASM: Tubercular
COMPARISONS: Scrophularia nodosa, Bryonia alba, Natrum muriaticum, Iodium purum, China officinalis, Ledum palustre, Nux vomica.

ARNICA MONTANA (LEOPARD'S BANE)

This is a favorite remedy of mine in every potency and also made into an oil (soaked).

Arnica—when not in homeopathic form—is **not to be taken internally** and should be used with care on an open wound as it can be an irritant to tissues, especially mucus membranes. Use for trauma and its effects, long ago or recent—from blows, falls, injuries, contusions, bruises, sprains. Amazingly effective where there has been bleeding into soft tissues. Use post-operative for pain and to promote rapid healing. Excellent remedy in labor and immediately postpartum.
KEYNOTES: Influenza with bruised muscles; severe mental stress or shock, particularly following an injury; restless in bed; can't get comfortable, everything feels too hard; wants to be left alone; insists that he is fine; use in women for labor pains that are weak and intermittent and the woman feels as if she is bruising and swelling internally.
SANKARAN MENTALS: Great fear of being hurt, mentally as well as physically; fear of being approached or touched lest he be hurt even worse; fear of approaching others.
MIASM: Acute
COMPARISONS: Bellis perennis, Baptisia tinctoria, Rhus toxicodendrom, Calcarea phosphorica, Ruta graveolens, Bryonia alba, Sulphur, Pyrogenium, Opium.

BELLIS PERENNIS (DAISY)

Trauma, similar to Arnica in many respects; injuries to the deeper tissues after major surgery; septic wounds; use for sore bruised feeling in pelvic area; migraine headaches with pain in the eyes; boils; prone to illness after a sudden chill or soaking.
KEYNOTES: Profound effect on female organs and complaints; varicose veins; predominantly left-sided remedy.
SANKARAN MENTALS: Controlling, or need to control, every potential problem; tidiness and punctuality considered extremely important.
MIASM: Cancer
COMPARISONS: Ruta graveolens, Arnica montana.

CALENDULA OFFICINALIS (POT MARIGOLD)

A remarkable healing agent, applied locally or taken internally. Treatment of wounds, abrasions, incisions, tears (vaginal in childbirth). Antiseptic to prevent infections—dramatic when taken internally in high potency. Astringent—will control bleeding used topically. Soothing for skin conditions.

KEYNOTES: Great tendency to catch cold, especially in damp weather; tendency to vaginal tears during childbirth. Heartburn.

SANKARAN MENTALS: Fear that something terrible will happen suddenly; always anticipating a shock or trauma.
MIASM: Acute
COMPARISONS: Staphysagria, Arnica, Arsenicum album, Bryonia, Licata, Carbo animalis, Carbo vegetabilis, Hamamelis, Hypericum, Ledum palustre, Nitricum acidum, Phosphorus, Rhus toxicodendron, Symphytum officinale.

CHAMOMILLA VULGARIS (GERMAN CHAMOMILE)
Hypersensitivity to pain. Patient seems to feel, and complain about, more pain than the situation warrants. Commonly used as a remedy for childhood disorders—if there is anger, complaining and irritability present. Difficulty and diarrhea when teething. Whining and clinging to mother.
KEYNOTES: Feet hot, must kick off the covers; restless sleep, wakes often; better for complaining Ailments from being insulted or humiliated—insults and humiliates in return; body feels cold but the face is burning hot
SANKARAN MENTALS: Constant fretting, and suspicion that he may have been insulted, or in the case of children, left alone.
MIASM: Typhoid
COMPARISONS: Cina maritima, Calcarea phosphorica, Antimonium crudum, Pulsatilla nigricans, Sulphur, Hepar sulphuris calcareum, Nux vomica, Colocynthis.

CINA MARITIMA (WORMSEED)
The first remedy for worms and other parasites. KEYNOTES: does not want to be touched or even have someone come near; ailments occur at the same time each day.
KEYNOTES: Extreme irritability; child cannot be quieted; capricious; angry; tantrums, to the point of convulsions; tantrums or convulsions from being disciplined; constantly picks at nose.
SANKARAN MENTALS: Feels that he is being persecuted by insults and emotional injuries.
MIASM: Malaria
COMPARISONS: Chamomilla vulgaris, Arum metallicum, Medorrhinum.

ECHINACEA ANGUSTIFOLIA/PURPUREA (PURPLE CONE FLOWER)
Blood and immune disorders; blood poisoning; septic conditions; gangrene; lymphatic clogging; bites of poisonous or venomous animals and insects; slowness in speech, action, pace; vertigo; headache with pale face; sleepiness with confusion and weakness.
KEYNOTES: Chilliness with nausea; achiness in limbs.
SANKARAN MENTALS: Feeling shattered by trauma; feels sense of self has been destroyed.
MIASM: Syphilis and Vaccinosis
COMPARISONS: many, the closest is Baptisia tinctoria.

EUPATORIUM PERFOLIATUM (BONESET)
There is another Eupatorium—purpureum (gravel root)

Influenza; recurrent fevers; malaria; also used for pain of fractured bones; great thirst followed by chilliness and aching of bones; hoarseness and cough with soreness in the chest; worse at night.
KEYNOTES: Tremendous aching in the bones, especially lower back; chilliness, but craves cold drinks.
SANKARAN MENTALS: Feels unable to cope with impending acute threat because of some deficiency in himself. Very anxious.
MIASM: Malaria
COMPARISONS: Bryonia alba, Pyrogenium, Natrum muriaticum.

ARCTIUM LAPPA (BURDOCK)
Diarrhea alternating with arthritic symptoms; gas; bloating; belching; uterine displacement; worse from wet and cold and from lying on right side; cold sweat with a sour smell.
KEYNOTES: Sour stomach. All food turns sour in stomach; vomiting.
SANKARAN MENTALS: The Leprosy miasm is just one degree less desperate than Syphilis. Includes feelings of worthlessness, hopelessness, even suicide. Sensation is a feeling that she must take all abuse and protect others from harm in order to be of value as a person.
MIASM: Leprosy
COMPARISONS: Arnica montana, Calendula officinalis, Cina maritima, Bryonia alba, Sepia succus.

ACHILLEA MILLEFOLIUM (YARROW)
Often used if an injury has not responded to Arnica; affects capillaries, particularly in the lungs; use for wounds that bleed profusely; nosebleeds; painful varicose veins during pregnancy; kidney stones—including pain after removal of stones: blood in the urine; ill effects of operations; sadness alternating with irritability and even violence; piercing thrusts of pain in the head; severe bruises from falling; wounds that bruise.
KEYNOTES: Continued high temperature; profuse bleeding—hemorrhages.
SANKARAN MENTALS: Feels isolated and oppressed by injuries and insults; hopelessness.
MIASM: Leprosy
COMPARISONS: The Composites generally. Arnica montana, Belladonna, Calendula officinalis

SENECIO AUREUS (GOLDEN RAGWORT)
Aversion or dislike of family and of self; self-centered; selfish; sadness; depression; marked effect on female and urinary organs, especially the bladder; backaches of congested kidneys; enlarged prostate in males.
KEYNOTES: Amenorrhea and other menstrual disorders; wavelike dizziness; sharp pains over left eye and through the left temple; constant urging of urine.
SANKARAN MENTALS: Avoiding hurt, insult, and injury by covering up and/or hiding himself.
MIASM: Sycotic
COMPARISONS: Caulophyllum thalictroides, Sepia succus, Arnica montana, Calendula officinalis, Pulsatilla nigricans, Bryonia alba.

TARAXACUM OFFICINALE (DANDELION)
Impatient and irritable, then talkative, laughing and merry; food tastes sour; gallstones; neuralgia of the knees; profuse night sweats; sleepiness in daytime; nausea with an inclination to vomiting from fatty foods; nausea with headache.
KEYNOTES: Cold fingertips; headaches due to liver disturbances; tongue coated or mapped
SANKARAN MENTALS: The ringworm miasm alternates between despair with inability, and great activity and struggle against perceived hurt. Taraxacum's sensation is struggling against injury, hurt and insult. Sometimes able to avoid it, and sometimes just accepting it, but never aggressively fighting back.
MIASM: Ringworm
COMPARISONS: Bryonia alba, Chelidonium majus, Hydrastis canadensis, Lycopodium clavatum, Nux vomica, Arsenicum album.

Conifers (Pine - Fir - Cypress)

MAIN THEME: The main theme is brittle, meaning easily broken or snapped. Sensations are feelings of being fragile, broken, connected then disconnected, empty then full, cut off from others. Passive reactions are feelings of lassitude, fearfulness, and weakness. Active reactions are being very rigid or hard. Compensates by showing great strength and being protective of others who are as brittle and fragile as they often feel.

ABIES NIGRA (BLACK SPRUCE)
As if something hard was lodged in the cardiac end of the esophagus; wakeful at night with hunger; digestive problems of the elderly, with functional heart symptoms; low spirits and unable to think or study; lungs feel as if they cannot be fully expanded.
KEYNOTES: stomach disorders—pain in the stomach always occurs after eating; constipation; tachycardia.
SANKARAN MENTALS: A sense of being more fragile than most, accompanied by intermittent attacks of panic due to the possibility of being broken or disconnected from things that are important to them.
MIASM: Ringworm
COMPARISONS: China officinalis, Bryonia alba, Pulsatilla nigricans, Nux vomica, Kali carbonicum, other conifers such as Thuja occidentalis, Sabina officinalis.

AGATHIS AUSTRALIS (KAURI TREE)
Mental power increased; memory for past events very good; restlessness and irritability; mistakes about left and right sides; bulimia; quarrelsome with family; boring pain, extending to right shoulder; constant urging to urinate; thirsty; burning pain in sternum, pressure aggravates; the face is generally pale; appetite increased with menses; tension headaches; photophobia during headaches; coldness at night in bed; unrefreshing sleep that is disturbed by dreams; floaty feeling with a tendency to fall forward.
KEYNOTES: Suddenness and violence of symptoms; moods are changeable, weeping and laughing at the same time.
SANKARAN MENTALS: Feeling that they have been suddenly broken into pieces.
MIASM: Acute

PIX LIQUIDA (PINE TAR)
Pine-tar has always been considered a stimulating expectorant for use in chronic bronchitis and tuberculosis; acts on the mucus membranes; alopecia; constant vomiting of black fluid with great pain in the stomach; cracked skin which itches intolerably and bleeds when scratched; sleeplessness because of the itching; eruptions on the back of the hands; often cures the bed-wetting of children; psoriasis and scaly eczema.
KEYNOTES: Chest pain; stomach pain, itching; vomiting; spitting up of sputum from the lungs that has an offensive odor and taste; constant vomiting of black fluids with pain in the stomach.
SANKARAN MENTALS: Feeling held back and oppressed because he is more fragile and brittle than others.
MIASM: Tubecular
COMPARISONS: Terebinthiniae oleum, Pinus sylvestris, Kreosotum, Myrica cerifera, Theridion curassavicum.

SABINA OFFICINALIS (SAVINE)
Fibroids with pain from the sacrum to the pubis; desires peace and quiet; in childbirth, retained placenta with intense pain; arthritic pain in joints; dry hacking cough with tickling in the trachea; sensation and dreams of falling; hemorrhages during menopause; hot flashes.
KEYNOTES: Dysmenorrhea; excessive menstruation; hemorrhages; miscarriages; warts; music is intolerable.
SANKARAN MENTALS: In control of the situation and of self even when broken or disconnected.

MIASM: Cancer
COMPARISONS: Calcarea carbonica, Trillium pendulum, Ipomoea purpurea, Achillea Millefolium, Thuja occidentalis, Sepia succus, Hamamelis virginiana, Nitricum acidum, Caulophyllum thalictroides, Cantharis to promote expulsion of foreign bodies from the uterus, Secale cornutum, Platinum metallicum for dark hemorrhage, Sabina officinalis for bright red hemorrhage, Belladonna, Rhus toxicodendron, Spongia tosta.

TEREBINTHINIAE OLEUM (OIL OF TURPENTINE)

Loathing of life; suicidal disposition; distention of the abdomen; burning and tightness across the chest; voice sounds unnatural to self, humming like a seashell; vertigo with loss of vision and nausea; poor equilibrium.
KEYNOTES: Inflammation of the kidneys; irritable bladder; burning pain in kidneys; odor of violets.
SANKARAN MENTALS: Demanding a connection with others or an organization, and demanding it right now!
MIASM: Typhoid
COMPARISONS: Alumen crudum, Secale cornutum, Cantharis vesicatoria, Nitricum acidum
Thuja occidentalis (arbor vitae).

Profound loneliness or emptiness; cannot concentrate; aversion to company; anxious dreams; left-sided headaches with pain as though pierced by a nail; fingernails are brittle, and distorted, or soft, distorted, and crumbling; cracking in joints when stretching them; hemorrhoids; urine stops several times before the bladder is emptied; chronic sinus infection; brown spots on hands and arms; skin eruptions but only on covered parts; chilly from least change of weather.
KEYNOTES: Exhaustion and emaciation; warty growths; depression, feels isolated and alone; self-contempt, thinks she is ugly; fear of germs, diseases, and infections; ovarian cysts; asthma in children.
SANKARAN MENTALS: Doing everything possible to avoid feelings of brittleness and emptiness.
MIASM: Sycotic, a well-known remedy. Vaccinosis, never well since a vaccination.
COMPARISONS: Many different remedies; has a rapidly changing mental picture;
An interesting symptom: for those who think that any bad thought they think will then come to pass.

Euphorbiaceae Family (Spurge)

MAIN THEME: Prejudiced, narrow-minded, inflexible, or unyielding; Sensations are that of being tied or untied, bound or unbound, held in like a prisoner. Passive reactions are tied and cannot possibly do anything because motion or change of position aggravates everything. Active reactions are a great desire to break free and intolerance of clothing. Compensates by managing somehow in a limited space or breaking out so that one no longer feels bound and held in.

CROTON TIGLIUM (CROTON OIL SEEDS)

Eyes feel drawn backward; drawing pain through left chest when child nurses; pain above right eye; weight of hat or headband causes headache; neck and shoulders painful; better after sleep; many symptoms are worse at night; intense itching, but to scratch is very painful.
KEYNOTES: Antidote to poison oak and ivy rashes; helpful for skin disorders; burning in the esophagus; drawing pain through left chest and into the back.
SANKARAN MENTALS: Feels that things are happening suddenly that will bind him or tie him down.
MIASM: Acute
COMPARISONS: Rhus toxicodendron, Anacardium, Sepia succus.

MANCINELLA VENENATA (MANGANEEL APPLE)

Weeps a great deal; dermatitis; forgets what she wishes to do next; anger brings on symptoms; backache with nausea; painful stiffness in small of the back and the neck after sleeping; eyelids heavy and sore; craves cold water; pressure in region of heart; palpitations in the evening or when turning in bed; worse from cold and cold drinks, though craving them.
KEYNOTES: Homesickness; blindness; sudden vanishing of thoughts; skin disorders; fear of becoming insane; used for mental disorders that include delusion, hysteria, or great fear.
SANKARAN MENTALS: Feels suddenly bound and that his life might be in danger; must find or demand release immediately.
MIASM: Typhoid
COMPARISONS: Crotalus horridus, Cantharis vesicatoria, Anacardium orientale.

STILLINGIA SYLVATICA (QUEEN'S ROOT)

Chronic arthritis; severe cramping of the abdomen followed by the passage of gas; used for bone diseases; raw feeling in chest down entire length of sternum; eyes inflamed and watery; urine contains deposits of white sediment; aching pains in bones of limbs and back; unusual drowsiness all day with general malaise and headache; better in the morning.
KEYNOTES: Gloomy forebodings; depressed; feels something bad is about to happen; hoarseness when speaking.
SANKARAN MENTALS: Totally destroyed by any situation in which he feels bound, tied, or held in.
MIASM: Syphilis
COMPARISONS: Syphilinum, Medorrhinum, Mercurius solubilis, Kali iodatum, Phytolacca decandra, Staphysagria.

Hamamelidae Family (Walnut and Bayberry)

MAIN THEME: Heavy, dragged down, limited. Sensations are shut-in, confined, compressed, or the opposites of open, expanded, flying or floating, feeling light and free. Passive reactions are dullness with no enthusiasm, drive or ambition; aversion to motion—all movement ceases, almost paralyzed. Active reactions are desire to move and be in the open air rather than in closed confined spaces; a lot of fantasizing and imagination. Compensates by adapting to living within a confined, limited space and learning a sense of balance, neither high nor low.

CANNABIS INDICA (INDIAN MARIJUANA)

Sudden loss of memory; pain across shoulders and spine, cannot walk erect; extreme sensitivity to noise; involuntary shaking of the head; pulse very slow; burning, scalding, or stinging pain on urination; grinding of teeth while sleeping; dryness of the mouth and lips.
KEYNOTES: Exaggeration of concepts of time and space, seconds seem like ages; forgetful, cannot finish sentence; uncontrollable laughter; craves sweets; thirsty for cold drinks; feels as if the top of the head is opening and shutting; very exhausted after a short walk.
SANKARAN MENTALS: Accepting of the limitations that are.
MIASM: Sycotic
COMPARISONS: many—Cannabis sativa, Belladonna, Hyoscyamus niger, Stramonium, Lachesis muta, Silica terra, Sulphur, Thuja occidentalis, Medorrhinum, , Valerian officinalis, Zincum metallicum.

CANNABIS SATIVA (MARIJUANA)

Fear of going to bed; easily frightened or irritated; voices, including her own, seem to come from a far distance; pressure from back of eyes, forward; palpitations of the heart with painful tension; pulse is slow and weak; cramps in the hands and fingers; cramps in the thighs and the calves of the legs; difficulty in breathing and palpitations, then must stand up; sleepy but cannot sleep; more tired in the morning than the night before; burning heat over the whole body at night.

KEYNOTES: Dragging heaviness, especially around the kidneys; very forgetful; everything seems unreal, as if in a dream; desires sweets and cold drinks; burning while urinating.

SANKARAN MENTALS: Not allowed to move; no space to move or escape the mounting pressure, will be attacked with no place to go.

MIASM: Malaria

COMPARISONS: Cannabis indica, Thuja occidentalis, Medorrhinum, Cantharis vesicatoria, Sarsaparilla (Similax regelii), Mercurius solubilis, Sulphur, Sepia succus, Rhus toxicodendron, Sabina officinalis, Apis mellifica, Cimicifuga racemosa.

HAMAMELIS VIRGINIANA (WITCH HAZEL)

The chief action of this remedy is on the veins and blood vessels, making it useful for venous congestions, varicose veins, hemorrhoids and hemorrhages of all sorts (menstrual right through nosebleeds); sore pain down cervical vertebrae; thirsty, but water makes him sick just to think about it.

KEYNOTES: Bruises; hemorrhoids; varicose veins and venous ulcers; nosebleeds

SANKARAN MENTALS: Forgetful; wants "the respect she is due"; worse from pressure applied; worse in open air

MIASM: not mentioned by Sankaran for any miasm.

COMPARISONS: Arnica montana, Calendula officinalis; Lachesis muta, Pulsatilla nigricans, Nux vomica, Nitricum acidum, Cimicifuga racemosa, Euphorbium officinarum, Terebinthiniae oleum.

JUGLANS REGIA (WALNUT)

Excited, as if intoxicated, in the evening; sharp pains in the forehead; peevishness; stitches in sacral region; styes in the eyes; l oss of tone of sphincter of bladder with involuntary dribbling.

KEYNOTES: Feeling as if the head were floating in the air; skin eruptions; sharp occipital pain.

SANKARAN MENTALS: Feels that confined, restricted situations or feelings are leading to their destruction mentally and physically.

MIASM: Syphilis

COMPARISONS: Rhus toxicodendron, Graphites naturalis, Rumex crispus, Mercurius solubilis.

MYRICA CERIFERA (BAYBERRY)

Tenacious mucus in the throat; used for combined liver and heart disorders; feelings of fullness in the organs of the abdomen; desire for sour things and acids; pain and stiffness in nape of neck; pulse is slow, feeble, irregular; better from open air, eating breakfast; worse from warmth of bed, worse after sleep; drowsiness but insomnia when it comes time to sleep; weakness; muscular soreness; aching in limbs; sharp pains around the heart with increased, audible pulsations, but slow pulse.

KEYNOTES: Insomnia; jaundice; gloomy; despondent; irritable; indifferent; dull heavy aching in temples and forehead on waking in the morning.

SANKARAN MENTALS: Similar to Cannabis sativa: not allowed to move; no space to move or escape the mounting pressure; will be attacked with no place to go.

MIASM: Malaria, Acute

COMPARISONS: Chelidonium majus, Leptandra virginica, Kali bichromicum, Hydrastis canadensis, Digitalis purpurea.

URTICA URENS (STINGING NETTLE)

As you might surmise from the plant it is derived from, Urtica urens is useful for conditions exhibiting stinging, burning pains; primarily thought of for skin rashes and for burns; gout; rheumatism; malaria and other recurring fevers; bee stings (Apis mellifica); kidney stones; first degree burns; *an antidote to shellfish allergy*; urinary problems accompanied by burning, stinging pains; hives; chicken pox
KEYNOTES: Burns; hives; gout; kidney stones; neuritis; urticaria.
MIASM: not mentioned by Sankaran for any miasm.
COMPARISONS: Apis mellifica, Natrum muriaticum, Rhus toxicodendron, Pulsatilla nigricans.

Labiatae Family (Mint)

MAIN THEME: The main theme seems to be pleasurable excitement that stirs the person to activity of some sort. The excitement may be nervous, mental, or sexual. Sensations are excitement, exhilaration, rush of ideas. Passive reactions are lack of excitability and reaction to external things, numbness. Active reactions are vivacity, irritability, fright, and anxiety. Compensates by learning to remain calm.

AGNUS CASTUS (CHASTE TREE)

More properly placed in the Verbenaceae family but fits here best because of pattern of excitability. Itching in all parts, but especially the eyes; sadness with a fixed idea of death; worn out, usually from overindulgence and excess; abdomen extended after meals; sprains and strains from lifting a little too much; mouth very dry; only the most simple foods agree; nausea in pit of stomach after eating; chronic diarrhea.
KEYNOTES: hormonal disorders; premature aging; sexual weakness; sprains; changeable moods; sadness with a fixed idea of impending death; infertility.
SANKARAN MENTALS: Must keep his (sexual) excitement totally controlled.
MIASM: Cancer (The combining of the sycosis and the syphilis miasm is clearly seen here).
COMPARISONS: Selenium, Conium maculatum, Natrum muriaticum, Sepia succus, Sabal serrulata, Camphora, Lycopodium clavatum

COLLINSONIA CANADENSIS (STONE ROOT)

Alternates between gloomy and excited; congestion in the pelvic organs; said to be of value given before a surgery to prevent constipation; depressed arterial tension; chronic nasal, gastric and pharyngeal catarrh; palpitation, faintness, oppressed feeling in cardiac regions seeming to be nerve related; yellow discoloration around the eyes.
KEYNOTES: Painful bleeding hemorrhoids and constipation; constipation of children—bowel lacks tone and peristalsis; hemorrhoids; cough from excessive use of the voice.
SANKARAN MENTALS: Balance in this family is pleasurable excitement. This remedy has the sensations of being stuck in a position where there is no pleasure and no passion; feelings of being persecuted and attacked at the same time.
MIASM: Malaria with aspects of the acute miasm,
COMPARISONS: Aesculus hippocastanum, Aloe socotrina, Hamamelis virginiana, Lycopersicon esculentum

MENTHOL (MADE FROM ESSENTIAL OIL OF PEPPERMINT PIPERITA)

Acute nasal and eustachian catarrh; laryngitis; colicky pains and vomiting; migraine headaches; pain over frontal sinus, extends to eyeballs, asthmatic breathing with congestive headache.
SANKARAN MENTALS: Sudden intense excitement.
MIASM: Acute
KEYNOTES: Itching; affects the spial nerve; plurus; neural paine

Leguminosae Family (Pea)

MAIN THEME: The main theme of the pea family is that of the opposite aspects of being either split apart or, alternatively, bound together. Peas and beans are bound together by their pod, but once the pod is broken, they become scattered. This is similar to the splitting or coming apart, scattered and fragmented, or bound tightly together sensations that are typical of this remedy. Sensations can be described as coming apart or being bound too tightly together. Passive reactions are feeling confused, scattered, split apart from things, split up or not together. Active reactions are getting things together. Compensates by creating situations in which he feels unified and together.

BAPTISIA TINCTORIA (WILD INDIGO)

Cannot keep his mind together; feels a wild wandering feeling, especially with eyes closed; indifference, doesn't want to do anything; parts of the body feel separated; eyelids feel heavy; headache, fever and delirium, septic fevers; sense of suffocation; putrid offensive breath; can only swallow liquids; offensive diarrhea; sleepless and restless; vertigo with severe nausea.
KEYNOTES: Has been used successfully in epidemic influenza; indescribably sick feeling all over; great muscular soreness.
SANKARAN MENTALS: Feeling scattered—must get all the pieces together immediately. Desperately trying to put all the pieces together—if he can just do it, he will be fine.
MIASM: Typhoid
COMPARISONS: Echinacea is the nearest match. Gelsemium sempervirens, Arnica montana, Arsenicum album, Pyrogenium may be needed as follow-up remedies. Also Baptisia tinctoria, Rhus toxicodendron, Hyoscyamus niger, Lachesis mutas, Nitricum acidum.

COPAIVA (BALSAM OF COPAIVA)

Chief action is on the genito urinary organs and rectum; also affects the mucous membranes of the respiratory organs and the skin, producing a nettle-like rash; painful urination with burning pressure; disfiguring acne; flushes of blood to the head and face; sensitive scalp; food seems too salty; chronic catarrh of the throat; painful cough with heat and oppression of the chest; burning in the lungs.
KEYNOTES: Chronic bronchitis; mucus colitis; hives.
SANKARAN MENTALS: Avoids any kind of splitting apart or disharmony in any relationships and hides and covers up any problems that are occurring.
MIASM: Sycotic
COMPARISONS: Santalum album, Cannabis indica, Cantharis vesicatoria, Apis mellifica, Vespa crabro, Senecio aureus, Sepia succus.

LATHYRUS SATIVUS (WILD VETCH)

Lack of inner strength of mind; hypochondria; sense of being trapped by circumstances; suppressed emotions; colic; back pain so severe that it prevents movement; frequent urge to urinate, must hurry; stiffness and lameness of the ankles and knees; impotence; tip of the tongue burns; continuous yawning and sleepiness, vertigo when standing with eyes closed.
KEYNOTES: Excessive rigidity of legs with spastic gait; lower limbs emaciated; infantile paralysis.
SANKARAN MENTALS: Being destroyed by the splitting or coming apart of any aspect of their lives.
MIASM: Syphilis
COMPARISONS: Secale cornutum.

MELILOTUS OFFICINALIS (SWEET CLOVER)

Irritable; impatient; discontented; fault-finding; shyness and blushing; broken sensation in back, always moving to get relief; very hungry about 10:00 a.m. with frontal headache; nose is stopped up and dry; periods of wakefulness during the night.
KEYNOTES: Great fear of danger; panic and fear; suspicious; engorgement of blood to any part or organ; face is intensely flushed and red; violent throbbing headache; profuse and frequent nosebleeds.

SANKARAN MENTALS: Acute threat from being suddenly split up or pulled away from something; attempts to, or wants to, run away.
MIASM: Acute
COMPARISONS: comparison remedies for certain symptoms, nothing for full range.

PHYSOSTIGMA VENENOSUM (CALABAR BEAN)

Spinal irritation; cramping sensation up and down spine; sharp shooting pains in the ears; food has a flat taste, nothing satisfies; sore feeling in area of kidneys; bladder feels distended; irresistible desire to sleep; cold, clammy skin; hands feel cold and dirty; vertigo, especially while going up stairs.
KEYNOTES: Used in endometrial cancer; loss of muscular power; weakness; headache, cannot bear to raise eyelids; fluttering of heart felt in the throat; contraction of pupils; myopia.
SANKARAN MENTALS: Stretched beyond one's capacity to hold things together. This is demonstrated by the feeling that there are too many possessions or things in the room, and constantly trying to create order from the perceived chaos by moving things around or throwing them out.
MIASM: Cancer miasm
COMPARISONS: None

Liliflorae Family (Lily)

MAIN THEME: The two poles of being forced out and hanging on tightly. The theme of feeling excluded must have its opposite reaction of a desire to be included. Sensations are being forced out, excluded, or left out. Passive reactions are holding on tightly, refusing to be excluded. Active reactions are moving on to someone or something else. Compensates by being more attractive, more useful, doing things to be included.

ALOE SOCOTRINA (COMMON ALOES)

Sensation of fullness in parts with a dragging down feeling; sadness in morning, but better later in the day; bloated abdomen, more on the left side; tends to a sedentary lifestyle, with poor habits and poor diet; pain deep in the eye sockets; headaches above forehead with heaviness in eyes, helps to partially close them; headaches are worse for heat but better for cold.
KEYNOTES: Sense of insecurity; dissatisfied and angry about himself; aversion to people; small hemorrhoids, like a bunch of grapes, which bleed profusely; itching of the skin that appears each year as winter approaches.
SANKARAN MENTALS: Feeling that he is being forced out and excluded because he is somehow not good enough.
MIASM: Leprosy. The Leprosy miasm includes an intense desire to change things, even to the point of suicide or homicide if it gets bad enough.
COMPARISONS: Sulphur, Camphora, Lycopodium clavatum, Nux vomica.

COLCHICUM AUTUMNALE (MEADOW SAFFRON)

Weakness of memory from fatigue; violent headache comes on in the evening and lasts till morning; symptoms worse for cold damp weather of autumn and worse sundown to sunrise; sleeplessness from restlessness of limbs; vertigo.
KEYNOTES: Depressed, irritable and sensitive; distention of abdomen with colicky pains; abdomen feels cold; intense boring pain in ovary; gags from mere mention of food; heart disease with violent palpitations; rheumatism; kidney failure with high uric acid, gout in the big toe.
SANKARAN MENTALS: Feels persecuted because others exclude him; wonders if or is sure, that he is deficient somehow.
MIASM: Malaria
COMPARISONS: Carbo vegetabilis, Arnica montana, Arsenicum album, Cocculus indicus, Kali carbonicum, Veratrum album.

HELONIAS DIOICA (UNICORN-ROOT)
Profound melancholy and depression; cannot tolerate the least criticism; finds fault with everyone; pain and weight in the back; frequent desire and urging to urinate; loss of appetite, food is tasteless; fullness and painful congestion of the stomach; headache that is better for exercise; all symptoms worse during pregnancy; feels hot when tired.
KEYNOTES: Prolapse and other mal-positions of the womb; uterine atony; can tell where the kidneys are because of the burning feeling in the area; menses too frequent and too profuse.
SANKARAN MENTALS: Must avoid being excluded. Accomplishes this by hyponchondria becasue illness keeps everyone focused on him.
MIASM: Sycosis
COMPARISONS: Lilium tigrinum, Pulsatilla nigricans, Senecio aureus, Stannum metallicum, Agrimony Bach Flower Essence.

LILIUM TIGRINUM (TIGER LILY)
Acts primarily on the heart and the female organs; strong sexual desire, lessened by keeping busy; neck aches, worse if tired; pains in left breast and left ovary; bearing down pains; palpitations during pregnancy; constant pressure on bladder with constant desire to urinate; urine feels hot and burning; feels suffocated in a warm room.
KEYNOTES: Mental and physical symptoms alternate; hurried, wants to do several things at once; restless and nervous; snappish; profound depression; heavy dragging down feeling; congestion of uterus; sensation of heart being gripped in a vise.
SANKARAN MENTALS: The feeling that he must cover up inadequacy centers around religious themes and saying the wrong thing; must be careful and cautious about behavior in order to escape exclusion; makes these people great to be around, but it is kind of a sad situation as they struggle to feel accepted
MIASM: Sycosis
COMPARISONS: Lilium tigrinum is the closest, but Sepia succus is also very like Lilium. Cactus grandiflorus, Helonias dioica, and Pulsatilla nigricans are also comparable in many ways.

ORNITHOGALUM UMBELLATUM (STAR OF BETHLEHEM)
One of main actions of this remedy is on the pyloric sphincter; considered a cancer remedy, particularly for gastric or pyloric cancer; also for stomach ulcers or a history of stomach ulcers followed by stomach cancer; depressed, possibly suicidal—cancer is sometimes an acceptable form of suicide to the subconscious mind; constipation/diarrhea; waking drenched in perspiration at night; legs and feet go to sleep on sitting; restlessness with creepy feeling in feet.
KEYNOTES: Flatulence; heartburn; gastric ulcer; cancer; pain increases when food passes pyloric outlet; stomach feels as if it is full of water; extreme restlessness.
SANKARAN MENTALS: Feeling that one must be in total control of self at all times; behavior and life circumstances must be perfect or they are sure they will be excluded by others.
MIASM: Cancer, which has parts of both sycosis and syphilis
COMPARISONS: Allium cepa, Abies nigra, Chamomilla vulgaris, China officinalis, Carbo vegetabilis, Lycopodium clavatum.

SABADILLA OFFICINALIS (CEVADILLA SEED)
Imagines that there are things wrong with his body; nervous; timid; thinking produces headaches and sleeplessness; affinity for the mucus membranes of the nose; hay fever; chilliness; burning sensation in chest; thirstless; itching and tickling inside of nose; mucus that is copious, thin and flowing.
KEYNOTES: Red, burning eyelids; desire for hot things; worse from cold air; spasmodic sneezing with running nose; oversensitive to odors.
SANKARAN MENTALS: Feeling that there is something incurable and unfixable (not necessarily fatal, however) wrong with them; if others are allowed to know their weakness or see what is wrong with them, they will be excluded—absolutely cannot let this happen!
MIASM: Sycosis
COMPARISONS: Colchicum autumnale, Nux vomica, Bryonia alba.

SARSAPARILLA OFFICINALIS (WILD LICORICE)
Despondent, gloomy without any cause; sensitive, easily offended; urine passes in thin feeble stream; pain at conclusion of urination; pains from occiput to eyes; pains cause depression; offensive breath.
KEYNOTES: Dwells on past bad occurrences and recalls old grievances; blood disorders; cystitis; kidney stones; itching and eruption on forehead; skin lies in folds as if the person is emaciated; dry itchy rash that comes on in the spring.
SANKARAN MENTALS: Feels excluded and is trying hard to come in and be included; resents being excluded.
MIASM: Ringworm
COMPARISONS: Berberis aquifolium, Lycopodium clavatum, Natrum muriaticum, Sassafras officinalis.

VERATRUM ALBUM (WHITE HELLEBORE)
This remedy is often used for head injuries, especially with violent pain driving the person to despair; profoundly affects the mind, nerves, abdominal area, heart, blood, blood vessels, respiration, vertex and digestive system; all effects of this remedy are violent and sudden; cold feeling in abdomen; thirst for cold water which is then vomited is a keynote; cold sweat on forehead; icy coldness of tip of nose and face; this is a polycrest remedy for influenza, especially if the illness has come on suddenly.
KEYNOTES: Leading remedy for hyperactive, disobedient children; sullen indifference; feels that misfortune is impending; exhausted states, usually, but not always, accompanying serious illness; extreme coldness (even the sweat is icy) is always a keynote symptom for this remedy; extreme evacuation (vomiting, diarrhea, saliva, sweat) is also present; fainting from emotions and from least exertion.
SANKARAN MENTALS: Having been suddenly forced out—created by a situation such as a job loss or divorce; fears losing social position as a result; literally desperate and thrown into a panic; his desperation and resultant behavior actually hastens and makes his exclusion worse.
MIASM: Acute
COMPARISONS: China officinalis, Camphora, Chocolate, Cuprum metallicum, Carbo vegetabilis. For disobedient children.
COMPARE TO: Tarentula hispanica, Anacardium orientale, Stramonium.

Loganiaceae Family (Strychnine)

MAIN THEME: Best described by the word "shattered", meaning to break or burst suddenly from a violent blow. This destruction can be physical or mental. Sensations are the range from let down and disappointed to ruined, torn to pieces, paralysed. Passive reactions are fainting, or being so paralyzed that they can neither move nor cry. Active reactions are frantic, beside oneself, excitable to the point of convulsions. Compensates by remaining composed and calm even in the most desperate situations. "I didn't dare scream. I felt if I once began it, I would never be able to stop."

CURARE WOORARI (ARROW POISON) exact composition unknown
Seems to be made from Curare, Cocculus toxiferous, and a new species of Strychnos.)

Action is on the muscles, causing paralysis; weakness, numbness with tingling; piercing, sharp pains; mind shows indecision, no longer wants to think or act for herself; forgetful; can be either depressed with desire to be alone or excited and in a hurry; stiffness of muscles of neck and shoulder, more often on the right side; instant giddiness while standing or walking.
KEYNOTES: Reflex action is poor; chest sore to pressure or touch; respiratory system feels paralysed.
SANKARAN MENTALS: Intensely shocked, shattered, and disappointed as the result of being abandoned by his own relatives and family; curare is in the leprosy miasm, but some of the mental symptoms are almost desperate enough to be described as syphilitic.
MIASM: Leprosy
COMPARISONS: no close ones for entire picture, some for individual symptoms of the whole

GELSEMIUM SEMPERVIRENS (YELLOW JASMINE)
This is a polycrest remedy—the symptoms go on for pages; leading remedy for recovery from "flu", whether epidemic (great record here) or ordinary, seasonal types; chief complaint is weakness, by itself or accompanying other problems; weakness can be seen on all levels (physical, emotional, mental); neurological damage, particularly to the left side; headache beginning at occiput and radiating to the forehead; congestive heart failure with accompanying keynote symptoms; use for stage fright by taking 20-30 minutes before performance; trembling of extremities from slight exertion; chills running up and down the back.
KEYNOTES: Never well since influenza; apathy regarding their illness; dread of being in a public place or going to a doctor; anxiety; debility; fatigue; fright; muscular weakness; neuralgias; paralysis; bed-wetting in nervous children; earache from cold.
SANKARAN MENTALS: Feels that it takes great strength, more than he has, to face situations of shock. Reaction is to avoid, in any way possible, the situation that might produce a torn, shattered, ruined feeling.
MIASM: Sycotic, because of attempt to avoid all shock and disappointment.
COMPARISONS: Caulophyllum thalictroides, Causticum, Ferrum phosphoricum, Phosphorus, Bryonia alba, Hypericum perforatum, Ignatia amara.

IGNATIA AMARA (BITTER CANDYTUFT)
One of the 3 famous grief remedies (others are Natrum muriaticum and Phosphoricum acidum).
Marked action on the heart; palpitations with vertigo and choking; heart symptoms made worse by going up stairs or hills; undemonstrative in grief, often bears intense suffering without complaining or uttering a word (see Loganiaceae family description); predominantly a women's remedy; pathological disorders brought on by grief or romantic disappointments; inflammation of the joints or twitching of the muscles.
KEYNOTES: Superficial and erratic character of symptoms; symptoms arising from grief or disappointment; pulse full, irregular, intermittent; convulsions in children after a fright.
SANKARAN MENTALS: A very deep need—an absolute must—to keep control during shock, grief, disappointment, bad news of the sort that would make most people feel shattered, torn to pieces, and ruined.
MIASM: Cancer
COMPARISONS: Spigelia anthelmintica, Digitalis purpurea, Cactus grandiflorus, Belladonna, Crataegus oxyacantha.

NUX VOMICA (POISON NUT)
This is an antidote for nearly all remedies!!! Cannot bear noises, odors, light, touch, music; impatient when spoken to, gets angry and violent without any provocation; stomach pains, worse for anger; cramping or sharp pains in abdomen; constipation with constant urging; cystitis with constant urging; back pain, worse at night in bed; insomnia, wakes between 3-4 am and cannot sleep due to worry about work or how to get tasks accomplished; craves stimulants but is worse for them.
KEYNOTES: The popular concept of "type A personality" describes the Nux vomica personality. Impatient; competitive; ambitious; successful; focused on work; argumentative; irritable; easily offended; workaholic; compulsive; weight and pain in stomach; sour taste and nausea in the morning; better after a nap; constipation; worse if sleep is disturbed; cramps and spasms of limbs.
SANKARAN MENTALS: Shattered and torn to pieces; must make rapid and immediate efforts to recover. These efforts will be zealous and fiery. Underlying feeling that someone has occupied his space or comfortable place.
MIASM: Typhoid
COMPARISONS: In Murphy's Materia Medica there is a list of comparisons half a column long—simply to many to list effectively here. There are a lot of variations on the type A personality and a multitude of remedies that fit them specifically. Many of these comparison remedies seem to fit the cancer miasm.

SPIGELIA ANTHELMINTICA (PINKROOT)

Mental exertions are difficult; weakness of memory; abdomen hard and painfully tight—contact and pressure of clothes is unendurable; severe pain around the eyes, worse for turning them; eating disorders such as bulimia and anorexia; foul odor from mouth.
KEYNOTES: Symptoms and diseases treated by this remedy are intermittent in nature; violent pains in the heart; migraines in which head feels too large; used for parasites; agitation and anxiety, with restlessness.
SANKARAN MENTALS: Stuck in a position where, from time to time, he is going to be shocked, shattered, disappointed, or torn to pieces. Because the situation is intermittent, this remedy is classified in the malaria miasm.
MIASM: Malaria
COMPARISONS: Nux vomica, Ignatia amara, Curare woorari, Aconitum napellus, Cactus grandiflorus, Cimicifuga racemosa.

STRYCHNINUM (STRYCHNINE) MAIN ALKALOID OF LONGANICEA FAMILY

Murphy's Materia Medica quotes both Cooper and Clarke as saying that "many cases of persistent cough recurring after influenza are met by Strychninum. The influenza cough has in it a strong spasmodic and asthmatic element, whether dry or not." Panic attacks; full and bursting headache with heat in the eyes; vertigo with roaring in the ears; very obstinate constipation; itching of whole body, especially nose; constant vomiting; nausea of pregnancy.
KEYNOTES: Pain and sensations come on suddenly and return at intervals; spasmodic rigidity of muscles; rigidity of the back, particularly the cervical area.
SANKARAN MENTALS: Suddenly being torn into little pieces. Acute sensation, rather than chronic.
MIASM: Acute
COMPARISONS: None that are very close.

Magnolianae Family (Magnolia)

MAIN THEME: Strange, bizarre feelings. Words which might be used to describe the sensations of this family group are: out of the ordinary, unusual, bewildering, confusing, disorienting. Passive reactions are withdrawn, floating, sleepy, fainting, collapsing. Active reactions are total withdrawal, shutting everything out, creating their own world where things feel familiar. Compensates by learning to, at least pretending to, adapt to strange, new, confusing or bewildering situations.

CAMPHORA (CAMPHOR)

Universal antidote for other homeopathic remedies. Serious cases of chronic fatigue or influenza, with almost total collapse; extreme coldness; very little vitality at all; diarrhea; heart disorders; fears to be left alone with his thoughts but does not like anyone near him; headache with occipital throbbing that is in sync with the pulse; persistent nosebleed; insomnia with cold limbs.
KEYNOTES: State of collapse; first stages of a cold with chilliness and sneezing; person is chilly but does not like to be covered up; violent convulsions.
SANKARAN MENTALS: Sudden intense threat and shock from something strange and bewildering. The reaction is to withdraw, run, and hide.
MIASM: Acute
COMPARISONS: Cuprum metallicum, Arsenicum album, Veratrum album, Aloe socotrina, Carbo vegetabilis, Dulcamara.

CINNAMONUM CEYLANICUM (CINNAMON TREE)
The leading feature is hemorrhage; heart weakness; retention of urine; flatulence with colic; toothache; offensive taste in the mouth; chilliness with trembling of limbs; fever in the evening; sore throat; hoarseness with cough.
KEYNOTES: Hemorrhages; postpartum hemorrhages, where the blood is bright red and clear; threatened miscarriages; menses early with profuse, prolonged, bright red bleeding.
SANKARAN MENTALS: Must avoid everything that is strange, bewildering, or confusing because they just can't handle any of it at all.
MIASM: Sycosis
COMPARISONS: Ipomoea purpurea, Phosphorus, Silica terra.

MYRISTICA SEBIFERA (BRAZILIAN UCUBA)
Useful for abscesses from splinters and foreign objects, especially under the nails; inflammation of the skin; restless sleep; dizziness in the morning; vertigo with swaying toward the left; mentals include indifference, heedlessness, carelessness; concentration is difficult; disturbed by a song that keeps running in his head.
KEYNOTES: Injuries; abscesses; whitlows; wounds; excitable; alternating with chilliness; pain in the fingernails with swelling in the fingers.
SANKARAN MENTALS: Strange, bewildering situations oppress the person, and they must escape them in any way that they can.
MIASM: Tubercular
COMPARISONS: Silica terra, Nux moschata, Calcarea sulphurica, Pyrogenium.

NUX MOSCHATA (NUTMEG)
Confused mind and impaired memory; thoughts suddenly vanish while talking, reading, or writing; slow learning to talk; ailments from overtaxing mentally; enormously distended abdomen; great dryness of throat with thirstlessness.
KEYNOTES: Dreamy and bewildered; irresistible drowsiness; complaints cause sleepiness; extreme dryness of the mucus membranes.
SANKARAN MENTALS: Strange, bewildering situations make one feel like a child. They feel they will be OK once they tackle the situation. They must do so immediately to relieve these uncomfortable feelings.
MIASM: Typhoid
COMPARISONS: Myristica sebifera, Nux vomica, Rhus toxicodendron, Ignatia amara, Asafoetida.

Malvaceae Family (Mallows)

This family includes a variety, including a couple of forms of chocolate, an Indian lime, and some mallows, and some cotton plants.
MAIN THEME: Feelings of separation and the opposite feeling of being together. The sensations are being together but then separated, attached and then detached. Passive reactions are to feel estranged from family and society and to feel a great indifference to everything. Active reactions are communicative, affectionate, dreams of falling in love. Compensates by being independent, self-confident.

CHOCOLATE (COCOA)
Anxiety that something will happen; feels open and vulnerable; loss of interest in loved ones; self-conscious; painful cough from deep in the chest; buzzing or fuzziness in ears, worse in the left one; dry chapped skin; congestion in head; wandering pain in hands and feet, muscles, joints and small bones; dry mouth with bad taste; tension in the shoulders and base of neck; perspiration; sleepiness, yawning a lot.
KEYNOTES: Moods changeable with emotional lows and highs; hyperactive.
SANKARAN MENTALS: Panic when separated or estranged, especially from family.
MIASM: Acute
COMPARISONS: none

GOSSYPIUM HERBACEUM (COTTON PLANT)
Used mainly for complaints of the female organs; symptom picture includes the uncomfortable symptoms some women experience with pregnancy such as morning sickness; external chilliness, with internal heat.
KEYNOTES: Intermittent pain in ovaries; all pains of this remedy are generally better by rest.
SANKARAN MENTALS: Trying to become attached, or reattached, to someone or something.
MIASM: Ringworm
COMPARISONS: Lilium tigrinum, Sabina officinalis, Cimicifuga racemosa, Apis mellifica, Belladonna, Bryonia alba, Pulsatilla nigricans, Secale cornutum, Sepia succus.

STERCULIA/KOLA NUT (KOLA NUT)
Regulates circulation and heart rhythm; promotes the appetite and digestion; is a diuretic and antidiarrheal; gives the power to endure prolonged physical exertion without food and without feeling fatigue.
KEYNOTES: Asthma; nervous exhaustion with abnormal tiredness.
SANKARAN MENTALS: Feels detached and disgusted with himself, sure that he is repulsive.
MIASM: Leprosy
COMPARISONS: Cacao, Avena sativa, Lachesis muta, Nux vomica, Kudzu.

Papaveraceae Family (Poppy)

MAIN THEME: Sensitivity to suffering. The sensations of most remedies are intense pain and suffering, being punished, violence, fright and shock, states of agony. Passive reactions are fainting, coma, narcolepsy, hibernation, deep meditative states. Active reactions are rage, spasms, colic, convulsion, violence, and numbness alternating with pain. Compensates by showing great calmness in situations where there is great pain, by being unaffected by pain, suffering or pleasure, and by being peaceful, serene, tranquil.

There are four homeopathic remedies in this family but no polycrest remedies; they are very useful remedies when indicated, however.

CHELIDONIUM MAJUS (GREATER CELANDINE)
Primarily thought of as a liver remedy, but useful in a wide variety of right-sided complaints; useful for neonatal jaundice; right-sided headache; abdominal pain radiating to right scapular region; right scapular or shoulder pain; right-sided pneumonia; irritable and easily upset; vexed about every trifle; violent attacks or passionate outbursts of temper; headache that is better after eating.
KEYNOTES: Right-sided complaints; domineering people; craves cheese, warm drinks, milk.
SANKARAN MENTALS: Stuck in a situation, and very frightened when subjected to intense pain and suffering. The malaria is noted for intermittent situations like gallstones, etc., which are very painful, but the pain is rarely constant.
MIASM: Malaria
COMPARISONS: Lycopodium clavatum, Bryonia alba, China officinalis, Sanguinaria canadensis, Sulphur.

MORPHINUM ACETICUM/PURUM (AN ALKALOID OF OPIUM)
Only remedy listed for ailments arising from electric shock; great pain in the back; itching of eyes; pulse small and weak; suppression of stool and urine; cramps in several muscles at the same time; vertigo from the least movement of the head.
KEYNOTES: Extremely susceptible to pain; forgetfulness; hunting for words while speaking; indifference, apathy; shock induced by terror; profound depression; very dry mouth; alternation of tachycardia and bradycardia; palpitations; numbness.
SANKARAN MENTALS: Acute intense, severe, violent, sudden pain and terror.
MIASM: Acute
COMPARISONS: Apomorphinum, Opium, Nux vomica.

OPIUM (POPPY)

Opium is indicated for those conditions that would mimic an overdose of actual opium. These symptoms are much like a fully developed stroke. Opium is useful in ailments characterized by stupor; painlessness where there should be pain; heavy, deep sleep; labored breathing; useful for drug overdose; fright; stroke or injury; loss of consciousness; great weight of pain in back of head; head feels as if it would burst.
KEYNOTES: Palpitations after a stressful event; hot perspiration over whole body; involuntary stools after a fright; stertorous breathing; deep snoring with rattling.
Note: Opium has a "swing" side which is extreme excitability—more so even than Nux vomica. This effect could be produced by overdose of the homeopathic and is occasionally the indication for the need of this remedy.
Rarely needed, but extremely effective when well indicated - and nothing else is likely to work anywhere near as well. Mentioned for the final stages of suffering from cancer.
SANKARAN MENTALS: Must maintain control even in situations of pain and violence, such as war.
MIASM: Cancer
COMPARISONS: Baptisia tinctoria, Nux vomica, Belladonna, Alumen crudum, Calcarea carbonica, Coffea cruda, Lachesis muta, Arnica montana, Aconitum napellus.

SANGUINARIA CANADENSIS (BLOOD ROOT)

Allergies and allergic asthma where the person is very sensitive to odors, flowers, and airborne pollen; migraine headaches on the right side that are better for vomiting; veins and temples are distended; headaches if one has gone without food; bursitis, especially of the right shoulder; acrid belching, heartburn and reflux.
KEYNOTES: Right-sided remedy; feet hot at night—puts them out of covers.
SANKARAN MENTALS: Tries very hard to avoid any type of violence.
MIASM: Sycosis
COMPARISONS: Belladonna, Lycopodium clavatum, Ferrum metallicum, Chelidonium majus, Pulsatilla nigricans, Sabadilla officinalis, all Calcareas, Kali sulphuricum, Sulphur.

Rubiaceae Family (Coffee)

MAIN THEME: A very active mind which desires many things. Sensations are many desires, ideas, and imaginations. Passive reactions are fatigue, exhaustion, weariness, vanishing of thoughts. Active reactions are constant planning and theorizing, frantic pursuit of creative endeavors. Compensates by seeking tranquility and using meditation techniques.

CHINA OFFICINALIS (CINCHONA)

Quinine, which is derived from this bark, was used extensively for malaria—the disease, not the miasm. Unfortunately cinchona is a deadly poison. It was the first remedy proved by Hahnemann.
Use for periodic fevers, bloating, gall bladder attacks, hepatitis and to rebalance male hormones; irritable; sensitive and very touchy with a disposition to hurt other people's feelings; ringing in the ears; intense throbbing of head and carotids; drenching sweats at night.
KEYNOTES: Irritable; "touchy"; fear of animals—even domesticated animals; in men, fantasize that they are heroic but feeling is that they really aren't acceptable as a man; (Sepia succus is more likely to be indicated for similar feelings in women).
SANKARAN MENTALS: Fixed idea that he is unhappy because he is being persecuted by enemies.
MIASM: Malaria
COMPARISONS: Nux vomica, Natrum muriaticum, Lycopodium clavatum, Ignatia amara, Arsenicum album, Carbo vegetabilis.

COFFEA CRUDA (UNROASTED COFFEE)

Coffea acts predominantly on the nerves creating over-excitement and over-sensitivity to any type of stimulation; insomnia—wakes from the slightest noise or is kept awake by racing thoughts; generally aggravated by stimulation, noise and strong emotions; pneumonia; cough of gastric origin.

Coffea cruda (and caffeine in any form) antidotes a great many homeopathic preparations. The stronger remedies (1M) and above are generally not affected by caffeinated drinks, at least not as drastically.

KEYNOTES: Over-excitability, over-sensitivity, insomnia.
SANKARAN MENTALS: Must come up with creative ideas quickly. There is a sense of tight deadlines to be met.
MIASM: Tubercular
COMPARISONS: Many for one symptom or another, but none for a good proportion of the whole picture.

GALIUM APARINE (CLEAVERS)

This plant, when used as an herbal remedy, is a popular remedy for cancers and ulcerative sores; the herb is also used as a diuretic and as a solvent for dissolving kidney gravel and stones; homeopathically it seems to act in much the same way; is also used for skin disorders and scurvy.

SANKARAN MENTALS: Responds to every stimulation; has hundreds of ideas bouncing around in his head; but must stay in control of himself and all the excitement.
MIASM: Cancer
COMPARISONS: None, not a lot of provings on record.

IPECACUANHA (IPECAC ROOT)

Migraine headache with severe vomiting; nausea not relieved by vomiting; uterine hemorrhage which starts suddenly with bright red blood, coming in gushes and often with nausea, vomiting and faintness; deficiency of ideas (an opposite reaction to above description); impatient and demanding, even childlike about it—doesn't actually know what is wanted but wants it right now.

KEYNOTES: Always consider when nausea and vomiting are a prominent characteristic no matter what other organ system may be involved.
SANKARAN MENTALS: Desires many things and demands instant stimulation and entertainment.
MIASM: Typhoid
COMPARISONS: Nicotiana Tabaccum, Kali carbonicum, Kali sulphuricum, Sanguinaria canadensis, Antimonium tartaricum, Pulsatilla nigricans.

Ranunculaceae Family (Hellebore)

MAIN THEME: Physical ailments can have emotional, often referred to as psychosomatic, roots and causes. Ailments in this family originate in fear, grief, and anger. The sensations are many and opposing: raw nerves, easily excited, morbid, overly sensitive, excessive irritability, anger with grief, feeling of guilt, annoyed, harassed, insulted. Passive reactions are numbness and a blunting of the emotions. Active reactions are nervous tension, many emotions all at once creating inner conflict, passionate outburst, brooding, tremors from emotions. Compensates by maintaining a calm and steady demeanor and attitude.

ACONITUM NAPELLUS (MONKSHOOD)

Use for shock following a violent or frightening event; earache with pain; eyes feel dry and hot with red and swollen eyelids; unquenchable thirst during fever; numbness and tingling; hot hands and cold feet; urine retention in infants or mothers right after delivery; use during delivery for women who feel they are about to die; acute, sudden and violent illness with high fever; influenza and colds.

KEYNOTES: All complaints, emotional or physical, come suddenly, with great intensity and anxiety, and usually follow exposure to wind, fright or shock; tremendous fear of imminent death.
SANKARAN MENTALS: Acutely and suddenly vexed.
MIASM: Acute
COMPARISONS: Belladonna, Phosphorus, Stramonium datura, Opium, Sulphur, Rhus toxicodendron, Ferrum phosphoricum, Arsenicum album, Bryonia alba.

ACTEA SPICATA (BANEBERRY)
Effects of over-exertion of the mind or from fright; fear of death; pain in upper jaw; pain from crown of head to between eyebrows; warm sweat on head; symptoms worse from changes in weather, worse from cold air, worse from slight exertion.
KEYNOTES: Arthritis pains in small joints such as wrists, fingers, ankles, and toes; shortness of breath, especially on exposure to fresh air.
SANKARAN MENTALS: Trying hard not to be vexed and impatient.
MIASM: Ringworm
COMPARISONS: Cimicifuga racemosa, Caulophyllum thalictroides, Ledum palustre, other members of Ranunculaceae family.

CIMICIFUGA RACEMOSA (BLACK COHOSH)
Fear that those in the house will suffocate her emotionally, or even kill her; thinks she is going crazy; stiffness and contraction in the back; shooting, throbbing pains in the head after mental worry; pulse weak, irregular, trembling, drops every third or fourth beat; suitable to the menopausal period of life; hypochondria.
KEYNOTES: Gloom and dejection, as if there is a black cloud over everything; pain across pelvis from hip to hip; displaced labor pains to back or hips; muscular and crampy pains; intolerance to pain.
SANKARAN MENTALS: Oppressed and trapped in a vexing situation.
MIASM: Tubercular
COMPARISONS: Caulophyllum thalictroides, Pulsatilla nigricans, Lilium tigrinum.

CLEMATIS ERECTA (VIRGIN'S BOWER)
Homesickness; confused feeling, better in open air; eyes are sensitive to cold and sunlight; urine stops and starts; swollen glands; herpes zoster; toothache, worse at night.
KEYNOTES: Acts especially on the glands; neuralgic pains; great sleepiness.
SANKARAN MENTALS: Destroyed by vexation, annoyance, and anger
MIASM: Syphilis
COMPARISONS: Many homeopathic remedies are similar for individual symptoms—whether skin, reproductive organs, or burning sensations—but no comparisons close overall.

HELLEBORUS NIGER (BLACK HELLEBORE)
Senses become blunt and responses are sluggish; sees, hears, and tastes imperfectly; muscles do not obey the will; gradual onset of diseases with progressive weakness; cystitis; constant desire to urinate.
KEYNOTES: Indifference to loved ones, family; indifference to everything; envious at seeing others happy; involuntary sighing; stupefying headache; automatic motion of one arm and leg.
SANKARAN MENTALS: Must shut out or "blunt out" the irritations of life or will surely die.
MIASM: Typhoid
COMPARISONS: Tuberculinum aviaire, Apis mellifica, Zincum metallicum, Opium, China officinalis, Cicuta virosa.

HYDRASTIS CANADENSIS (GOLDEN SEAL)
Absentminded; forgetful; weak memory; thick yellow discharges; irritability after dinner; obstinate constipation during pregnancy; constipation with hemorrhoids; weak digestion with debility; tongue looks yellow and dirty; chilliness or heat in flushes over whole body.
KEYNOTES: Herbally and homeopathically, hydrastis is well regarded for use in cancer. Clarke considers that more cases of more types of cancer have been removed with this remedy than any other remedy.
SANKARAN MENTALS: Vexed by everything; disgusted with self; despairing.
MIASM: Leprosy
COMPARISONS: Kali bichromicum, Conium maculatum, Arsenicum iodatum, Phytolacca decandra, Pulsatilla nigricans.

PULSATILLA NIGRICANS (WIND FLOWER)

This is the same plant and remedy that Sankaran refers to as pratensis.

This remedy is useful both as constitutional and an acute. Need is often indicated by a few keynotes, the chief among these and the most confusing is the "changeableness" of the symptoms. All symptoms build to a pitch and then suddenly subside. The symptoms may begin on one side of the body but then move to the other side. There may be no symptoms at all when a person first goes to bed but symptoms quickly develop on whichever side is lain on. Movement brings only temporary relief as the symptoms begin again on the side that is now being lain on.

Pulsatilla nigricans people (constitutional or acute) tend to inward suffering and silent resentments, but feel better for whining or being sympathized with; predominantly a female remedy; particularly useful for tearful, clingy, whiny infants and children.

KEYNOTES: Symptoms are many and varied, as is fitting for "wind flower" people; a polycrest remedy and well worth studying in detail. Other keynote symptoms are irritable, "touchy," fear of animals—even domesticated animals. In men, there are often fantasies that they are heroic, but their true feeling is that they really aren't acceptable as a man.

SANKARAN MENTALS: Avoids situations that cause vexation or anxiety. Intense need to be alone.

MIASM: Sycosis

COMPARISONS: Kali bichromicum, Kali sulphuricum, Sulphur.

RANUNCULUS BULBOSUS (BUTTERCUP)

Muscular pain along the lower margin of the shoulder blade; various kinds of pain and soreness in the chest; intercostal arthritis; herpetic eruptions; cold air brings on many of the ailments; there is oppressed breathing with a great desire to draw a deep breath; pains in stomach; nausea in afternoon or evening, sometimes accompanied by headache.

Ranunculus, like shingles, is a remedy that has often proven helpful with shingles.

KEYNOTES: Anger alternating with discontentment; neuralgias; shingles; burning and intense itching.

SANKARAN MENTALS: Feels vexed and quarrelsome, letting these feelings occupy his mind for days. Eventually, since he doesn't want to be that way all the time, just settles into feeling discontented. These two states alternate in his life or until the pattern is dealt with and eliminated.

MIASM: Malaria

INCOMPATIBLE WITH: Sulphur, Staphysagria, alcohol, wine, vinegar—antidotes this remedy.

STAPHYSAGRIA (STAVESACRE)

Staphysagria is a polycrest remedy, meaning a remedy that is often indicated and effective for a lot of people in a wide variety of complaints.

Staphysagria certainly shows the family theme of suppressed anger, humiliation, or grief. A person who would benefit from this remedy is usually of a sweet and compliant temperament, but is suppressing a lot of anger or grief over perceived or real humiliations. This is especially a remedy for abused women, or the children of domineering parents (whether that domination was real or perceived). This remedy may give them the strength to end bad marriage or to take the responsibility to care for themselves. Used for styes or tumors on the eyelids; cystitis that began with first sexual encounters and may happen after every instance thereafter.

KEYNOTES: Some keynotes are: ailments are usually brought on by the suppressing of emotions; the person is sleepy all day but sleepless at night; has a tendency to throw things when angry; is worse from taking a nap in the afternoon.

SANKARAN MENTALS: Great fear of losing self-control; must keep complete control of self no matter how vexing, or just plain dreadful, the situation becomes.

MIASM: Cancer

COMPARISONS: Pulsatilla nigricans, Silica terra, Natrum carbonicum, Causticum, Natrum muriaticum, Nux vomica.

Scrophulariaceae Family (Figworts and Snapdragon)

MAIN THEME: Bonds and connections between people or between people and things. Bonds and connections are not, or do not feel, strong enough, so they want to hold on very tightly. If the connection is perceived as broken, great fear and mis-perceptions often occur. Passive reactions are indifference to and detachment from people and things. Active reactions are sticking to or attaching oneself to people and things, and to amorous feelings. Compensates by not needing any bonds or connections at all.

DIGITALIS PURPUREA (FOXGLOVE)
This remedy is a heart remedy; also affects liver, lungs, stomach, and genitourinary organs; slow pulse while reclining, becomes irregular on sitting up; better when stomach is empty; blue color of the lips and eyelids; thirst but little appetite; coldness of hands and feet; enlarged liver; jaundice with heart disease; starts from sleep; neuralgic pain in stomach.
KEYNOTES: Doubtful of his soul's welfare; embarrassment in the presence of strangers; cardiac muscular failure; great weakness; anxious about future; sudden sensation as if the heart has stood still; mitral valve disorders; pulse weak and quickened by the least movement.
SANKARAN MENTALS: If I do something wrong and am discovered, some important connections will be broken; I must be careful so that these connections do not break. I could not stand it if these connections were broken.
MIASM: Sycotic
COMPARISONS: Crataegus oxyacantha, Spigelia anthelmintica.

EUPHRASIA OFFICINALIS (EYEBRIGHT)
Cramp-like, pressing pains in the back; catch just under the sternum when breathing in; eyes are very sensitive to light and air; scanty menses flow that lasts only a day and comes late; shooting pain in the temples and in the forehead; numbness in the arms and hands; shortness of breath, even when seated; stammering; constipation; chilly, but sweating at night.
KEYNOTES: Eyes water all the time; thick yellow discharge from the eyes; allergies and hay fever.
SANKARAN MENTALS: Loss of connection to people that seemS to come on suddenly, right out of nowhere. Feels a great need to repair and restore the connection immediately.
MIASM: Typhoid
COMPARISONS: Allium cepa, Arsenicum album, Gelsemium sempervirens, Sabadilla officinalis.
ANTIDOTED BY: Pulsatilla nigricans.

LEPTANDRA VIRGINICA (CULVER'S ROOT)
Acts on the right side of the body and also on the liver; internal hemorrhages due to liver disorders; gloomy, despondent; weary, can hardly walk; irritable all day long; great distress in stomach and intestines; burning ache over liver and near the gallbladder area; chilly sensation in shoulders and down the back; dull frontal headache; drowsiness; red or orange colored urine; pain in sciatic nerve, on the left side, that is worse for sitting.
KEYNOTES: Jaundice; black, tarry stools.
SANKARAN MENTALS: A lot of despair and hopelessness. Being destroyed by, cannot recover from, the disconnection that he feels from others.
MIASM: Syphilis
COMPARISONS: Podophyllum peltatum, Iris versicolor, Bryonia alba, Mercurius solubilis, Myrica cerifera.

VERBASCUM THAPSIS (MULLEIN OIL)

Has a marked effect on the nerves, especially those of the face; also effects on the respiratory tract, the bladder, and the left side of the body; bed-wetting; ear pain; urinary incontinence; worse for drafts and changes in temperature; earache.
KEYNOTES: Trigeminal nerve pain, face feels as if it were being crushed by tongs; soreness of joints of lower limbs; salty saliva; voice hoarse.
SANKARAN MENTALS: Feels an urgent need to establish new connections without which he will face destruction.
MIASM: Tuberculosis
COMPARISONS: Causticum, Platinum metallicum, Stannum metallicum, Spongia tosta, Sulphur.

Solanaceae Family (Potato and Tomato)

MAIN THEME: Sudden violence and sudden spasms. The sensations are of things bursting, exploding, tearing, pulsating, jerking, and of being choked or pursued. Passive reactions are to feel faint, almost unconscious, sluggish, cowardly, with a lack of irritability and reactions. Active reactions are panic, rage, need to flee or fight back hard, spasms, acute senses, need to hurry through everything. Compensation is to show great courage in the face of danger.

ATROPINUM PURUM (ATROPINE—ALKALOID OF BELLADONNA)

Affinity for the pancreas; hypersensitivity of the sensory nerves; corneal ulcers; irritability of the eyes; dim vision with dilated pupils; deep red distorted face, especially when angry; congestion of kidneys; periodical headache of different kinds that comes on suddenly; vomiting, sometimes extremely violent; constant burning in back; sad, preferring solitude to time with friends; rambling speech.
KEYNOTES: Internal coldness with external burning heat of the whole body.
SANKARAN MENTALS: Suffocated by the violence around them.
MIASM: Tuberculosis

BELLADONNA (DEADLY NIGHTSHADE)

Hallucination; sudden explosive anger; acute and chronic vertigo; migraine aggravated by light and noise; ear congestion; suppurating tonsils; swelling of glands of the neck; earache is severely painful with eardrum bulging; child cries out in sleep; spasm, shock, jerks, and twitching; constrictions in various parts of the body
KEYNOTES: Cold hands and feet but face hot; aggravation at 11am and/or 3 pm; affected by change in temperature; aggravation from motion, flushes of heat; right-sided complaints; intense heat in the affected part; the heat can be felt by practitioner.
SANKARAN MENTALS: Sudden, violent, bursting explosions of rage or terror.
MIASM: Acute
COMPARISONS: Glonoine, Hyoscyamus niger, Stramonium, Calcarea carbonica is often required as a follow-up to Belladonna.

CAPSICUM ANNUUM (CAYENNE PEPPER)

Acts with great intensity on the mucus membranes; also has an affinity for the bones, especially the mastoid bone (just behind the ears); burning pains and general chilliness; muscle pain and jerking of muscles; neuralgias; pain felt in distinct parts of the body when coughing.
KEYNOTES: Homesickness, with sentimental, nostalgic moods; swelling and pain behind the ears; great thirst, but drinking causes shuddering and nausea; bleeding from hemorrhoids.
SANKARAN MENTALS: Stuck in a situation where they are exposed to attacks of violence. Reaction is periodic outbursts, discontentment, being critical of other people, and a longing for home as a means of escaping the current situation.
MIASM: Malaria
COMPARISONS: Arnica montana, Belladonna, Bryonia alba, Cantharis, Psorinum, Lachesis muta

DULCAMARA (WOODY NIGHTSHADE)
Mental confusion, cannot concentrate; cannot find the right word; pain in the small of the back; pain in left chest; hay fever with watery discharges; cough worse after exertion or getting chilled; vertigo on waking in the morning, giddy and dizzy, with trembling and weakness.
KEYNOTES: worse from cold and damp; arthritis, worse for and induced by cold and damp; enlarged glands; getting chilled brings on urge to urinate.
SANKARAN MENTALS: Alternates between avoiding and succumbing to rage and violence.
MIASM: Ringworm
INCOMPATIBLE Belladonna, Lachesis muta.
COMPARISONS: Aconitum napellus, Arsenicum album, Chamomilla vulgaris, Helleborus niger, Nitricum acidum, Pulsatilla nigricans, Staphysagria, Sulphur.

HYOSCYAMUS NIGER (HENBANE)
Profound effects on the mind, brain, and nervous system; profoundly disturbed, as though the mind is overcome by diabolical forces; mania; quarrelsome; sometimes obscene; muttering delirium, hallucinations and delusions; lightness and confusion of head; sensations as if heart and chest were torn up; heart's action becomes violent, tremulous, irregular; carotids beat violently; muscle twitches; toothaches.
KEYNOTES: Nervous agitation; tremulous weakness and twitching of tendons; inclined to laugh at everything; very suspicious; dry, spasmodic cough at night; involuntary urination.
SANKARAN MENTALS: The mentals of this remedy center around business concerns. Sudden intense threat of someone's rage or violence, with a great desire to reach or achieve a position of safety.
MIASM: Typhoid
COMPARISONS: Belladonna, Camphora, Stramonium, Agaricus phalloides, Gelsemium sempervirens

STRAMONIUM (JIMSON WEED)
This is a remedy of the mind, and symptoms are driven by the mind; includes references to raving mania, manic depression, paranoia, schizophrenia, terrifying hallucinations, night terrors, religious insanity, deliriums with a desire to escape, and terror.
KEYNOTES: Must have light and company; dreads the darkness; anxiety when going through a tunnel; aversion to all fluids; headache from the sun; violent pain in left hip; stammering.
SANKARAN MENTALS: Sudden rage and violence as a result of fright or terror.
MIASM: Acute
COMPARISONS: Hyoscyamus niger, Belladonna.

NICOTIANA TABACUM (TOBACCO)
Mental confusion and fatigue; slow perception; forgetful; indifferent; desire for company in evening; nervous and restless; pain in small of the back, worse lying down; dry cough, helped by swallow of cold water; eyes sunken, blue around them; morning sickness of pregnancy; angina pectoris with nausea; profuse salivation.
KEYNOTES: Feels very despondent; fainting; giddiness; nausea; motion sickness; vertigo; headache with nausea and vertigo; chill with cold sweats.
SANKARAN MENTALS: Must always keep calm and in control with no panic even in situations of violence and rage.
MIASM: Cancer
COMPARISONS: Lobelia inflata, Ignatia amara, Sepia succus, Nux vomica, Phosphorus, Camphora, Veratrum album, Arsenicum album.

Umbelliferae Family (Carrot/Celery)

MAIN THEME: Sudden, unexpected violence and attack in any form. Sensations are of stabbing, blows, vertigo, fainting, accidents. Passive reactions are numbness, indifference, sadness, and profound exhaustion. Active reactions include violence, convulsion, furious attack, fits of emotion, mania, and escape. Compensates by remaining icy calm in situations where there is violence or a sudden attack of some sort.

ASAFOETIDA (GUM OF THE STINKSAND)

Dissatisfied with one's self; irritable; magnifies her symptoms; craves sympathy; decay of bones; aching bone pains which change places and are better by touch; irritability during menses, alternating with indifference; headache that is pressive pain from within pushing outward.
KEYNOTES: Offensive discharges; reverse peristalsis; diarrhea; over sensitivity, mental and physical; spasmodic tightness in the chest.
SANKARAN MENTALS: Avoidance of unexpected blows or stabs. They see themselves as weak, so they avoid violent and dangerous situations.
MIASM: Sycotic, according to Sankaran; others mention Syphilis, but, in my opinion, the remedy lacks the deep despair and destructiveness that is characteristic of Syphilis.
COMPARISONS: Aurum metallicum, China officinalis, Lachesis muta, Mercurius solubilis, Valerian officinalis.

CICUTA VIROSA (WATER HEMLOCK)

Concussions; convulsions; epilepsy; head injuries; cerebrospinal meningitis; tetanus; spasms; colic with convulsions and vomiting; twitching of facial muscles; craves to eat chalk and many other strange things; trembling palpitations of the heart; nightmares after movies or sad stories; hiccups.
KEYNOTES: Anxiety about the future; suspicious; aversion to company and people in general; contemptuous; neck muscles are contracted; rigid limbs.
SANKARAN MENTALS: Suspicious, mistrustful, feels both attacked and shunned; reaction is to hate and shun people back.
MIASM: Leprosy
COMPARISONS: Natrum muriaticum, Arsenicum album, Belladonna, Arsenicum album, Bryonia alba.

CONIUM MACULATUM (POISON HEMLOCK)

Acts primarily on the nerves and muscles anywhere in the body—useful for a great many complaints if general and keynote symptoms match; cataracts; weakness of body and mind; paralysis of some sort; trembling; progressive debility marks this remedy; this remedy is often indicated following injury or bruising where the affected part becomes hard, swollen, or inflamed.
KEYNOTES: Strange symptom of sweating when sleeping, or even just closing one's eyes; noted for menstrual problems in women where keynote symptoms (particularly swollen breasts before period) are present; also noted for use with cataracts.
SANKARAN MENTALS: Must be in control even when unexpectedly attacked.
An example: Socrates, even though poisoned by deadly hemlock, maintained total control of his faculties. He continued his philosophical lectures with great calmness and showed no fear of coming discomfort or death. He chastised his followers and asked them to leave his bedside if they broke into tears or lost control of their emotions. Perhaps this was the poison taking effect on his mental state as well as his physical body.
MIASM: Cancer
COMPARISONS: Hydrastis canadensis, Kali phosphoricum, Hyoscyamus niger, Curare woorari

CORIANDRUM SATIVUM (CORIANDER, COMMONLY KNOWN AS CILANTRO)

Cough; fever; chills; blocked sinuses; hypoglycemia; throbbing pain in temples; water retention; dreams about evil and being unsafe; vertigo from motion in peripheral vision.
KEYNOTES: Extreme fatigue; body feels like a dead weight; headache; cravings for sweets; feeling disconnected from people; anxious; depressed; overwhelmed; spacey; makes silly mistakes in writing and speaking.

SANKARAN MENTALS: Destroyed by violence.
MIASM: Syphilis
COMPARISONS: None. There is only one proving done by Louis Klein (R.S. Hom). Not near enough known about this remedy.

Violaceae Family (Violets & Melons)

MAIN THEME: Two-fold main theme and sensations. Mentally, the feeling is aversion to the disquietude or distress of mind caused by humiliation or annoyance. Physically, the feelings are of being cut or stabbed. Passive reactions are complete prostration, deep sadness, avoidance of people, aversion to being disturbed, wants total rest and quiet. Active reactions are irritable when questioned or disturbed, restlessness, maliciousness, violence and rage. Compensates by cultivating quietness, calmness, stillness.

BRYONIA ALBA (WILD HOPS)
A frequently used remedy for acute conditions; affects mucus membranes such as the pleura, the synovial membranes of joints, the gastrointestinal membranes, the meninges, by drying them out; headaches over left eye or forehead extending to the occiput and then the whole head; fractures, sprains, or arthritis with severe pain from slightest motion; this remedy is a polycrest with many symptoms.
KEYNOTES: Deep fears of many things; marked aggravation from motion; symptoms related to the dryness found throughout the system; overwhelming fear of poverty; irritable and wants to be left alone.
SANKARAN MENTALS: Working busily to reach a position of authority and comfort so that life will be free of vexations and disturbances and peace and quiet can finally be found.
MIASM: Typhoid
COMPARISONS: Kali muriaticum, Aconitum napellus, Belladonna.

CISTUS CANADENSIS (ROCK ROSE)
Listed for bone disorders; glandular swelling; cancers; herpes zoster; pyorrhea.
KEYNOTES: Extreme sensitivity to cold; coldness in various parts; throat is very dry; throat becomes sore if least bit of cold air is inhaled.
SANKARAN MENTALS: Being suffocated by disturbances, needs to get out and away.
MIASM: Tuberculosis
COMPARISONS: Angentum, Nitricum, Belladonna

COLOCYNTHIS (BITTER CUCUMBER)
Lamenting and complaining day and night; ailments after anger, with silent grief; impatient, easily annoyed when in pain; sensitive to misfortunes of others—equally sensitive to own pain and grief; many symptoms in the abdominal area and head (neuralgic, cutting-type pains usually on the left side); colic remedy; worse after cold drinks, when over-heated and following anger (generally irritable people who anger easily); neuralgia with chilliness; sounds re-echo in the ears; contractions and cramps in muscles.
KEYNOTES: Pain in abdomen causes the person to bend over double, is better for hard pressure; sciatic pain, better for pressure and heat; persistent bitter taste in mouth; ovarian cysts.
SANKARAN MENTALS: Feels that people are doing disturbing things deliberately to annoy him.
MIASM: Malaria—this miasm falls between the acute miasm and the sycosis miasm and has characteristics of each. The malaria miasm is fitting because there is the desire to escape (acute miasm) uncomfortable situations that are uncomfortable only because the person perceives that they have some flaw in their character (sycosis miasm) that make them unworthy or unable to cope with the situation.
COMPARISONS: Dioscorea villosa, Chamomilla vulgaris, Cocculus indicus, Mercurius solubilis, Magnesia phosphorica, Staphysagria.

VIOLA ODORATA (SWEET-SCENTED VIOLET)
Marked affinity for the wrists; neuralgias; tension in muscles of the neck; feels as if a weight on chest.
KEYNOTES: Emotions subjected to the intellect; must keep tight control of emotions at all times; cancers; headaches across the forehead; pains in the joints of the fingers.

SANKARAN MENTALS: Must keep in control even though disturbed and upset.
MIASM: Cancer
COMPARISONS: No really good comparisons. An unusual remedy.

VIOLA TRICOLOR (PANSY)

Action on skin, scalp and urinary organs; principal use of this remedy is for eczema in childhood; tendency to sleep in the afternoon; awakens frequently at night without cause; sore throat in the evening; vertigo and dizziness when walking; perplexed and bewildered.
KEYNOTES: Copious urine with an offensive odor; impetigo or ringworm on the scalp.
SANKARAN MENTALS: Trying to be quiet and at peace and not disturbed.
MIASM: Ringworm
COMPARISONS: Lycopodium clavatum, Chamomilla vulgaris, Viola odorata.

Vegetable Kingdom Remedies (One In Each Family)

ALLIUM CEPA (ONION)

The symptom picture is what you would expect with an onion—cold-like symptoms from either a cold or a seasonal allergy. (A word of warning here: overuse of this remedy for colds and allergies may suppress the minor annoying symptoms while they develop into asthma. Setting up this energetic asthma picture takes serious over dosing, but the possibility needs to be mentioned.) Allium cepa, while an excellent "acute" remedy, needs to be followed by a deeper acting remedy once the acute symptoms have been relieved!
KEYNOTES: profuse watery discharge from nose—like a faucet; hay fever made worse from flowers and warm rooms; is mostly on the left side; worse in the evening; headache aggravated by closing the eyes.
COMPARISONS: Sabadilla officinalis, Euphrasia officinalis.

COCCULUS INDICUS (INDIAN COCKLE)

This remedy mainly affects the central nervous system; usually includes some type of vertigo. Early symptoms are over-excitability, restlessness, dizziness, anxiety and agitation; later problems with conduction along the nerves. Senses become distorted (confusion) and delayed (full second delay before perceiving a pin prick).
KEYNOTES: Intense concern for the welfare of another—so intense it leads to a breakdown of the nervous system; true vertigo (must lie down); motion sickness.

DIOSCOREA VILLOSA (WILD YAM)

This is a remedy for many kinds of pain, colic and severe abdominal cramping—often accompanied by acute diarrhea; should always be considered for gallbladder problems and gallstones.
KEYNOTES: The colic pains of Dioscorea are better for stretching out and by moving about (Colocynthis is better for bending over and holding still).

HYPERICUM PERFORATUM (ST. JOHN'S WORT)

Frequently used for general depression, but only really successful when other keynote symptoms are present—not a palliative for all types of depression; excellent remedy for injury to nerve-rich areas such as fingers, toes, eyes, spine, or tailbone; consider for all puncture wounds as a prevention for lockjaw. (Here is a strange and unique symptom—use for stye on left, lower eyelid);
KEYNOTES: Shooting pains from injured part; spasms of muscles after injury is also a keynote.

LYCOPODIUM CLAVATUM (CLUB MOSS)

This is one of the most fundamental, often used remedies—classed with Sulphur and Calcarea and used in a triad regimen. Mental picture is pronounced and characterized by feelings of inferiority and lack of self-esteem (this may manifest as either shyness or egotism and bragging); lack of self-control—craving sweets

and things that are not good for them is another hallmark. Large remedy, usually with pages and pages in remedy guides—check it out! The list of uses is long and important!!
KEYNOTES: Symptoms begin on the right side and then move to the left and are worse from 4 to 8 pm.

PHYTOLACCA DECANDRA (POKE ROOT)
This remedy acts on the glandular system with a particular affinity for breast tissue and the glands of women and is specific for breast cancer and cancer of the uterus and rectum. Phytolacca is specific, both in herbal form and homeopathically, for mastitis. In addition, Phytolacca decandra has a powerful effect on the throat, muscles of back and neck, all fibrous tissue, tendons and joints (tendonitis) and the digestive tract. Phytolacca is indicated for certain types of dental pain associated with clenching the teeth.
KEYNOTES: cannot endure pain, it is simply intolerable; worse for damp cold weather; (compare to Mercurius solubilis) Never forget this one for nursing mothers with mastitis.

RUTA GRAVEOLENS (GARDEN RUE)
One of the chief remedies for injured or bruised bones and sprains—usually used following Arnica. It is often difficult to distinguish between the need for Ruta graveolens and the need for Rhus toxicodendron, the other leading remedy for injuries and sprains. Ruta graveolens is often of benefit in back pain where the vertebrae slip out of place easily, particularly in situations where the original cause was injury or strain. Other symptoms include eye-strain, particularly with headache, ganglion of wrist, sore thighs, and weak knees.

SABAL SERRULATA (SAW PALMETTO)
Considered a homeopathic catheter for the retention of urine due to prostate enlargement; nearly always indicated for enlarged and weakened prostate; interestingly, it is useful in women for undeveloped breast glands (usually with dysmenorrhea) and for sharp pains in mammary glands; consider for bedwetting, particularly in older gentlemen if the "mentals" match. This is a valuable remedy but is not considered a polycrest because its actions are so specific.

SAMBUCUS NIGRA (ELDER)
I needed this remedy many years ago. I had not previously realized that Sambucus nigra was elder and I found the connection between the herbal and homeopathic uses very interesting at that time. Asthma, chest oppressions, choking, coughs, croup, where a constant state of fretfulness is present are part of the symptom picture. A keynote symptom is profuse sweat over entire body, or dry burning fever while sleeping with copious sweating on waking up. Another keynote is edema and dropsical swelling in various parts of the body, especially in the legs and feet. The feeling is that of being pushed out.

SYMPHYTUM OFFICINALE (COMFREY)
There has been very little "proving work" done on Symphytum so the list of uses is very small. However, it is of such enormous value as a first-aid treatment for injuries to the eye and for broken bones that it should be in everyone's homeopathic kit. In cases of bone fracture, it is helpful both for pain and for improving the knitting together of the bones.

TRIFOLIUM (RED CLOVER)
This is a very little used or studied remedy. I include it here for three reasons: 1) I love the herb and find it useful as a blood purifier and many other things 2) Strongly indicated for anyone whose family history includes cancer (Is there anyone nowadays whose family history does not include cancer?), and 3) It is indicated for whooping cough and certain other types of respiratory illnesses and hay fevers.

CUNDURANGO (MARSDENIA CUNDURANGO—EAGLE VINE)
This is a fairly recently proven remedy. It is indicated for a wide range of digestive complaints. Cundurango's symptom picture includes vomiting of food with constant burning pain, loss of appetite, stricture of esophagus, pain behind sternum where food seems to be stuck, and cracks or sores at the corners of the mouth. There are reports of Cundurango being used successfully in the treatment of stomach cancer.

Chapter Nineteen - Animal Remedies

In the homeopathic world, nearly everything that isn't human, plant, or mineral is considered to be an animal remedy. This category includes ocean mammals, spiders, insects, and snakes and (most likely) some species I have not thought to list here. Animal remedies share the common issues of survival, hierarchy (place in this world), and competitiveness.

Many of the animal remedies, except insects and some spiders, have symptoms in the areas of heart, lungs, blood, nerves, and circulation. They are also characterized by over-stimulation of some kind. The over-stimulation and over-excitement may occur in the nerves, the electrical system of the heart, the emotions, the respiratory system, or all of these at once.

The insect remedies share a common affinity for the kidneys and for the stinging pain of any type of burn. In fact the insect remedies all include stinging and burning pains of any type.

The first few pages of this chapter contain some information about a few common animal remedies. Following that are descriptions of some remedies in each of the major family groups with the symptoms of major organs described and compared.

BLATTA ORIENTALIS (INDIAN COCKROACH)

This remedy is useful for asthma, especially when associated with bronchitis, difficult breathing, and a great accumulation of mucus—it follows Arsenicum album well in these cases. Chronic inflammation of bronchial tubes; shortness of breath; pneumonia; bronchitis; worse from dust, wet weather, and winter; chest feels as if a great weight were pressing on it; often clammy, cold sweat on the body.

BUFO RANA (TOAD POISON)

The symptoms of an epileptic seizure are a close perfect description of the symptom picture of Bufo rana.

Other symptoms include confusion; loss of memory; anxiety about health; sadness on waking; violent colic; headache that feels like tight bands around the head; heaviness in region of the heart; palpitations with nausea after eating; burning pains in kidneys; congestion of lymph fluid with red streaks under the skin; constant licking of the lips; profuse sweat that feels oily in the head and face or cold and clammy sweat on hands and arms; burning like a fire in the lungs.

MALANDRINUM (GREASE OF HORSES)

This remedy is often used to counteract the negative effects of vaccinations (this use has an interesting history! There is a short synopsis of some of these statistics below.)

Skin symptoms include red spots on legs; impetigo covering back of head and extending down the back to the buttocks; dry, scaly skin that cracks on hands and feet in cold weather or from immersion in water; slow suppuration, never ending: as one heals another always appears. Other symptoms include dizziness and dullness of mind; dread of any mental exertion; lack of concentration; frontal and occipital headache; pains in limbs and joints; dreams of quarrels and troubles with other people.

These symptoms can often be tracked as starting shortly after a vaccination. Interesting history of use during smallpox epidemics and to counteract the effects of smallpox vaccines. When Malandrinum was given along with the vaccine, no scar occurred (a scar indicates that the vaccine "took"), but neither did any one using the Maladrinum with the vaccine contract smallpox. Interesting statistics!! Hopefully we will never meet smallpox, but remember this one for other vaccinations. Very deep acting remedy even in low potency; not meant to be repeated at close intervals.

MEPHITIS PUTORIUS (SKUNK SECRETION)

One of the major areas of action of this remedy is in the lungs and throat. Description of symptoms include sudden contraction of the glottis, making swallowing and exhaling nearly impossible; severe chest pains when coughing or sneezing; spasmodic cough; whooping cough; violent, suffocative, nervous cough that is worse at night or when attempting to talk; cough with vomiting after eating. Symptoms also include great hunger alternating with absence of appetite and painful weariness and desire to sleep after a meal.

Milk Remedies (Various Types of Milks—Animal and Human)

Milk contains within itself a wide range of cells from the tissues and salts of the animal from which it is taken. The symptom picture of any milk remedy must include the pictures of the various salts, glands, and tissues common to life. For example, the symptom picture of Natrum muriaticum (potassium chloride) can be seen running through all of these remedies, as can the pictures of the other tissue salts and glandular remedies such as raw thymus and Thyroidinum.

LAC CANINUM (DOG'S MILK)

The remedy guides contain several pages of symptoms for this remedy. I will list only a few of them here. Mind: despondent; oversensitive to touch; lack of self-confidence; fits of weeping; fears to be alone; fear of snakes—even dreams of snakes. Physical: pressure and swelling in abdomen; severe backache and stiffness of neck; mastitis in nursing mothers; ear infection that alternates from ear to ear; ringing in the ears; sensation of reverberation, like speaking in a large empty room; eyes watering and discharging; menses flows in gushes; craves milk and drinks it even though it aggravates; headache with blurred vision, nausea and vomiting; headaches that alternate sides; migraines; arthritic pains which move from joint to joint and side to side; sore throat; tonsillitis; tongue coated, whitish grey, brown, or yellow matter; difficulty in reading because the letters seem to run together; tendency of eye to retain the impression of objects and colors; symptoms are better from cold drinks and open air; worse for touch, pressure, or motion; symptoms are often worse for rest.

LAC DEFLORATUM (SKIMMED MILK)

Many people develop symptoms such as severe constipation and violent headaches when ingesting milk. This remedy is particularly helpful for these types of disorders, whether caused by milk or not. (Remember it is the symptom, not the cause, that determines homeopathic treatment.) Other symptoms include: restoring of scanty milk flow in nursing mothers; restoration of menses that is suppressed when hands or body is put in cold water; intense throbbing headache with nausea; pressure around the heart; persistent constipation; skin very sensitive to cold; person always feels chilly; vertigo that is worse lying on left side; feeling of faintness when extending arms over the head; headaches in anemic women.

LAC VACCINUM BUTYRICUM (BUTTERMILK)

Mind: deep depression—the future looks dark and hopeless. Physical: dullness of hearing, as if ears were full of water; rumbling in abdomen with loose stools; eyeballs are sensitive to pressure; scanty urine with involuntary dribbling; irritation and coughing; feeling of adhesion between lung and the pleural lining; canker sores on inside of cheeks and lips; groups of pimples that are sore to touch and itchy; sleepy during the day with very great drowsiness; wakes at 4 a.m. with no desire for further sleep.

Arachnid Remedies (Spider)

The symptom pictures of remedies from the arachnid family (usually referred to as spiders although there are other member of the family than just spiders) have some common characteristics and some characteristics that are unique to each remedy. The three remedies which are made from spiders are more similar to one another than are the other remedies. Of the five listed here, one is made using a tarantula and the other (Buthus australis) is made from scorpion venom.

Similar physical symptoms: The true spider remedies have a marked effect on the heart, nervous system, and lungs. Spider bites, and the remedies made from them, also affect the composition of the blood, with coagulation problems and hemorrhages of varying degrees being a common symptom. Addictions and addictive behavior patterns are among the mental/emotional keynotes of the remedies of web-building spiders. A keynote of arachnid remedies in general (not just the spiders) is symptoms of over-stimulation in the affected organs and systems. This, of course, means that these remedies alleviate these symptoms where they are present. There is also a great restlessness with constant movement, jumping, climbing and continual movement of the hands.

Similar mental symptoms—arachnid family in general: sensitivity to noise, music, vibrations; extreme busyness; need to hurry because time is passing too quickly; jealous; seeks revenge; fear of death; heightened sexual feelings or desires.

Similar mental symptoms—web-building spiders: feeling of being trapped or caught in a situation; feeling isolated; feelings of being powerless or weak; cunning; conniving, deceitful; uses flattery or trickery to get one's way.

LATRODECTUS MACTANS (BLACK WIDOW)

OVER-STIMULATION: Occurs predominantly in the electrical system of the heart. The heart symptoms can be very frightening and very similar to the classic symptoms of a heart attack.

HEART: Latrodectus overstimulates both the heart, predominantly the electrical system, and the nervous system. Heart symptoms resemble those of a *classic heart attack* and include violent chest pains radiating out to the shoulders and down to the fingertips, usually of the left arm but can be both arms on occasion; partial paralysis of, usually, the left arm; symptoms are accompanied by restlessness, a feeble but rapid pulse, and great fatigue and prostration.

LUNGS: Gasping for breath; respiration very slow; pulmonary edema; cough with thick yellow sputum; great fear of suffocating.

BLOOD: Blood becomes very thin and watery with poor coagulability; chronic hemorrhage and bruising.

NERVES AND MENTAL: Intense anxiety, anguish, and fear of imminent death; inability to think clearly or make logical deductions; speech becomes hesitant; nervousness; depression; extreme mental fatigue; sensitivity to noise; tendency to complain, mostly to companion and close friends.

KIDNEYS: Urine reddish with burning pain; proteinuria; diminished levels of nitrogen in urine.

GENERAL: Severe abdominal pain with nausea; colic; abdomen hard but without additional pain when touched; pain on swallowing; pain in the lumbar region of the back, in the neck, and in the back of the head; headache, worse between 2 and 3 pm; black, tarry vomit and stools; burning on the soles of the feet; hair loss; anxious sleep; vertigo.

MODALITIES: Better when sitting quietly; feels less restlessness and anxiety when lying on the right side with the head slightly raised; worse from the slightest movement—often worse from moving just the hands.

Latrodectus mactans symptoms are those of a classic heart attack. This remedy should be considered, or tried as a first response, whenever a heart attack is suspected.

THERIDION CURASSAVICUM (ORANGE SPIDER)

OVER-STIMULATION: Occurs predominantly to the nerves and to the heart. Nerve symptoms are particularly pronounced, with great sensitivity to noise; increased talkativeness; hilarious; hysterical.

HEART: The heart symptoms of Theridion are less severe than those of Latrodectus. They include cardiac pain with anxiety about the heart; sharp pain radiating to the left arm and shoulder. The pulse is slow and there is vertigo, chilliness, and nausea.

LUNGS: The predominant symptom here is difficult breathing or shortness of breath when going up stairs. At rest or when coughing there is a sensation of too much air entering the chest cavity. Coughing causes the body to draw together with the head going forward and down and the knees being drawn upward.

BLOOD: Issues show up as violent burning pain in the region of the liver and stinging pain over the spleen.

NERVES AND MENTAL: Sensitivity to noise, which penetrates the entire body settling into problem areas and seems to resonate in the teeth; easily startled; noise causes chills and nausea; restlessness; taking pleasure in nothing while continually moving from one thing to another; lack of self-confidence; confusion; aversion to work; feels and looks as if dying, but is able to hear and understand what is going on around them; desire to please others but a great desire to live their own lives which often creates tension and stress.

KIDNEYS: Unusual stimulation of the kidneys and bladder during the night with frequent need to urinate but very little passage of urine during daytime hours.

GENERAL: A keynote of Theridion is bone decay and pain; bones feel broken; spine is ultra sensitive to pressure and jarring—the person often sits sideways to avoid pressure on the spine; sensitive areas between the vertebrae; headaches with pain over the root of the nose; itching with stinging and stabbing pains all over the body; internal coldness with the interior of the head feeling hot and congested.

MODALITIES: All symptoms are better from rest in a horizontal position; warmth improves symptoms with warm water improving nausea; worse from touch, pressure, stooping, rising, walking, travel, from noise, with eyes closed, and from going up and down stairs.

LOXOSCELES RECLUSA (BROWN RECLUSE)

OVER-STIMULATION: Over-stimulation occurs mostly to the nerves and to the mental state and is followed almost immediately by a depressed and collapsed state.

HEART/BLOOD: *The symptoms of this remedy lack the frightening heart and hemorrhagic/blood symptoms that occur with other spider remedies. There are heart symptoms but they are usually not severe.* Symptoms include feelings of excess energy in the heart, as if large quantities of caffeine had been consumed; heart palpitations occurring after frightening dreams; accelerated pulse; mild pain in sternum.

LUNGS: Accelerated breathing seems to be the only lung symptom for this milder spider remedy.

NERVES AND MENTAL: Over-stimulation to the nerves manifests first as over-sensitivity and rudeness, then rage, and finally deteriorates into deep, even suicidal, depression; sudden anger followed by quick remorse; feels forsaken; forgetful; difficulty concentrating; apathy; obstinate; lack of self-confidence; a confusing symptom of Loxosceles reclusa is, unlike Theridion curassavicum, the person may show an industrious almost manic attitude toward work.

KIDNEYS: Urine is very scanty, bright yellow in color with a strong odor; bed-wetting.

GENERAL: Alternating coldness and heat; cramping pain in the abdomen; backache in the lumbar region; stiffness in neck and back; eyes are bloodshot in the mornings; frontal headaches that throb and pulse with burning pressure behind the eyes; joint pains; sciatica that is better for walking; heartburn; belching; nausea

MODALITIES: Symptoms are worse in the early evening but better during the night and worsening again in the morning or waking.

TARENTULA HISPANICA (TARANTULA)

Tarentula is the most proven and best understood of the spider remedies. It is listed in the Materia Medicas as a possible remedy for multiple sclerosis, Parkinson's disease, and Meniere's disease. It is also said that Tarentula palliates the agony and pains of the dying process.

OVER-STIMULATION: The symptoms of over-stimulation in the nervous system are particularly pronounced. Symptoms appear suddenly and often violently. This is the most hurried of all homeopathic remedies.

HEART: Angina pectoris—the heart muscle not getting the blood that it needs due to partial obstruction of the arteries; mitral valve damage; violent palpitations; thumping and trembling sensations in the region of the heart; sensation that the heart is twisting around in the chest or jumping suddenly; heart feels as if it is squeezed or compressed; heart suddenly skips a few beats; oppression in the chest when lying down, when raising the arms, or when lying on left side; pulse is hard, irregular, and infrequen.

LUNGS: Feelings of suffocation, feel they must have fresh air immediately; panting with oppressive feeling in the chest; symptoms worse with coughing.

BLOOD: Profuse menstruation; dark red or purplish coloration of the skin and tissues.

NERVES AND MENTAL: Lacks emotional control; destructive impulses; selfish and demanding; impatient and irritable; sudden fits of throwing things away; discontented; anger and despair at the same time; fits of nervous laughter followed by yelling; anxious and full of fears; erratic moods; obstinate; wildly hyperactive; great sensitivity to music; aversion to bright colors, particularly black, red, yellow, and green.

KIDNEYS: Foul urine with sandy sediment; sensation of constriction and pressure in the bladder; leaking of urine when laughing or coughing; excessive urine with violent pains in the back and even paralysis of the legs; diabetes mellitus; cystitis.

GENERAL: Twitches and jerking motions; restless leg syndrome; numbness in legs; restless sleep; *heart and ovarian diseases occurring together;* uterine fibroids; eczema; loss of appetite or desire for highly seasoned food; cravings for sand; intense pain in the head as if a thousand needles were pricking the brain; violent crushing headaches; copious perspiration which is worse when excited; chilliness alternating with heat; general feeling of heat but with cold feet; vertigo.

MODALITIES: Better in open air; better from music; mental symptoms are often better right after eating; worse by putting hands in cold water; worse for unrequited love, bad news, scolding, or punishment; unusual reoccurrence of symptoms periodically—yearly and at the same time of the day.

BUTHUS AUSTRALIS (SCORPION)

OVER-STIMULATION: Over-stimulation of the lungs and the heart; the over stimulation of this remedy tends to focus on the mental symptoms more than on the physical.

HEART: Feeling of heat in heart; feeling as though a piece of wood has been nailed between heart and lungs.

LUNGS: Difficult breathing, often with palpitations; fear of not being able to breathe.

NERVES AND MENTAL: Lack of confidence with an intense need to prove themselves as clever, brilliant, and sophisticated; tend to become complainers, suspicious, and hypochondriacal and see themselves as victims; often feel like outsiders; indecision and worry; intellectual work is difficult and tiring; alternating moods relating to speaking—sometimes taciturn and at other times feeling an irresistible need to speak.

GENERAL: Pains and stiffness in the neck; throbbing headaches; trembling of the limbs; pain when walking; red spots on the skin; sensation of coldness with icy needles pricking the skin; sleepiness and insensitivity; constriction in the throat; vertigo when walking; symptoms reappear with yearly periodicity.

MODALITIES: Better from rest and eating; worse from effort and intellectual work; worse in the late afternoon.

A Comparison of Spider and Snake Remedies

A comparison of the arachnid/spider remedies and the snake venom remedies to the concepts of yin and yang in eastern medicine can shed a little light on both families of remedies. Spider remedies more closely resemble yin energy while the snake remedies are definitely more yang in nature and attributes. The spider remedies represent a focus that is more inward on personal change and quiet growth rather than a need to compete and conquer the environment and themselves that is a basic component of snake remedies.

Yin energy is the shady side of the hill with its dampness and quiet, tending to linger near home. Yang energy, on the other hand, is the sunny side of the hill with light and warmth and a tendency to strike out when threatened. Spiders typically prefer to find dark spaces near their webs to hide themselves in, while snakes come right out and lie in the sun, reacting only when their territory has been invaded. The energies of yin and yang are also reflected in the chilly nature and in the fiery hot passionate natures of the snake remedies and in the alternating cold and hot aspects of spider remedies.

The remedies of the arachnid family which are true spiders and build webs share some common themes among themselves that are not present in the rest of the arachnid family or in the snake remedies. When out of balance, the patterns of these remedies include using cunning or trickery to accomplish their goals. These spider remedies include themes of emotionally devouring those close to them or feelings of being devoured emotionally themselves.

The emotional pattern of snake remedies in relationships is completely different. People needing snake remedies are usually intelligent, powerful, and fascinating. Their passion and fire draws us to them and yet frightens and repels us a little at the same time. Perhaps we recognize, on a subconscious level, that snakes move, by choice, from the light and sun of earth to the dark of cracks, crevices and the "underworld." his dynamic is important in understanding that snake remedies often manifest with themes of deliberate evil, succumbing to temptation, periods of aberrant sexuality that sometimes includes themes of female dominance (a demonstration of yang depleted and yin out of balance in proportion). Twisted religious practices are sometimes seen.

Spider remedies include themes of entrapment—trapping others or being trapped themselves. The emotional pattern often includes feelings of abandonment. Snake remedies, on the other hand, are more about betrayal—betraying or being betrayed, often deliberately and with intent and self-rationalization.

Among the homeopathic remedies of the web-building spiders there is also a theme of compulsiveness, addictions, and addictive behaviors. They simply must spin that web! There is also an element of "hiding dark secrets" that is common to addictive behavior patterns and to the spider remedies.

A common theme among both spider and snake remedies is the periodicity of symptoms, with some symptoms reoccurring in yearly cycles. In spiders, the more regular and precise the pattern of the web the more pronounced is the tendency for symptoms to reoccur in cyclical patterns.

Spider remedies, as one might expect, show a great industriousness, moving about quickly and efficiently. Spider remedies show a love of intrigue and a fascination with politics and political scheming.

Snakes can also be very quick in their movements, striking almost faster than the eye can follow. Yet there is something effortless, almost lazy, about their movements. Their slithering seems to occur without effort, almost other worldly and supernatural in its seductiveness.

The venom of both spiders and snakes is destructive. Snake venom is generally more destructive and more likely to be lethal than the venom of spiders and there is a remorselessness in snake venom and snake remedies that is not present among the emotional patterns of the spider remedies.

Spiders tend to hide when possible, leaving the fight for another day or biting without warning. Snakes rarely run away or hide themselves. They strike when provoked but generally give warning first. These patterns are reflected in the emotional patterns of both families of remedies. Snake remedies appear to belong to the syphilitic miasm.

Snake Remedies

Like the spider remedies, those made from snakes and snake venom share several common primary affinities. The first of these commonalities are in the blood and manifest as coagulation and bleeding problems, hemorrhages, and heart disease. Other commonalities are susceptibility to neurotoxins, kidney issues, lung problems, necrosis of tissues, and paralysis. Emotionally, snake remedies are concerned with survival and hierarchy issues. Excellent at camouflage, there is a tendency to hide behind an image, giving an impression of shyness and high moral values (accurate or not). Consistent with the colorful and appealing coloring of many snakes, clothes, money, and jewelry are important in their attractiveness to others.

A snake's body enlarges to accommodate the prey that it has swallowed. Interestingly, a primary theme among snake remedies is the sensation of, or actual enlargement, of body parts along with feelings of constriction, especially round the neck. Snake remedy symptoms are almost universally worse when sleeping or upon first waking up. The symptoms of the more aggressive snakes are predominantly left-sided, while the less aggressive snakes have symptoms manifesting more on the right side of the body. Respiratory problems are also common, as are throat chakra issues such as speech impediments and trouble speaking either too much or too little.

LACHESIS MUTA (BUSHMASTER)
NOTES: In the medicas, Lachesis is listed as a remedy to fight bubonic plague, yellow fever, and cancer.

HEART: High blood pressure; visible palpitations worse in a warm room; palpitations in morning on waking (symptoms representative of coming out of hibernation are a common theme of snake remedies); the heart seems to stand still and then starts with a tremendous bound (like a snake still and then striking suddenly); feeling that the heart is enlarged (enlarged body parts are common in snake remedies and reflects the snake expanding to swallow their prey); feelings of constriction in heart; palpitations with pain and fainting spells.

BLOOD/HEMORRHAGIC: Rapid bleeding from even a small wound; nosebleeds; bloody urine; flushes of heat and rushes of blood; hemorrhages are thin, containing dark patches that seem like charred material; scanty menstrual flow produces pain; troubles at menopause, hot flashes; capillaries that are dilated and appear purplish in color; purplish hemorrhoids that protrude and become constricted.

KIDNEYS: Pressure in bladder with frequent urging but scanty urine; urine is dark brown with gravelly sediment; bloody urine; dribbling after urination; sharp pains; burning after urination; kidney stones.

LUNGS: Sensations of suffocation; breathing seems to almost stop on falling asleep; feels the need for frequent deep breaths; can breathe freely only in an upright position; pneumonia; cyanosis; large quantities of ropy mucus that is difficult to expectorate.

PHYSICAL/GENERAL: Pain in the coccyx, worse on standing up after sitting for a while; stiff neck with movement of the jaw being difficult; lumbar region of back feels weak and tender; earache with sore throat; ears sensitive to wind; congestive headaches with rush of blood to the head; headaches from the sun; headaches with menses and menopause; *useful for paralysis after a stroke if other symptoms match;* liver region sensitive; gnawing pressure in the stomach that is better by eating; toothache pain that extends to ears; sore throats that are worse on the left side and aggravated by hot drinks; left-sided, aggressive symptoms; malignant or septic states; gangrene; slow healing of diabetics; cellulitis with blue color of skin.

MENTALS: Nervous and excitable; talkative, jumping from subject to subject very rapidly; sarcastic; wants to be going somewhere constantly; sadness in the morning; manic-depressive; mental confusion; jealousy; mistrust, interrupts train of own conversation with another story; often speaks of or seeks revenge; volent anger and behavior; religious mania; delusions and hallucinations.

MODALITIES: Symptoms are relieved by the appearance of discharges—menstrual blood or mucus; better from open air, cold drinks, and eating; worse from any extremes of weather; worse from hot drinks; worse after sleep, especially in the mornings; worse from closing the eyes and from motion; cannot tolerate the pressure or constriction of clothes, particularly around the neck or the waist.

CROTALUS HORRIDUS (TIMBER SNAKE)

NOTES: The timber rattlesnake, though quite poisonous, is not very aggressive. Most symptoms of this remedy are right sided. Another interesting note—like Lachesis, Crotalus horridus is listed as a remedy to fight bubonic plague, yellow fever, and cancer—particularly stomach cancer.

HEART: In the Materia Medicas there are a lot of heart symptoms listed but none are highlighted as keynotes. Symptoms include the heart beating rapidly, but feebly; heart tender when lying on left side; pain in heart felt through left shoulder and down left arm; palpitations.

BLOOD/HEMORRHAGIC: Hemorrhages from every part of the body; hemorrhages are slow, oozing dark thin blood with clots; retinal hemorrhages (suggested for absorption of eye hemorrhages).

KIDNEYS: Nephritis; painful retention of urine; urine copious and light colored.

LUNGS: Asthma accompanied by heart disease: asthma with great prostration, a blue puffy countenance, and cold sweats; quick labored breathing with weak pulse and nervous agitation; pneumonia with a tendency to serious destruction of lung tissue and/or hemorrhage.

PHYSICAL/GENERAL: Profound nervous shock; septic conditions with the sloughing of tissues; infection of the lymph vessels; tired on the slightest exertion; tissues rapidly decomposing; intestinal hemorrhage; violent pain in left side near last ribs; sensitivity to light; in females, sensation as if uterine would drop out (see Sepia); menopausal symptoms such as hot flashes and sweating; miscarriages due to septic conditions; diseases related to alcohol abuse; headache with severe pain in the center of the forehead; vertigo; nosebleeds with black, stringy blood.

MENTALS: Aversion to family; poor memory; forgets words, figures, names, and places; mistakes in writing; suspicious about friends; melancholy; readily moved to tears; indifference; thoughts dwell on death continually; sensitivity to certain people; nervous agitation with paleness and cold sweats; impatient; irritable; infuriated by least annoyances; alternating suspicion and snappishness with quiet indifference.

MODALITIES: Like most snake remedies, symptoms are worse in the morning on waking; symptoms are worse on the right side; worse from alcohol; worse in a yearly cycle; better from rest, motion, and light (except eye symptoms); head and stomach symptoms are better from open air.

BOTHDROPS LANCEOLATUS (YELLOW VIPER)

NOTES: Murphy's Materia Medica states, "After being bitten in the little finger of one hand, paralysis began in the fingertips of the **other hand** and extended over the whole of that side. Intolerable pain in right great toe (this patient was bitten in the left thumb). **Marked diagonal course of symptoms**." Interesting!

HEART: Pulmonary congestion; fainting spells; rapid pulse.

BLOOD/HEMORRHAGIC: Hemorrhages from every orifice of the body; blindness from hemorrhage into the retina; hemorrhages from wounds; blood clots; thrombosis.

KIDNEYS: Blood in urine.

LUNGS: Pulmonary congestion; oppressed breathing with bloody expectoration; spitting of blood.

PHYSICAL/GENERAL: Necrosis of bones; septic conditions; lung and lymph congestion; septicemia; day blindness; lockjaw; one-sided headaches; phlebitis; swollen veins; gangrenous ulcers; inability to articulate words; nervous trembling; clammy sweats; skin bluish, looks as though bruised; swollen or infected lymph glands; tendency to sleep; coma that becomes deeper and deeper until death occurs; necrosis of bones; easy bruising; one-sided paralysis; paralysis following a stroke.

MENTALS: Mental symptoms after a stroke; inability to articulate; forgetful of words; uses wrong words; considered a kind of super Lachesis - very egotistical.

MODALITIES: Worse on the right side even though this snake is said to be very aggressive.

ELAPS CORALLINUS (CORAL SNAKE)

NOTES: Elaps is a predominantly right-sided remedy. The snake is not very aggressive but the venom is extremely poisonous. This snake remedy is listed as a remedy for cancer, particularly breast cancer. Many other factors are at play in any cancer. Snake remedies predominate because of their miasmatic relationship. As always, a remedy—snake or otherwise—should be chosen based on the totality of symptoms of the individual person having the cancer.

HEART: Palpitations with anxiety and trembling of the hands; sensation as if the heart has been lacerated; sharp pain and soreness of the chest when touched; oppression of chest when going up stairs; feeling of a heavy load on the chest; soreness across chest moving from right to left armpits.

BLOOD/HEMORRHAGIC: Hemorrhages that are dark black; sensation as if all the blood were collecting in the head; black ear wax; black discharges from the lungs.

KIDNEYS: Urine red colored with cloudy sediment; discharge of mucous from urethra.

LUNGS: Pneumonia—each indrawn breath produces a crackling sound in the lungs; cough with terrible pain through lungs; hemorrhage from lungs that is black and watery; sharp pain in left side of chest, worse breathing; stitching pain in apex of right lung.

PHYSICAL/GENERAL: Spasms followed by paralysis, usually on the right side; internal coldness with cold feeling in the stomach; acid stomach with feeling of faintness; stomach pain better lying on the abdomen; bowels feel knotted and twisted together; painful pressure on the right side in liver area; pressure between the shoulders; pain and chilliness in the back; buzzing noises in the ears; eyeballs feel as if they are sticking to the lids; in females, discharge of black blood between menses; sensation as if something has burst in the uterus, then continuous stream of dark colored blood (cysts or fibroid tumors?); violent headache extending from forehead to base of skull; headache worsens with mental exertion; severe sharp pain in forehead; cold perspiration all over; skin hot and dry; drowsy all day, no sleep at night; red blotches in the throat; vertigo when stooping; dirty red spots or a red bar between eyes.

MENTALS: Fear of being left alone; feels separate from others; fear that causes chattering of the teeth and trembling; depressed; tolerant of touch unless feeling restrained; vibrant; attractive; can be confident when well-balanced; articulate, or struggling here; aggression towards others; struggles with parenthood and parental instincts; desire to be independent sparring with a desire to be connected to home.

MODALITIES: Cold things disagree causing a cold feeling, first in the stomach and then in the chest.

NAJA TRIPUDIANS (COBRA)

NOTES: Naja is not a hemorrhagic or septic remedy in the same way that other snake remedies are. The disorganization of the blood is often the *result* of a septic or infectious state rather than the cause of it. Naja is said to relieve the terrible pains of cancer; consider the Euphorbiums in conjunction for this

Although the cobra is one of the most poisonous snakes in the world, the left-sideness of the symptom picture reflects its centuries of contact with humans.

HEART: Damage to the heart after infectious disease; inflammation of the inner layer of the heart usually involving the valves and sometimes turning septic; heart is enlarged; heart lesions; low blood pressure; visible palpitations; palpitations cause choking and prevent speech; nervous excitement with resulting heart disorders; sharp pain in region of heart extending to neck, left shoulder and arm accompanied by anxiety and fear of death; heart symptoms with pain in forehead and temples; irregular heart beat that is slow, weak, and tremulous; in females, pain in groin, abdomen, or left ovary moves up into the heart; chest pain is worse when breathing in; tenderness over sternum and in throat

BLOOD/HEMORRHAGIC: Except for the spitting of thin blood from the lungs that shows no tendency to coagulate, there are no marked hemorrhagic symptoms with this remedy

KIDNEYS: Pressure in bladder; urine is dark colored and full of red sediment, gravel, stones, and mucus

LUNGS: Difficult breathing that is labored; slow, shallow breathing; suffocative spells when sleeping; dry or empty feeling in left lung; spitting of blood which shows no sign of coagulating; irritating dry cough; dry, hacking cough with spitting of blood; inability to cough because of the pain that it causes.

PHYSICAL/GENERAL: Headache pain in left temple and on left side of the head; severe headache with intense depression; feeling as if the head has taken a blow from behind; sleepiness and weakness in the evening; long, vivid, and disturbing dreams; flushes of heat in face, worse on the left side; vertigo followed by astounding pain in right side of head.

MENTALS: Nervous, excited and tremulous; brooding, usually over imaginary troubles and diseases; feels the anguish of others personally; fear of death, disease, accidents, misfortune and fear of rain; aversion to talking; often feels that everything has gone wrong and cannot be fixed; ailments from grief; feels he is a failure, has neglected his duty; feels that he has been injured by others.

MODALITIES: Very sensitive to cold; better from being in the open air (common among snake remedies); worse from stimulants and alcohol; great relief from pain and labored breathing by lying on the right side with all symptoms worsening from lying on the left side; many symptoms are worse in the week before menses begins; headache worse about 3 pm.

Comparison of Mental/Emotionals of Naja and Elaps

NAJA TRIPUDIANS	ELAPS CORALLINUS
Grey color; large in size	Brightly colored; small in size
Strong maternal instincts	Little maternal instinct; aggressive towards others
Has greater contact with people	Hides; avoids contact with others
Feels duty towards family and community; Feeling of secure place in family and community	Feels separate and apart from family and community; Strong desire to be connected
Sense of personal failure: a lot of self-blame	Feels that he was prevented from succeeding by others; blames others with no blame put on himself
Hatred towards those he feels have hurt or offended him in any way	Lack of feeling for those who have hurt or offended him; just walks away and leaves them behind
Tendency to stay in abusive relationship	Independent, intolerant of those who don't support him or benefit him; once again, just walks away
Defensiveness, but very controlled reactions	Uncontrollable, explosive rage
Bound by family and community ties	Freedom and travel are of prime importance

CENCHRIS CONTORTRIX (COPPERHEAD SNAKE)

NOTES: Cenchris is a deep acting and restorative remedy and has the main features that belong to all snake remedies but with little hemorrhagic symptoms inissues with the kidneys.

HEART: Heart feels distended or enlarged, filling the entire chest; hard aching with sudden sharp stitching pain in heart; throbbing or fluttering under left scapula; shortness of breath; strongly conscious of the beating of the heart.

LUNGS: Hard, dry, tickling cough that gets worse in the afternoon, even causing escape of urine.

PHYSICAL/GENERAL: Swelling of upper lip; increased sexual desire; pain in right ovarian region; intolerant of tight clothing, particularly over the abdomen; swelling like bags over eyes and under the brows; left eye waters; eyes ache with dimness of vision; itching of eyes, beginning with the left eye and spreading to the right eye; headache on left frontal eminence going down into the teeth; vivid horrible dreams that cannot be shaken off even during waking hours; nausea better by ice but water causes vomiting; diarrhea early in the morning on waking; thick tough mucus in the throat.

MENTALS: Alternation of moods; great foreboding followed by laughter and joy; forgetful; absent-minded (gets into the wrong car, drives past destination); sensation of time passing very slowly; anxiety and presentiments of death; jealousy; quarrelsome; suspicious; vivid dreams; anxiety, especially in the evenings with feelings that they are going to die suddenly and without warning.

MODALITIES: Worse lying down, and from pressure; symptoms are worse on waking, getting better with the day's movements but get worse in the afternoon, staying all evening and into the night; relief is short-lived as symptoms will be worse again when first waking in the morning.

BITIS ARIETANS/CLOTHO ARIETANS (PUFF ADDER)

NOTES: Bitis is a left-sided remedy; Bitis "puffs" itself up when threatened; does not slither like other snakes but moves with a caterpillar-like movement; venom is extremely cytotoxic, destroying blood and tissues

HEART: Constriction in chest; low blood pressure.

BLOOD/HEMORRHAGIC: Bleeding into tissues with necrosis of the tissues.

KIDNEYS: Pain before and during urination; uncontrollable urge to urinate; pain in lower abdomen from putting off urination; ineffectual bearing down pains with no urine flow.

LUNGS: Asthma; needs to sit up to breathe; feeling of a weight on the chest which does not allow the chest to expand enough allow breath to be taken in; lungs congested; feeling of coldness in lungs and airways.

PHYSICAL/GENERAL: Single irritating scab on back of head (like I inherited a tendency for from my Grandmother); vertigo even sitting worsened by turning the head, bending forward, closing the eyes, concentrating; headache made worse by cold food or drink; throbbing temples, sometimes oscillating from side to side; sinuses congested; nose full of crusts; cannot breathe through the nose; lips and mouth dry but no thirst; uncontrollable hunger with need to eat at short intervals—hunger increases late in the day; sore feeling in head after the headache has passed; aching in left side of nose, in the bone, with dull headache; one large dry scabby pimple on the scalp that is long and narrow; venous swelling; varicose veins, cellulitis.

MENTALS: Suspicious of others, fears they are going to hurt him; fear of death; irritable; angry at trifles; keeping busy keeps anger under control; lonely; feels deserted by family; intolerant of contradiction; wants to cry and be comforted; claustrophobic around people; insecure; lacking in confidence; untidy; mouth seems disconnected from brain; conflict between heart and mind and between male and female sensitivities; mind races then becomes lethargic then races again; wants to talk but feels no one cares.

MODALITIES: Better from exertion and exercise; cravings for cheese but cheese aggravates digestive system; better for fresh air; craving for chocolate.

VIPERA BERUS (GERMAN VIPER)

NOTES: Bites from the viper are excruciatingly painful but rarely fatal; the symptoms can resemble the symptoms of polio; great periodicity with Vipera—the symptoms may return annually for years; may experience an increase in reflexes along with the negative symptoms.

HEART: Hardening of the veins; pain in heart; faintness; pulse may be rapid, irregular, or slow and weak.

BLOOD/HEMORRHAGIC: Greatly swollen veins; cerebral hemorrhage; inflammation of blood vessels; affected part (usually legs) feels as if it is about to burst; if untreated the veins become ulcerous and gangrenous; in females, bright red flow with large clots usually indicative of a fibroid tumor; continuous bleeding for many weeks after childbirth; nosebleeds; hemorrhages at menopause.

KIDNEYS: Blood in urine; urine bright yellow as in jaundice conditions; involuntary urination; sticking pain in the back and in the loins.

PHYSICAL/GENERAL: Painful, very swollen varicose veins; phlebitis (tender veins); impaired circulation; faintness, collapse; this remedy is associated with premature aging and with slow development in children; enlarged liver with violent pain; paralyses beginning in lower limbs then ascending; great chilliness; will do almost anything to avoid the cold; anorexia.

MENTALS: Dazed; unhappy, sad, depressed, especially during very warm weather; confusion; restlessness, nervousness; speech hesitant or incoherent; talks to himself; great rage progressing to delirium and vomiting which is then replaced by lethargy.

MODALITIES: Better from elevating the legs; worse from change of seasons; worse yearly.

HYDROPHIS CYANOCINCTUS (SEA SERPENT)

NOTES: Hydrophis is a snake that has adapted to survive and thrive in a marine environment. They have many of the characteristics of snakes—except for hemorrhagic symptoms—but they also reflect their watery environment and have many of the symptoms common to the sea realm. The venom of this snake attacks the peripheral nerves, producing polio-like symptoms. It is speculated that the fundamental action of the venom, and the homeopathic remedy, is on the muscles as well as the nerves. Hydrophis is recommended as a treatment for the side effects of schizophrenia medications, poliomyelitis, muscular dystrophies, diphtheria, and injuries from accidents. Hydrophis is a left-sided remedy.

HEART: Chest and heart pain that is worse for lying flat; feelings of abnormal dryness and burning in the chest; extra contraction between regular heart beats (systole); arrhythmia; valvular diseases; coronary arthritis-like inflammation; septicemia.

BLOOD/HEMORRHAGIC: Menses abundant; blood-streaked vaginal discharge; fibroid tumors; none of the serious hemorrhagic symptoms of other snake remedies.

LUNGS: Inflammation of the trachea; bronchitis; shortness of breath.

PHYSICAL/GENERAL: Paralysis without loss of sensation in the affected parts; stinging pains in the limbs and in the left hip; dry throat; numbness in the limbs; shingles; earache; deafness in left ear; vaginitis; headache with beating in the temples and sensation of tight band around head; headache particularly bad on the left side and in the front; headache worse in the morning and worse from heat; mouth very dry in the morning; toothache in the molars on the left side; painful swollen hemorrhoids; dry skin with chapped hands; skin itching on different areas of the body; disturbed sleep with nightmares between 2 and 4 am which produce a feeling of anguish; pain in the upper part of the abdomen, worse after meals; profuse sweating without body heat; fever with shivering; tonsillitis; hoarseness worse in the morning and after speaking; dryness in the larynx; fatigue; tenderness in the muscles.

MENTALS: The young of sea serpents are born alive and must swim immediately to the surface to breathe. They must do this entirely on their own, independently, with no parental assistance or care at all. This need to "do it themselves" is reflected in the remedy.

There is also an element of overcompensation for any inadequacies, whether emotional or physical. If there is something wrong (an injury from which they should never walk again, for example) the person will work and work as hard and as long as it takes to conquer or compensate for the deficiency. The opposing symptoms of depression or disgust for life also exist, of course, and are severe to the same degree that the more positive symptoms appear.

Other mental/emotional symptoms include a state of euphoria followed by a period of sadness with tears; depression; likes, and is better, for consolation from others; irritable; lethargic; lacks initiative; forgetful; difficulty concentrating; anxiety about the future (sometimes with clairvoyance about what is to come)

MODALITIES: Worse at night; worse in the morning; worse from heat; worse lying flat; worse lying on left side; worse before menses; worse from speaking (hoarseness and dryness of the throat).

Ocean Remedies

Ocean remedies form a large and very diverse category. Within this family are subcategories that include the water itself, ocean growing plants, mammals that have adapted to a watery environment, invertebrates, vertebrates of many varieties, true fishes, sponges, corals (skeletal structures), even a reptile or two, and others that I haven't thought to mention. Nevertheless, there are some themes common to these remedies, mostly because they all belong to the realm of the sea.

The most obvious of these connections is to the watery environment of the womb in which we all began our mortal development. There are some core themes of suspension, safety, peace, potential, and possibilities. For some the ocean represents calm and tranquility but, as with anything in the world and with all homeopathic remedies, the polar opposites of any emotion or physical symptom are also possible.

Common keynotes of these remedies are principally emotional and include universal fears relating to survival, abandonment issues, feeling of persecution, and fear of violence or tendencies to violent behavior.

The family of ocean remedies contains both the polar opposites of feeling the stillness and calm of the immortal sea and the fierce, implacable, often destructive forces of nature. Ocean remedies can bring a sense of connection with humanity and all of creation when we are feeling isolated or betrayed in our relationships.

AQUA MARINA (SEA WATER)

NOTES: Sea water contains all of the minerals of the periodic table and is particularly useful for great weakness and for lack of reaction to other homeopathic remedies. It is like a massive elemental combination homeopathic in one remedy. This last rubric, lack of reaction to remedies, brings to mind the psora miasm which is common to all mankind and indicates a strong connection to birth and birth traumas.

Not surprisingly, this remedy is often effective for thyroid problems; it may condition the body for the uptake and more efficient utilization of iodine as well as other minerals.

One homeopathic practitioner mentions Aqua marina for its rapid action with newborn infants suffering from malnutrition and gastroenteritis.

This remedy is specific for treatment of diseases of the skin, kidneys, lungs, and intestines.

BLOOD: Aqua marina is one of the foremost remedies for purifying and revitalizing the blood.

SEASICKNESS: Used for sensitivity to the ocean, fear of the ocean, ailments worsened by living near or visiting the sea, and for seasickness.

PHYSICAL/GENERAL: Hypersensitive people with congestion of veins and mucus membranes; general fatigue in the morning.

Arthritis of the spine, scapula, and shoulder; stiffness and pain in neck and along the spine; pain at nape of neck with difficulty turning the head; stinging pain in the right ear; headaches with vertigo; localized pain in the forehead and occiput; buzzing in ears with visual disturbances; morning cough with a rusty taste at the back of the throat; early tuberculosis; itching of the toes, inner side of thighs, and at the bends of arms and legs; eczema of the palms; rectal bleeding; pin worms; fetid smelling perspiration of the hands and feet; feeling of a hair or fish bone stuck in the throat.

PHYSICAL/EMOTIONAL: Unstable, nervous dispositions; anxiousness that is aggravated by talking or being with people; intellectual concentration difficult; absent-minded; slow and apathetic; delusion of being watched or spied upon.

MODALITIES: Unusual symptom of increased appetite and thirst, often about 11:30 am with the appetite and the thirst still there, or increasing, after eating; aversion to eating fish; desires salt—salt makes symptoms better in some people and worse in others as does the drinking of cold water; generally worse for pressure and heat; worse in the afternoon and evening; usually better for eating and from resting.

SEPIA SUCCUS (CUTTLEFISH INK)

NOTES: Sepia is one of the top 10 polycrest remedies; counting just women, it is among the top 3 remedies. Most women will show symptoms, and would be benefitted by this remedy at some time in their lives.

FEMALE: Disturbances in the necessary fluctuations of hormones throughout a lifetime; never well since puberty, childbirth, weaning a baby, taking hormone therapies; hot flashes and other symptoms of menopause; bearing down sensation as if everything is falling down and out; affects circulation, primarily to the female pelvic organs; menses either too early and profuse or too late and scanty; prolapse of the uterus or vaginal wall; tendency to miscarriage from the fifth to seventh; extreme morning sickness; retained placenta; infertility; aversion to sex and low sex drive; acne before menses; hair falls out at menopause; constipation and hemorrhoids during pregnancy.

FOOD: Desires chocolate, sweets, vinegar, acids, and pickles; nausea at the smell or thought of food; typical pattern of the food cravings of pregnancy.

PHYSICAL/GENERAL: Feels cold even in a hot room; weakness in the small of the back; weak or prolapsed bladder; bed wetting during first part of the night; yellowish brown discoloration of the nose and cheeks; irregular circulation; congestion of the blood vessels; restlessness in all limbs; limbs go to sleep easily and constantly; liver area sore and painful but relieved when lying on right side; shooting pains in rectum and vagina; prolapsed anus; bleeding gums; black points or spots before the eyes; intolerance of reflected light from bright objects

HEART: Circulation irregular: wakes with violent beating of the heart and sensation of beating in all arteries; nervous palpitations, especially when lying on left side; congestion of blood vessels; violent intermittent palpitations; palpitations with anxiety; pulse accelerated by motion or being angry.

PHYSICAL/EMOTIONAL: Feels mentally and physically worn out—displays as indifference and disconnectedness; demands of family viewed as burdens and are met with irritability and anger followed by feelings of guilt; tearfulness; depression; weeping, worse when talking or trying to explain feelings and symptoms; aversion to both sympathy and company when depressed or discouraged; postpartum depression; loss of sex drive; sensitive; easily offended; doesn't take criticism or contradiction well at all; anger and irritability first thing in the morning, especially sensitive to noises, especially music playing in the background.

MODALITIES: Symptoms worse when tired or working too hard (motherhood?); better from exercise or vigorous motion; better after some sleep; better from warm bed or warm applications; better from cold drinks; better sitting with legs crossed; better when sleeping with legs pulled up; worse from cold air or dampness; worse before thunderstorms; worse in the morning; worse in the evening with a "second wind" of energy or strength late at night; worse after sex; worse from being touched or rubbed absentmindedly

AMBRA GRISEA (MORBID SECRETION OF WHALE)

NOTES: This is a remedy specific to the nerves. It is especially indicated for those who are anemic, experiencing abnormal coldness, weakened by age or overwork, and whose symptoms are aggravated by music or by slight or unusual things.

PHYSICAL/GENERAL: Keynote of bashful bladder and bowel—unable to urinate or pass stool if others are anywhere present; tearing pains at crown; headache pains so bad that hearing is impaired; bleeding gums; palpitations with pressure in the chest as if an abnormal lump was lodged there; cramps in hands and fingers when grasping something; arms numb; nervous spasmodic cough; cannot sleep because of worry; coldness and twitching during sleep; anxious dreams; sweat on slight exertion; bleeding between periods—lying down aggravates the bleeding; distention of stomach and abdomen; feeling of coldness in abdomen

PHYSICAL/EMOTIONAL: Dwells on unpleasant things; slow comprehension; forgetful; cannot understand what is being read; bashful, blushes easily; jumping from one subject to another, never waiting to have a question answered before moving on the next one.

MODALITIES: Worse from the presence of others; worse from any change in routine; worse in the morning

ASTERIAS RUBENS (RED STARFISH)

NOTES: Asteria was used by Hippocrates in uterine diseases and has a pathogenic relationship to the great polycrest remedy, Sepia succus. Asteria was also used anciently as a remedy for stroke and epilepsy. Asteria is said to have been used successfully with ulcerative breast cancers where the pain is worse nightly with sharp pains that radiate down the arms and make the nipples feel drawn. Asteria rubens is a predominantly a left-sided remedy.

PHYSICAL/GENERAL: Eyes sensitive to light; twitching of eyelids; acne of adolescence; red face with throbbing carotids; sensation as if head would burst, sometimes a precursor to a stroke; severe pressure in forehead; boring pain above the left eye; pulse hard, full, and frequent; gait unsteady with the muscles refusing to obey; insomnia at night, but tends to fall asleep after reading for a moment; sudden attacks of vertigo, like shocks in the head.

PHYSICAL/EMOTIONAL: Sense of impending misfortune; fears that bad news is coming; cries from least emotional upset; irritated by criticism or contradiction; unwilling to think or work; indifference to life; sadness, depression, anxiety with heart palpitations; irritability with the need to quarrel with someone.

MODALITIES: Worse from stimulants; worse at night and from cold damp weather.

CORALLIUM RUBRUM (RED CORAL)

NOTES: Corallium affects the mucus membranes, especially those of the respiratory tract.

RESPIRATORY SYSTEM: nosebleeds, ulceration within the nostrils; whooping and spasmodic coughs; violent suffocative coughing attacks, with complete exhaustion afterwards; coughs with spitting of blood; face becomes purple from coughing; pain between shoulder blades when coughing; air passages feel cold when breathing deeply; mucus dropping through posterior sinuses.

PHYSICAL/GENERAL: Congestion of blood to head when bending over; pressing pain in forehead aggravated by breathing cold air, especially through the nose; nausea with dry mouth and violent headache; constipation followed by passing of mucus with stool; teeth feel as if they are sitting too close or as if something is lodged between them; feels chilly but skin feels abnormally warm; throat sensitive to cold air.

PHYSICAL/EMOTIONAL: Fear of suffering and pain; cross; fretful; quarrelsome; tends to scold others or become abusive when not feeling well; great restlessness, nervousness, and tossing about during sleep; feels unaccustomed to his life and unable to cope.

MODALITIES: Worse from inhaling cold air; worse moving from a warm room to a cold one; worse towards morning; worse being uncovered at night.

SPONGIA TOSTA (ROASTED SPONGE)

NOTES: Spongia tosta is a remedy of renown for acute respiratory infections and coughs—no remedy that I know of covers more types of coughs. This is an important remedy for asthma and cardiac disorders—specifically heart valve problems. Oceanic remedies are often useful for thyroid disease, glandular problems, and lymphatic congestion. This is certainly true of Spongia tosta.

PHYSICAL/GENERAL: Hoarseness and dryness of the throat; vertigo and giddiness; paralytic muscle pain; spasmodic clenching of the bronchial tubes; dry chronic sympathetic cough of heart disease

PHYSICAL/EMOTIONAL: Instinctive movement away from danger and discomfort; constantly seeking a safer environment; timid; fearful; full of terror and anxiety; panic attacks; fears death; grudges (like the holding of a grudge is emotionally supportive to them); awakes in fright with feeling of suffocating; attacks of heat with extreme anxiety; a tendency to replace a relationship if they feel unsupported; cannot tolerate being, or feeling, alone; immature; dependent on others, go into the water when stressed or ill.

MODALITIES: Better lying horizontal, head low; better from eating or drinking, especially warm food or drink; better in cold weather; worse from exertion, sweets, touch or pressure, motion, lying on the right side.

HOMARUS GAMMARUS (LOBSTER DIGESTIVE FLUID)

NOTES: A little lobster poison put into warm milk causes the milk to become a hard mass within 10 minutes. It is interesting that all symptoms of this remedy are worse for milk and milk is listed as the cause of the various ailments.

PHYSICAL/GENERAL: Headaches with sharp pain that is mostly frontal and temporal, worse on the left side; headache with soreness in the eyes accompanied by dizziness; burning pain in the stomach that is usually better for eating, although even a light meal in the morning is not tolerated well; sudden itching of the skin, worse at night; itch is better for scratching but immediately upon relief itching reappears somewhere else; strange dull feeling all over; is better for movement but finds it difficult to begin moving; great chilliness all over; feet feel cold and damp but then suddenly begin to burn; grinding pain just above the elbows; knees become weak and tremble; pain and lameness in various parts of the body; stinging and burning in nasal passages extending into the throat; nose stopped up in the morning; allergic reactions—burning and swelling in the throat with swelling spreading to lips, nose and eyes accompanied by difficulty breathing; sleep disturbed by illusive pains all over.

PHYSICAL/EMOTIONAL: Frightened and nervous but with an even greater dread of moving away from the perceived threat.

CONCHIOLINUM (MOTHER OF PEARL)

NOTES: There is not a lot of information about this remedy in the medicas and I can find record of no useful provings to glean a picture of symptoms from. I mention Conchiolinum here because it does have a wide range of action in disorders of the bones, especially when growth plates at the end of bones are involved. Calcarea and Calcarea phosphorica are its closest symptomatic relatives.

BONES: Inflammation and swelling at the ends of bones with intense pain coming on suddenly and then becoming intermittent. The swollen areas are very painful to the slightest touch or pressure. Bones most often affected are the lower jaw, scapula, humerus, radius, ulna, tibia, fibula, tarsal, and metatarsal bones (jaw, shoulders, legs and feet). Thirst, loss of appetite, sleeplessness, dark colored urine with sediment accompany the bone pain.

RESPIRATORY: Symptoms of mucus and inflammation of the respiratory organs.

PHYSICAL/EMOTIONAL: Suffering from long held and very deep emotions and emotional scars; feels a loss of connection to others; enormous pride; need for perfection and absolute purity in everything; inflexible; rigid.

CALCAREA CARBONICA (CALCIUM CARBONATE-OYSTER SHELLS)

NOTES: This remedy has characteristics common to both mineral remedies (where it is usually classified) and oceanic remedies. Calcarea carbonica is discussed in depth in other places throughout this book.

HYDROPHIS CYANOCINCTUS (SEA SERPENT)

NOTES: This remedy has characteristics of both snake remedies and oceanic remedies. It is discussed in the section on snake remedies.

Insect Remedies

Insect remedies, like any group of remedies drawn from a specific class or family, have similarities to each other. With the insect remedies, the commonalities are quite extensive and easily recognized.

EMOTIONS COMMON TO INSECT REMEDIES: Feels small, tiny, powerless, helpless and vulnerable. Feels that others trap, corner, step on them, and invade their territory. People whose emotions fit the symptom picture of insect remedies in general are busy to the point of hyperactive, move suddenly flitting from place to place. The need to get things done quickly rules their lives. Those needing insect remedies often express that they feel inferior, dirty, or creepy. Many times, when feeling particularly vulnerable, they can be mean, nasty, greedy, rude, or sarcastic. Among insect remedies there is a strong focus on food, reproduction, and basic needs. There is also a fascination for, or love of, bright colors.

All insect remedies have the characteristic of sensitive to touch, and skin conditions predominate.

PHYSICAL CONDITIONS COMMON TO INSECT REMEDIES: Insect remedies are among the leading polycrests for burns; for ailments that contain burning, stinging, biting pains and for anything related to the urinary tract.

When any insect remedy is called for you will usually find the pace of the case quite rapid. Symptoms develop rapidly, respond quickly to a remedy and then move on to new symptoms almost immediately.

APIS MELLIFICA (HONEYBEE)

NOTES: Polycrest for stings and allergies. Apis acts on the cellular tissues of the eyes, face, throat, ovaries and on the serous membranes of the heart, brain, and pleura creating edema, inflammation, and intense swelling.

SENSITIVITES AND SKIN CONDITIONS: Allergic reactions to bee or wasp stings with burning, stinging pains and excessive swelling, allergic dermatitis, hives, intolerable itching at night, nettle rash, sudden puffing up of the whole body; sensitivity to touch

KIDNEYS: Severe bruised feeling over kidney area; acute nephritis (inflammation and pain); burning when urinating, especially with the last few drops; scanty, dark colored or milky urine; profuse amounts of urine according to liquid consumption (an indication of kidney compromise); cystitis; leaking of urine, worse at night and when coughing; retention of urine in a newborn.

TEMPERATURE/FEVER: Thirstless during fever; burning fever but becomes chilly when moved; afternoon chills with great thirst; chills alternating with great heat; desire to be uncovered; heat of one body part with coldness in another part

PHYSICAL/GENERAL Burning pain in coccyx and sacrum worse when sitting down; dragging pain in lumbar region with ovarian and uterine problems; burning and stinging pains throughout entire chest region; hydrocephalus; stinging pains; numb, tired headache which is better from pressure (unusual since other symptoms are worse from pressure); feels a great need for sleep but cannot still himself enough to rest; kicks off covers during sleep; cancer of the tongue; pulse weak, thready; cyanosis.

The symptoms of Apis are the classic allergy symptoms of puffy, red, burning eyes and eyelids; redness, burning, and swelling of face, nose, eyes, lips, mouth, tongue, and throat—throat swelling can be scary.

REPRODUCTIVE: Premenstrual syndrome with water retention and great emotional upset; ovarian cysts or tumors accompanied by stinging pains; toxemia of pregnancy; tendency to miscarry during early months; uterine hemorrhage during pregnancy.

MENTAL/EMOTIONAL: Anxious; restless; fidgety; constantly busy; hard to please; weeping, cannot help crying all day and night with no apparent cause; constant whining in children; cannot bear to be left alone.

MODALITIES: Better from cool air; worse from heat of any kind—warm room, warm bath, hot drinks; worse from touch, even touching hair; worse after sleep; worse on right side.

CANTHARIS VESICATORIA (SPANISH FLY)

NOTES: Cantharis is a leading remedy for *burns* of any type from sunburns to very severe burns from any cause. I used this one when my husband was severely burned in a gasoline explosion. A keynote of this remedy is that the inflammation and swelling are rapidly destructive to the tissues. This rapid destruction of tissue is seen in the burned tissues but also can occur from other causes. This destruction of tissue is sometime seen in the gastro-intestinal canal, and in the large intestine.

SENSITIVITES AND SKIN CONDITIONS: Great remedy for burns, dermatitis, vesicular eruptions; small wounds tend to infection, larger wounds tend to gangrene; slightest touch aggravates all symptoms; stomach, throat, esophagus, rectum are hypersensitive and easily damaged by any issue.

KIDNEYS: Constant intolerable urge to urinate; nephritis with bloody urine; burning, with cutting pains when urinating; urine can only be passed drop by drop, dribbling; acute cyctitis; urine thick and jelly-like; kidney region sensitive to touch.

TEMPERATURE/FEVER: Terrible feelings of coldness and shuddering when passing stools; cold hands and feet; cold sweat; soles of the feet burn; has a burning thirst but is made worse by sipping cold drinks and stimulants

PHYSICAL/GENERAL: Burning in eyes; eyes have a fiery, sparkling, staring right at you appearance; heart palpitations; feeble pulse; weak ankles; tendency to fainting; tongue becomes furred with burning in mouth and throat; violent burning in the stomach; vomiting of blood-streaked membrane; violent retching and vomiting; great difficulty when swallowing liquids; very tenacious mucus in the throat.

REPRODUCTIVE: Retained placenta with painful urination (see Sepia for other types of retained placenta issues); menses too early and too profuse with black blood; cutting burning pain in ovaries; sharp tearing pains in os and coccyx; inflamed sexual organs; hemorrhages.

MENTAL/EMOTIONAL: Anxious restlessness which deteriorates into rage; despondent but crying aggravates; excessive sexual desire; acute mania related to sexual issues; insolent and contradictory; irritable and dissatisfied with everyone and everything; whining and complaining with anxious restlessness that unfortunately is made worse by motion (need to be made to lie quietly, if possible); sudden loss of consciousness with very red face.

MODALITIES: Better for application of cold; even though this is an insect remedy, the symptoms are sometimes made better by rubbing; worse from cold water or stimulants; worse from the sound of running water; worse from bright objects; worse from most touch, especially on the throat.

VESPA CRABRO (WASP)

NOTES: The uses for Vespa crabro almost always include seeking relief from the pain and symptoms resulting from stings. The pains are stinging and burning, as if pierced by red hot needles. The stinging sensation pierces deeply

SENSITIVITES AND SKIN CONDITIONS: Boils; stinging and soreness that is relieved by bathing with vinegar; intense itching and burning; sweating of parts lain on with intense itching.

KIDNEYS: Burning pain with itching on urinating; incessant bed wetting; blood in the urine

TEMPERATURE/FEVER: Feet continually cold except in summer when they burn like fire; very sensitive to hot weather.

PHYSICAL/GENERAL: Cutting shocks through joints; burning of a body part followed by swelling (just like a wasp sting); nerve and muscular excitement with trembling, quaking, and chattering of teeth; convulsion, loss of consciousness; burning conjunctivitis; swelling and liquid held in the membranes of the conjunctiva (white part of the eye); pulse rapid and feeble with violent beating of the carotids; heart's action barely perceptible; swelling of throat, tonsillitis with cheesy secretions; itching over whole body; dizzy, better lying on the back.

REPRODUCTIVE: Left ovary frequently affected with burning pain accompanied by excessive urination; erosion of tissues around external os; menstruation preceded by pain, pressure, depression, and constipation; swelling of scrotum and penis.

MENTAL/EMOTIONAL: Terrible anxiety and restless, especially when there is burning pain or itching; sadness and low spirits.

MODALITIES: Applying cold helps at first but then aggravates symptoms; worse from motion, from sleeping, and from eating.

COCCUS CACTI (COCHINEAL)
NOTES: This remedy is made from insects that infest cactus plants.

SENSITIVITES AND SKIN CONDITIONS: General sensitivity to touch and pressure mouth so sensitive that brushing teeth sometimes causes vomiting.

KIDNEYS: Lancing violent pain from kidneys to bladder; urine with brick-red sediment; kidney stones; blood in the urine; constant urging to urinate that is better for passing clots from the uterus

TEMPERATURE/FEVER: Most symptoms are worse from warmth, being in a warm room, or from the warmth of bed; teeth extremely sensitive to cold; catarrh worse with slightest exposure to cold; catarrh from autumn until warm weather returns.

PHYSICAL/GENERAL: Whooping cough attacks; coughing attacks ending in vomiting due to ropy mucus; pepper-like burning in mouth and nostrils; coughs from feeling of rawness in air passages; feeling that something is wedged under the eyelids; cracking in ears when swallowing.

REPRODUCTIVE: Menses too early with profuse bleeding, black and thick with dark clots; inflamed labia.

MENTAL/EMOTIONAL: Confusion that is better for fresh air; irritable; fretful; anxiety about the heart; sadness on waking; sadness again in the afternoon; a lively talkative mood.

MODALITIES: Better for cold drinks; better for washing with cold water; better for walking; worse after sleep; worse from pressure of clothing.

FORMICA RUFA (RED ANT)
NOTES: Formica rufa is an arthritis remedy, rather than one for burns or stings. Also affects the liver, kidneys and right side of the body; has an action on the formation and clearing of polyps.

SENSITIVITES AND SKIN CONDITIONS: Nettle rashes; hives that present in flat plaques; wounds that atrophy; nodes around the joints.

KIDNEYS: Paralysis of the bladder; urine is bright yellow, saffron colored, with no sediment; urine seems to need to be passed frequently; bloody albuminous urine with much urging.

TEMPERATURE/FEVER: Disagreeable sweat during the night, awakes with clammy skin; profuse sweat that brings no relief from the heat.

PHYSICAL/GENERAL: Arthritic and gouty pains which appear suddenly and dart from place to place; chronic; gout and stiffness in joints; paralysis and spasms of the spinal cord; weakness of lower limbs; pain in hips; itching in armpits in the morning; hands go numb; spasmodic twitching of the eyelids; would like to sleep but cannot find the right position; vertigo with everything moving about them; constant pressure at cardiac region of the stomach, with burning pain—homeopathic description of acid reflux.

REPRODUCTIVE: Menses scanty and pale with bearing down pains in the back; menses appears a full week before it should, ovarian cysts containing both water and blood.

MENTAL/EMOTIONAL: The emotional pattern of this remedy is that of being a slave—defenseless, weak, crushed, held down and needing to work very hard to prove to everybody their value and right to even exist.

MODALITIES: Unlike other insect remedies, the symptoms that match this remedy are usually made better by pressure and by being rubbed; worse for motion but also worse for sitting; worse from cold and damp.

CULEX MUSCA (MOSQUITO)

NOTES: This remedy presents as on fire, burning pains like the fires of Hades; itching and burning are present everywhere throughout this remedy; continually rubbing and scratching wherever the itching appears.

SENSITIVITIES AND SKIN CONDITIONS: Tormented by itching and burning heat; must scratch to relieve the constant itching, but scratching only aggravates the condition further; no comfort to be found anywhere.

KIDNEYS: No particular kidney or bladder symptoms, unless the incredible itching is somehow tied to the kidneys. This seems logical since there is also edematous swelling going on.

TEMPERATURE/FEVER: Hot flashes with a feeling that a chill will follow

PHYSICAL/GENERAL Dull frontal headache about 5 a.m. which goes away after lying awake for awhile; headache over the right eye accompanied by vertigo; boring pain in temple coming and going throughout the day; inflamed eyes, painful to keep open but just as painful when closed; margins of the lids sore and crusted over; inflammation of the lids with discharge of sticky fluid in the morning; restless unrefreshing sleep with much tossing about.

REPRODUCTIVE: Menses too soon with a dark clotty flow; violent pains in the uterus, relieved only by going to bed; horribly intense itching and burning in vagina—this symptom may return at intervals for years.

MENTAL/EMOTIONAL: The provings and notes of homeopathic practitioners are full of comments about people needing this remedy having found themselves in preposterous situations of having their possessions borrowed, taken, or moved about for someone else's convenience without their consent. The general feeling is of having one's space invaded, of being taken advantage of, and being manipulated. It is almost as though the expectation sets one up for the actual events. Restlessness; great impatience when interrupted; ready for a quarrel; fear of death; poor memory; doesn't feel like working.

MODALITIES: Worse in a warm room; better in the open air; worse for light pressure but better from firm pressure.

Butterfly Remedies

INTRODUCTION

As you might have noticed from the titles of my books and the name of the company I started (not to mention the decor of my house), I have had, since childhood, an appreciation and love for butterflies and what they symbolize. I have felt in my heart that homeopathic remedies from butterflies would be very powerful and amazing healers, but I could find only one butterfly remedy available for which there was any information at all (at least, in English).

About a year ago I came across the research of Patricia LeRoux and purchased her book on butterfly remedies. I would like to thank her and her team of friends, researchers and provers for their dedication to opening the world of butterflies to the homeopathic community. I would also like to mention the people that she thanks in her own forward. JP Janssen in Holland and Chetna Shukla in India, for their pioneering work with butterfly remedies.

I believe that the butterfly remedies match the changes that are occurring in our global society at this time (please see the information about the AIDS miasm in Section 3) in many important ways. I expect to see butterfly remedies become, if not polycrests, at least very useful in our day and time for the aberrations in physical and mental health brought about by both the global qualities and the feelings of disconnection brought about by this age of electronic communication.

GENERAL THEMES

METAMORPHOSIS/TRANSFORMATION/RESURRECTION: Butterflies are truly creatures who have accomplished the movement from the realm of the earth to the realm of the sky. (See chapter 12 for more information on realms and moving from one to another.) I find much symbolism in butterflies pertaining to the eventual move each one of us must make from mortality to immortality. Butterflies also represent to me the endless possibilities as we each strive to throw off the "natural man" and move toward a state of divine perfection. There is much in butterfly remedies about gender identity and dressing up.

A caterpillar places himself in his cocoon, symbolic to me of the grave. While in this confined and dark place, his body completely dissolves (for dust thou art and unto dust thou shalt return Genesis 3:19). From this darkness and destruction the butterfly emerges—a creature of the sky, free and so beautiful in its perfection. The caterpillar has, literally and figuratively, been reborn and given a "new heart", body and soul.

INNOCENCE: Because butterflies, unlike most other insects, do not bite or sting, they have become symbols in many cultures for kindness, compassion, and child-like innocence. In Japan, two butterflies together are the emblems of fidelity and a happy marriage.

WISDOM: The Aztecs used the symbol of a butterfly to represent the hand and the number 5, which they interpreted as the key to everything in the world.

UNDERSTANDING BUTTERFLY REMEDIES
BY UNDERSTANDING BUTTERFLIES

SYMBOLISM IN NATURE: Butterflies are magical, mystical and universally loved creatures. They are found fluttering over every continent of our world except the Antarctic, surviving everything from the cold of polar regions to the sweltering heat of the tropics.

There are over 160,000 species making the range of possible remedies very broad indeed. The research done by LeRoux and others include only about 10 remedies and includes both butterflies and moths. Butterflies are typically brightly colored and are creatures of the daytime. Moths, on the other hand, are nocturnal and their coloring is generally darker and more subdued. Moths tend to expend their energy on others, either worrying or serving. This trait is unlike butterflies.

THEMES AND SYMPTOMS COMMON TO BUTTERFLY REMEDIES

KEYNOTES: Those symptoms that, while common, manifest uniquely in each remedy and can be used to differentiate one remedy from another.

MENTAL ABILITY: Difficulties with memory and concentration; (butterfly remedies are excellent for hyperactive children/adults and for ADHD); hyperactivity and mental difficulties manifest very differently in different circumstances and are unique to each person—the symptom pictures of the remedies vary from one species to another, becoming a keynote for choosing one remedy over another.

SIGHT: Butterflies can see a wider spectrum of color than any other creature—perhaps this manifests in some people as psychic seeing, visions, dreams, and the ability to see auras. The type of dreams experienced varies from species to species with dreams of houses being common and sometimes having almost prophetic significance. House dreams generally have to do with the safety, physically or spiritually, of themselves and their children.

PROTECTION/DEFENSIVENESS: A great range according to species—scales and color on wings mimic to hide, look scary; some species develop the ability to eat noxious substances, making themselves toxic or nasty tasting to the animals that try to eat them (is there a correlation to energy toxic people that so deeply affect the energy of those around them?); do not respond very well to criticism or correction; some persons will wrap their arms around themselves when criticized or threatened.

GENERAL SYMPTOMS: *EMOTIONAL*

Note the preponderance of emotional symptoms—emotional/mental symptoms make up a great deal of what we know about butterfly remedies at this time

RESPONSIBILITY: Can be a lack of responsibility; light-hearted; careless about family responsibilities and about commitments made.

ABANDONMENT: Feeling abandoned or abandoning others emotionally or physically.

LACK OF LIMITS: Parents, perhaps also caught in the negatives of this or similar patterns, fail to provide guidance, direction, sufficient care, limits or boundaries (often seen in children but manifesting their whole life long). Lack of limits, as much as actual loss of a parent, seems to be the source of the feeling of abandonment in several of the butterfly remedies.

FEAR: Many symptoms, but especially abdominal pain, are brought on by fear.

SLEEP PATTERNS: Needs very little sleep but rarely feels fatigue; commonly sleep is deep and restful and wakes feeling refreshed; periodic sleepless nights—needs to sleep but does not feel tired; might as well stay up and get something done as sleep will not come just by going to bed.

AGITATED AND ENERGETIC: Inability to sit still; flitting everywhere; constantly in motion, like the energizer bunny; feels like dressing up and going somewhere and doing something.

FEELINGS: Feeling of lightness and well-being with opposite patterns of periodic sadness about random or unexplainable things.

FOOD: Desires sweets, rich foods, sugar—one remedy craves honey.

TRANSFORMATION (LOOKS): Loves to change their "look"—hair, makeup, clothes—example: long hair that can be braided, twisted, piled up, worn curly or straight); career or life-style: manifesting by changing careers, as soon as they are proficient or no longer learning in current career, feels a great urge to move on to something else.

APPAREL: Likes to dress in black with an accompanying color as an accent; likes color and movement.

SOLITUDE: Hiding/Being alone. This is a general animal symptom that manifests in butterflies as a requirement for time alone, not to rest and recuperate but to be very busy without interruptions; always better for being in open air or large, light-filled rooms; sometimes shows up as a negative sort of agitation.

CONSTRICTION: This applies to the clothes they wear, being in enclosed spaces, or even being indoors as in a schoolroom.

GENERAL SYMPTOMS: *PHYSICAL*

FRAGILE: Sensitive to environment and energy: affected by surroundings, temperature, humidity, light, foods, just about everything imaginable; small changes in environment affect them dramatically.

TEMPERATURE: Some form of coldness, with pain in extremities when they get cold.

FEMALE: Late start to menses; longer than average length of time between periods—up to six-week cycles.

PAIN: Pulsating pain in the back (the effect of constant wing fluttering?); headaches, aggravated by noise and light; not localized; feeling of floating.

KIDNEYS: Recurrent burning urine.

EYES: Most remedies have some sort of eye or eyesight issues; constant stuffiness of frontal sinuses.

SKIN: Problems with skin—eczema, psoriasis, and hives.

PROVINGS OF INDIVIDUAL REMEDIES
UNIQUE VARIATIONS OF BASIC THEMES

Patricia LeRoux points out in her book, <u>Butterflies: An Innovative Guide to the Use of Butterfly Remedies in Homeopathy</u>, that the criteria for provings today and for getting the results of those provings accepted and validated was beyond the scope of the private "provings" she has conducted. She says,

> *". . . it is necessary to consider that the following information is only minimal and calls for verification. This is only the beginning of a collection of data that can open the door to prescribing such remedies."*

Most of the information presented here is taken from Ms. LeRoux's work and from what little information is available from similar sources. Even the big homeopathic manufacturers who carry these remedies provide very little information (at least in English) that is not taken directly from LeRoux's writings.

The following information is not an attempt to write a complete description of each remedy such as you might find in a Materia Medica. There is simply not enough information available to do so. I hope to provide what information we have and to point out the unique aspects of each remedy so as to make it possible to differentiate between one remedy and another in prescribing.

ACHERONTIA ATROPOS (DEATH'S HEAD HAWKMOTH)

There are some outstanding similarities between this moth's life cycle and the symptoms shown in the provings and the symptoms that were ameliorated by this remedy when used in treatment protocols.

AFFIRMATIONS: (PIRATES) Provers of this remedy mentioned that their dreams were filled with pirates and pirate themes. Children who responded well to this remedy had a marked love of pirates, particularly dressing up in pirate costumes. This is very interesting because there are distinguishable skull markings visible both on the caterpillar and on the moth. *(Bees and Honey)* This large moth loves honey and will raid beehives to get it. This remedy has proven useful for allergic reactions to bee stings.

FOOD: Provers or persons benefited by this remedy either had or developed extraordinary love of and craving for sweets, particularly honey! Butterfly remedies, with a couple of exceptions, crave sweets. This remedy has a special affinity for honey.

ADHD/HYPERACTIVITY/LEARNING: Very restless children with mercurial temperaments; agitation; the need to be moving and to have others moving and getting things done—even manifested in dreams; difficulty concentrating—having to ask questions more than once; obsessed with details; great happiness, with a feeling of mental release.

ABANDONMENT/LACK OF LIMITS: There are the usual butterfly issues of abandonment and lack of limits; hiding—this caterpillar burrows down into the earth for its chrysalis stage, hiding in much the same way that a person needing this remedy would hide if only they could do it (hiding away, becoming a hermit); dreams of troubles and of being abandoned to take care of the problems all by themselves.

EMOTIONAL: Loss of self-confidence; feels a continual need to purchase pretty and colorful things; in spite of all the negative sensations listed above, provers described an overall sense of happiness, with a feeling of freedom and liberation.

PHYSICAL/GENERAL: Hives, eczema, angiodema (localized swelling, usually on the face, neck, hands, feet, genetilia, and deep tissues of the visera); itchy, swollen eyelids; tendency to ailments of the respiratory tract such as bronchitis.

SENSITIVITIES: Feelings of suffocation—interesting to note that these moths often die by suffocation by irate bees during raids on beehives; severe allergic reactions to bites, stings, and vaccinations; feelings of being trapped; dreams of 'fluttering' against a window but cannot get out.

SLEEP: Deep sleep, but only for short periods of time; waking exhausted or with headaches; vivid dreams interrupting normal sleep patterns.

APEIRA SYRINGARIA (LILAC BEAUTY)

Information based on one dream proving and one case history reported by Patricia LeRoux.

RESPONSIBILITY: This remedy is about taking too much responsibility rather than too little, as is common with butterfly remedies. The person's energy is spent caring for worrying about, and taking responsibility for others, and surviving the conflicts of life situations (parents, family members, co-workers).

SENSATION/EMOTIONS: Feeling is that of being crumpled with nothing left to give and no way out. Interestingly, this moth is light in color with crimped edges on its wings. It very much resembles a crumpled leaf.

PHYSICAL: Recurrent pain in the neck and shoulders which restricts arm movements; conjunctivitis; eruptions of eczema between the fingers (this prover was a harp player, making the fingers an interesting place for the skin issues of the butterfly pattern to manifest); bruises; clammy cold hands and feet (again, the hands); urine incontinence at night; vaginal discharge when immune system is low.

FOOD: Craves sweets but dislikes fatty foods, milk, eggs, anything unfamiliar.

BOMBYX LIPARIS CHRYSORRHOEA (BROWN TAIL MOTH)

This is one of the species of moths that have been domesticated as silkworms. Perhaps a study of the life cycles and habits of these moths, both domesticated and wild, would lead us to additional clues.

The only proving that I know of was done by Patricia LeRoux, MD, in December 2007 with a group of six medical students. Three of the students took the remedy and the other three took only a placebo. A 30C remedy was given twice, a week apart, and the results of the homeopathic provers collated. I am amazed at the depth of the reactions in the proving based on the lowness of the potencies used in this and in the other provings.

MENTAL/EMOTIONAL: Symptoms of balanced state—feeling of great freedom; independent; thrives and is energetic when moving from place to place; overall sensation of calm; feelings of amazing efficiency; feeling they want quiet rather than usual distraction of music playing *Out-of-balance state*—camouflaged/hiding—life is better when hidden away; shyness; desire for freedom that displays itself as a desire for travel and a need to experience new things and constant changes.

PHYSICAL/GENERAL: Eruptions on the skin of the wrists and knee joints that nothing ameliorated; burning pain in eyes with the lids very red and swollen; redness, aching, itching, and burning of the neck.

FOOD: The usual butterfly desire for sweet things but not necessarily for honey as the sweet (as in Acherontia).

SLEEP: No longer falling off to sleep as usual, need to either calm down first by reading or just go to bed later when more fatigued.

BOMBYX PROCESSIONEA (THE PROCESSION CATERPILLAR)

A proving was carried out by Dr. Grandgeorge, MD, in France in 1991, a double blind study with 20 provers and one additional volunteer. One case study quoted by Patricia LeRoux. This remedy, with information similar to the following, is found in Murphy's (and other) Materia Medicas.

MENTAL/EMOTIONAL: Unusual and strong sensation of being *attacked* from time to time; fingers pointing, as if to make him a scapegoat; victim mentality; agitated and aggressive.

PHYSICAL/GENERAL: Strange sensations as of a foreign body under the skin; itching all over the body, worse in the evening; dreamed of skin and muscles being shot through with an arrow; general burning pain; hives; fever; swelling of joints; nausea; asthma—recorded case of Bombyx curing asthma.

SKIN: Feeling of sand grinding away under the skin.

SLEEP: Interrupted by the itching; patterns of sleepwalking; sleepiness at inappropriate times.

NOTES: Several provers reported sensations of problems in male genitals, specifically symptoms of a twisted testicle. No actual problem on examination, only the sensation. There is a case history of a child with a twisted testicle who had been playing with caterpillars just before the problem arose. 3 grams of Bombyx homeopathic remedy brought down the swelling and eliminated the pain.

EUPHYDRYAS AURINA (MARSH FRITILLARY)

One proving by Patricia LeRoux at a working seminar for homeopathic doctors in 2007. Six provers took the remedy; six took a placebo. One case history of a small child.

SKIN: Eruptions of weeping plaques which itched, found particularly on the large surface areas of the body such as the back, stomach, thighs, which were ameliorated by warm water and by exposure to either sunlight or ultraviolet light.

EYES: Red and hot, as if they had been burned, with swelling of the eyelids.

HEAD: Headache as though the forehead was bound with a tight band; throbbing temples; head symptoms ameliorated by warm applications.

HYPERACTIVITY: Lively and cheerful but also restless and mercurial; can become very agitated.

FEELINGS OF ABANDONMENT: In the case study, the child had lost her mother at a young age but was being well cared for by loving extended family members. In spite of loving environment, further separations, such as going to school, aggravated the child's symptoms.

GENERAL: Symptoms were made better by warm applications and better in the sunlight.

TRANSFORMATION/METAMORPHOSIS: Liking to change their environment by redecorating, even as children.

FOOD: NOT the usual butterfly desire for sweets—desire was for spicy food, served warm/hot.

SLEEP/PROTECTION: The child in the case study slept on her stomach with arms folded under her like butterfly wings—a very protective pose.

GONEPTERYX RHAMNI (THE BRIMSTONE)

Proving done by Patricia LeRoux, double blind, 10 participants with five taking remedy and five taking the placebo. One dose, 200C, two times in a 24 hour period. One case history of an infant.

HYPERACTIVITY: Restlessness not constant as with other butterfly remedies—great ability to concentrate and display an unusual calm when something catches the attention or interests them. This was true even in a 9-month-old child. Sitting still is a very unusual symptom for a butterfly remedy—a keynote of this remedy.

SLEEP: Child in case study was very restless at night—may have been because of itching of skin or because she was naturally a restless child.

EMOTIONAL: Feelings of well-being and peaceful calm; perfect feeling of goodness, wanting to do good; not wanting to move—feeling that life is best when still; dreams are of beautiful things and great peace—one dream included a beautiful mother and baby, wrapped in swaddling clothes (a cocoon); feelings of abandonment (or real abandonment) and a need for protection that are common to all butterfly remedies.

PHYSICAL: Eruptions on the back of the hands, very itchy but not made better by scratching; eczema on face and around the joints such as knees and elbows; very aggressive, weepy conjunctivitis; headache, mostly in the forehead which lasted for 48 hours beyond the taking of the remedy.

COMMENTS: An outstanding characteristic is that, although they tend to be agitated and lively, they have a very great capacity to remain calm and still for very long periods of time.

GRAPHIUM AGAMEMNON (THE TAILED JAY)

Dr. Chetna Shukla, India, conducted this proving with provers who were mostly practising medical homeopaths. The homeopathic history and profile of each prover was known to Dr. Shukla so all new symptoms were easy to trace and link back to the Graphium remedy.

Patricia LeRoux placed a detailed description of the observations of one of the provers in her book. The following is a synopsis of that material. One single dose, at 30C potency, was given. *Amazingly strong and long-lasting reactions for such a dose.* It was noted, however, that her prover traditionally responded dramatically to homeopathic treatment.

SKIN CONDITIONS: Pustular eruptions on the cheeks but with no pain or itching (unusual)—unnoticed by the prover until pointed out by his wife.

MENTAL: *Balanced state*—felt less mental stress than normal, even though events of the day were stressful and hectic—not stressful because I was *enjoying* it; physically and mentally free; felt particularly good when doing a lot of physical and mental exercise (this is a bit different from other butterfly remedies).

Out-of-balance state—lack of concentration; moves to one toy or one project after another; appears lazy; attention span is short—wants to play instead of work; moving and fidgeting even when they are sitting down (just as the tailed jay flutters its wings ceaselessly, even when drawing nectar from a flower).

EMOTIONAL: Felt like spending a lot of money; felt a desire to go out and spend money—on others and self, just for fun; freedom from everything—a feeling of new beginnings; felt depressed and with a great need to cry from the weight of the world on his shoulders; felt the need for one season to end and a new one to begin—strongly desired a new beginning.

REACTIONS: Wanting things done quickly and efficiently; irritable when they are not done with efficiency; aggressiveness especially with those who have criticized him in some way.

HYPERACTIVITY: Restlessness that was usual for this prover was gone for a few days—able to sit calmly (useful for hyperactivity and ADHD?).

ABANDONMENT: Manifests, in this remedy, as a loss of self-confidence leading to self-criticism and disgust. Will be heard saying such things as "I'm worthless"; Feels that the adults in his life have betrayed and deserted him; if an adult, feels betrayal on every side; retreating into a depressive state but, like a butterfly emerging from a chrysalis, may emerge amazingly beautiful and productive after their hiding away period.

SLEEP: Woke feeling fresh and energetic—willing and able to take on the day's challenges; requiring less sleep than usual; sleep is sound and good.

FOOD: Eating for the enjoyment and the taste, particularly ice cream and sweet treats.

TRANSFORMATION/METAMORPHOSIS: A desire to wear black but with a color, usually bright, accenting it; a liking for colors that were previously disliked intensely (such as purple); generally a remedy for persons who are still in search of their own identity (or, as in my case, simply bored with things they already know and moving on in search of something new to learn and something else to do).

GENERAL: Wanting to converse and be listened to; very agitated and annoyed when not being heard.

REACTIONS: Desire for amusement, freedom, lightness and most strongly, a desire for speed and to spend money, quickly and without much thought.

COMMENTS: One case history included a young boy with a long-standing penchant for dressing up in girls clothing. This is a pattern among butterfly remedies. In this boys case, Graphium given a total of three times, cleared up the skin symptoms as well as putting an end to his dressing up as a girl.

Ten days after the remedy was taken, the mental and emotional symptoms the prover was experiencing were changing, but still very pronounced. He expressed that all restlessness was gone. The feeling of being ready and able to take on *all* challenges had been replaced by indifference to all things except *one* project, although he had always been able to do 5 or 6 jobs at the same time.

Sleep patterns had also changed. Felt tired and wanted to sleep but found sleep to be too boring to contemplate—wanted to get something done but felt little energy or inclination to do it. Felt himself watching a lot of movies, an unusual trait for him. It was a little more than two weeks after taking the remedy before the prover felt that he was returning to normal self.

NOTES: I took this remedy recently, because I didn't have the one that was a closer match. While the remedy cleared the symptoms I was aiming it at very well, I also experienced some interesting symptoms of the remedy as described above. It was as though I was proving those parts of the remedy that I was not experiencing at the time.

I felt less stress and more enjoyment of the work I was doing—my life is so hectic and full that sometimes I forget to enjoy it. I felt a desire to spend money (actually did and spent it on myself in one whirlwind shopping spree!) I also experienced the focus on only one project (this book) where before I was more able to tolerate multiple projects and interruptions better. This was also mentioned by the prover.

I found myself very annoyed and frustrated by a situation in which things were not done in an efficient and quick manner. I was quite aggressive in my disapproval and, yes, it was in a situation where I often feel that others are critical of me. Recent homeopathic theories claim that it is rare for the wrong remedy to produce symptoms in people (at least, at low potencies) unless the symptom was something they covered up or suppressed at a previous time. Reacting aggressively to criticism is certainly one of those areas for me. I thought I had that under control until this situation arose while taking this remedy. Thought provoking.

I experienced eruptions on my cheeks exactly as described by other provers (haven't had those in years but used to get them all the time). A few days later as the remedy wore off, I felt a great depression and need to cry (again exactly as described by the prover). The feeling was that too many people were relying on me and I simply couldn't do it all. This is actually a fairly common feeling for me, remedy or not, but the feeling was particularly intense.

I always like to wear black accented with color—I felt this compulsion less for the first few days after taking the remedy. In fact, I wore several outfits with no black at all and enjoyed them! This is consistent with homeopathic theory. This is a pattern for me, not necessarily a good one, and the remedy cleared it because it was present at the time.

INACHIS IO (THE EUROPEAN PEACOCK BUTTERFLY)

Patricia LeRoux conducted a proving at a seminar in Belgium in 2006 with 10 provers. Her description of the seminar included observations that everyone seeming to want to speak at once with conversations becoming confused and ever more confusing. Everyone felt good, full of energy, very active, and wanting to leave the room. Everyone seemed to be quite *agitated*. In a short time, the agitation settled into a general sense of well-being with expressions of appreciation of each other's color choices in clothes and style. Still lots of energy. Suddenly, one prover began to feel ill and the others began to feel a concern that the remedy they had ingested might be dangerous. Many of them expressed a need to leave the seminar. (attacked, need for protection, need to hide). Interesting descriptions of many of the basic themes of butterfly remedies.

SENSITIVITIES: Dreams, in more than one case, included the wearing of Venetian masks (the masks have a double face). These masks are considered by homeopathic practitioners to be symbolic of both the need to hide and the bi-polar aspects of this particular remedy.

ABANDONMENT: From the few recorded case histories, there seems to be a pattern in children of being raised in home environments where there are few rules and limits. The absence of authority can be the basis for the type of feelings of abandonment that are typical of this remedy. They want to be protected and given limits. They often act up to provoke the application of rules and boundaries in their lives.

PROTECTION/TRANSFORMATION: Feeling of threat hanging over them all the time; the metamorphosis aspects of butterfly remedies, in Inachis io, become ways to protect themselves from perceived threats. Even the manic and mild aspects of their personalities are ways to protect themselves and avoid trouble. The eyespots that give this butterfly its peacock name are only displayed when trying to frighten off predators. The flapping of their bright wings and a high whistling sound also help frighten off predators.

COMMUNICATION: Sound is a very unusual characteristic for a butterfly and is part of the picture of the overactive, disruptive child who wants to tell you about everything and gets very agitated when not listened to. This need for speech was seen in the provers' intense and confused conversations.

This butterfly, when flapping its wings furiously to display its bright "eyes" so as to frighten off predators, produces a high-pitched squealing noise. Sounds by butterflies are very unusual and this is the only remedy in which I found any indication of talking and speech being common in the provings.

PHYSICAL: Sour burps and belches; pressure and stitches in the chest; symptoms are often very different from right to left; some indication of asymmetry of facial features and of the body.

COMMENTS: This is a remedy that has proven useful for disruptive, disobedient children who simply cannot sit still in school. They are restless, talkative, and agitated.

LIMENTIS BREDOWII (CALIFORNIA SISTER BUTTERFLY)

Butterflies can symbolize lack of responsibility or can be a symbol of new beginnings and the emergence into a glorious new stage of being—beautiful, renewed, and no longer bound to earth.

RESPONSIBILITY/ABANDONMENT: Lack of responsibility shows more clearly in this remedy than in most of the other butterfly remedies. In adults, responsibility issues show up as a casual attitude toward their children and the responsibilities of parenthood. This pattern can become generational in the sense that the children of irresponsible parents often become irresponsible themselves or, conversely, display various issues of abandonment.

COMMUNICATION: Any communication by most butterflies is completely inaudible (to us, at least). Issues to do with communication seem to be a theme of this remedy and was also seen with Graphium. There are things that need to be brought out into the open and expressed, but which are never talked about for fear that it might upset someone or bring about criticism of themselves. The person feels that to speak up and create a problem might cause them to be even more unloved and unsupported. **SENSITIVITES AND**

SKIN CONDITIONS: Skin issues appear at this time and from what little we know to be limited to burning sensations, mostly in old scars and wounds which are also painful and red; there are also cracks at the corners of the mouth.

TEMPERATURE/FEVER: Warmth alternating with cold; clammy with cold hands and feet.

PHYSICAL/GENERAL: Easily bruised, even from just being held firmly; dull pain in left temple; pain behind the eyes; pain extending from left ear to the teeth; capricious appetite with indigestion; weak voice, whispery; asthmatic at night; palpitations at night; pain and stiffness in left cervical region of the back; pain in right knee that is better wen walking.

KIDNEYS: Bed wetting; urinary incontinence.

REPRODUCTIVE: Generally strong and well-grounded sexually but may show the patterns of early abandonment. Unusually fragile where reproduction and sexual relationships are concerned.

MENTAL: Little capacity for, or even a very strong aversion to, mental effort; feeling of dullness and disconnectedness after mental exertion; dislikes or has turned away from mental activity *(this is a little bit different from the typical butterfly pattern)*.

EMOTIONAL: This is a remedy for those just about to emerge into a new level of life and joy. Emotional patterns include being encased (chrysalis stage) in grief but wanting desperately to be free of it; craving solitude in the moment but also longing to be "flitting about" in the world without a care; anxiety about the future because they feel that there are no limits or guidance to protect them; inconsolable when criticized; affectionate; naive; spontaneous; can be cheerful, happy, with a feeling of lightness and joy.

Limentis is also a remedy for adolescence and for parents of adolescents. For parents/people who have plenty of love and compassion but are unable or unwilling to set limits for their loved ones. It is also a remedy for teens who have feelings of being without guidance, limits, or adequate protection and for teens who are unable or unwilling to set boundaries for themselves.

AGITATION: Panic or agitation when amid conflict.

MODALITIES: Is always better in the open air; attached to home, which represents the protection and limits that is always sought for by the Limentis personality.

COMMENTS: *Found this description on a web-site.* "Of all the butterflies, Limentis is the most beautiful, the most stable, the most down to earth, the most faithful." It is always nice to focus for a moment on the positive aspects of any homeopathic remedy; we spend so much of our time analyzing the negative aspects.

MACROTHYLACIA RUBI (FOX MOTH)
Proved by Nancy Herrik in 2001.

PHYSICAL: Hives, much like other butterfly remedies.

EMOTIONAL: A desire to spend money, even on useless things; lots of energy and sociability (as with most, but not all, butterflies)—wanting to chat with everyone.

ABANDONMENT: Once again, feelings of abandonment and the need for protection; forming or joining groups and achieving solidarity with others for protection; dreams of all sorts of protective things.

ADHD/HYPERACTIVITY: unable to concentrate; constantly moving from one thing to another.

SLEEP: Sleep disturbed by dreams and a desire for ice-cold water; constant waking up during the night—note the great amount of night-time activity of the female moths of this species; great energy on rising—wanting to do lots of things and do them at the same time; frequent dreams where people wear black (and look elegant); dreamers woke with a desire to dress up in black.

MORPHO PELEIDES (BLUE MORPHO)

The Blue Morpho butterfly is the loveliest butterfly in all the world, in my opinion. The top side of its wings are an amazing iridescent blue, while the underside is a dull brown. The blue color is created by light diffracting off millions of minuscule scales. When the wings are fluttered rapidly the color flashes, warning of predators. The brown underside is also a defensive strategy, acting as camouflage when set against the dead leaves of trees. When the Morpho is in flight, the contrast between the flashing blue color and the dull brown makes it seem that the butterfly appears and then disappears.

SENSATIONS: An interesting note is the "beauty is in the eye of the beholder" aspect seen in the provings of this butterfly—provers say that even things that aren't really attractive look good, or at least better to them; beauty is found everywhere in the provings; dual aspect in both physical and emotional symptoms—a reflection of the physical appearance of this butterfly, bright and flashing on one side, but dull on the other.

SENSITIVITIES: Opposite patterns of feeling that they are known, even liked, followed by the feeling that they have "disappeared" as far as others around them are concerned (see first paragraph, this remedy, above).

EMOTIONAL/ABANDONMENT: All provers experienced a sense of well-being followed by a let-down feeling that included feelings of abandonment; strong interest in pretty clothes and in dressing up.

PHYSICAL: A unique shimmering light effect in the eyes—in my experience this 'light show' precedes a headache of migraine proportions accompanied by the feeling that one is descending into darkness and obscurity; hyperactivity (as with all butterflies); dermatitis.

COMMENTS: LeRoux tells an interesting story of all the provers, who did not know what remedy they had taken, turning up the next day wearing blue.

NYMPHALIS URTICAE (SMALL TORTOISESHELL)

This butterfly feeds almost exclusively on nettles and there is a link between nettles and the skin rashes of this remedy if only in that the rash always looks like a nettle rash.

RESPONSIBILITY: Dislikes responsibility, would prefer to be a child again; anxiety about skill level or performance.

EMOTIONAL/ABANDONMENT: Strong feelings of well-being and lightness; as always with butterflies, feelings of abandonment; frightened of losing someone close to them.

PHYSICAL: Nettle rash skin eruptions on elbows and knees.

SENSATIONS: Renewed energy—can cope with anything (all butterfly remedies have this trait but it is particularly pronounced with Nymphalis); enjoys brightly colored clothes.

HIDING/PROTECTION: Hates winter, just wants to hibernate.

FOOD: Fruits and vegetables with love of sugar and fruits—the love of sweets seems less in this remedy.

PIERIS BRASSICAE (LARGE WHITE OR CABBAGE WHITE)

This butterfly is delicate, elegant, classy, and very pretty and these are the words that came in the dreams and preferences of the provers over and over again. There was a very definite theme of white and a love of white. The same wanting to dress up (transform themselves) as with other butterflies but the preferred color was always white. Children expressed a desire to dress up as white fairies.

PHYSICAL: The skin symptoms that are typical of all butterfly remedies.

ABANDONMENT: Sense of abandonment; loss of self; loss of security.

ADHD/HYPERACTIVITY: Difficulty concentrating and almost total inability to hold still.

FOOD: Unusual for butterfly people, the case histories show a love of green vegetables and a really strong preference for any form of cabbage, including broccoli.

Final Commentary

I was intrigued by the lowness of the potency of the remedies used in the provings, as well as by the low number of doses given. Butterflies are sensitive to their environment, sensitive to the weather, sensitive to energy, and sensitive to the presence of danger. This seems to be reflected in the reactions of provers and patients to homeopathic remedies in general and to butterfly remedies in particular. In each case and proving, they developed symptoms and achieved results that seemed way out of proportion to the potency of the remedy, in my experience. Perhaps, and this is speculation on my part, use of a butterfly remedy of any sort eliminates the psora pattern of "difficult to treat" that underlies so much of the pathology of humankind. If so, this is an amazing aspect of these unique remedies.

Miasmic Classification of Remedies

Bold Indicates Polycrest/First Choice Remedies
BOLD/ALL CAPS INDICATES NOSODE REMEDIES
Nosode remedies should be taken intercurently with a matching symptomatic remedy

ACUTE
Aconitum napellus
Agathis australis
Arnica montana
Belladonna
Calendula officinalis
Camphora
Chocolate
Collinsonia canadensis
Colocynthis
Croton tiglium
Hydrogen
Melilotus officinalis
Mentholum
Morphinum aceticum/purum
Myrica cerifera
Stramonium
Strychninum
Veratrum album

TYPHOID
Baptisia tinctoria
Byronia alba
Chamomilla vulgaris
Euphrasia officinalis
Helleborus niger
Hyoscyamus niger
Ipecacuanha
Mancinella venenata
Nux moschata
Nux vomica
Podophyllum peltatum
Rhus toxicodendron
Terebenthiniae oleum

PSORA
Alumen crudum
Ammonium carbonicum
Antimonium crudum
Argentum metallicum
Argentum nitricum
Arsenicum album
Borax veneta
Carbo vegetabilis
Causticum
Cereus bonplandii
Conium maculatum
Digitalis purpurea
Graphites naturalis
Hepar sulphuris calcareum
Lachesis muta
Lycopodium clavatum
Magnesia carbonica
Magnesia muriatica
Natrum carbonicum
PSORINUM
Sarsaparilla officinalis
Secale cornutum
Sepia succus
Silica terra
Sulphur
Thuja occidentalis
TUBERCULINUM BOVINUM
Zincum metallicum

MALARIA
Berberis vulgaris
Cactus grandiflorus
Cannabis sativa
Capsicum annuum
Chelidonium majus
China officinalis
Chinuinum arsenicosum
Cina maritima
Colchicum autumnale
Collinsonia canadensis
Eupatorium perfoliatum
Myrica cerifera
Ranunculus bulbosus
Rhus radicans
Spigelia anthelmintica

RINGWORM (POLIO)
Abies nigra
Actea spicata
Calcarea fluorata
Calcarea silicata
Colocynthis
Dulcamara
Gossypium herbaceum
Magnesia sulphurica
MEDORRHINUM
Niobium Metallicum
Taraxacum officinale
Sarsaparilla officinalis
VARIOLINUM
Viola tricolor

SYCOSIS

Agnus castus
Asafoetida
Cannabis indica
Caulophyllum thalictroides
Cinnamonum ceylanicum
Copaiva
Digitalis purpurea
Gelsemium sempervirens
Helonias dioica
Lilium tigrinum
MEDORRHINUM
Natrum sulphuricum
Nitricum acidum
Ornithogalum umbellatum
PSORINUM
Pulsatilla nigricans
Pyrogenium
Radium bromatum
Sabadilla officinalis
Sanguinaria canadensis
Sarsaparilla officinalis
Senecio aureus
Staphysagria
Tarentula hispanica
Thuja occidentalis
VARIOLINUM

VACCINOSIS

Anthracinum
Antimonium crudum
Apis mellifica
Arsenicum album
BACILLINUM TESTIUM
Baptisia tinctoria
Belladonna
CARCINOSIN
Carbolicum acidum
Chamomilla vulgaris
Crotalus horridus
DIPHTHERINUM
Echinacea angustifolia
Graphites naturalis
Gunpowder
Hepar sulphuris calcareum
Kali muriaticum
Lachesis muta
Ledum palustre
LEPROMINIUM
LYSSINUM
Malandrinum
MEDORRHINUM
Mercurius cyanatus
Mercurius solubilis
Mezereum
Phosphorus
Sabina officinalis
Sarsaparilla officinalis
Sepia succus
Silica terra
Sulphur
Thuja occidentails
TUBERCULINUM BOVINUM
VACCININUM
VARIOLINUM

CANCER

Agnus castus
Anacardium orientale
Argentum nitricum
Bellis Perennis
CARCINOSIN
Conium maculatum
Euphorbium officinarum
Galium aparine
Ignatia amara
Nitricum acidum
Nicotiana tabacum
Opium
Ornithogalum umbellatum
Physostigma venenosum
Sabina officinalis
Staphysagria
Viola odorata

TUBERCULOSIS

Abrotanum artemisia
Arsenicum iodatum
Atropinum purum
Baryta carbonica
Calcarea carbonica
Carbo animalis
Cereus bonplandii
Cimicifuga racemosa
Cistus canadensis
Coffea cruda
Lathyrus sativus
Myristica sebifera
Phosphoricum acidum
Phosphorus
Pix liquida
Sanguinaria canadensis
Silica terra
Stannum metallicum
TUBERCULINUM BOVINUM
Verbascum thapsus

LEPROSY
Aloe socotrina
Anacardium orientale
Cicuta virosa
Curare woorari
Hydrastis canadensis
Kola Nut
Arctium lappa
LEPROMINIUM
Achillea millefolium
Mandragora officinarium
Ocimum sanctum

SYPHILIS
Agnus castus
Asafoetida
Aurum metallicum
Baryta carbonica
Berberis aquifolium
Clematis erecta
Coriandrum sativum
Echinacea angustifolia/purpurea
Fluoricum acidum
Juglans regia
Leptandra virginica
Mercurius solubilis
Ocimum sanctum
Stillingia sylvatica
SYPHILINUM
Nicotiana tabacum

AIDS
Aconitum napellus
AIDS nosode
Arsenicum album
Arsenicum iodatum
Baptisia tinctoria
CARCINOSIN
Echinacea angustifolia
Ferrum phosphoricum
Gelsemium sempervirens
Lycopodium clavatum
MEDORRHINUM
Mercurius solubilis
Phosphoricum acidum
Phosphorus
Pulsatilla nigricans
Pyrogenium
Silica terra
Symphytum officinale
Thuja occidentalis
TUBERCULINUM
X-ray

ALZHEIMER'S
Agus casus
Aluminum oxydata
Anacardium orientale
Argentum nitricum
Arsenicum album
Aurum iodatum
Aurum metallicum
Baptisia tinctoria
Baryta carbonica
Belladonna
Bryonia alba
Calcarea phosphorica
Cannabis indica
Conium maculatum
Crotalus horridus
Hyoscyamus niger
Ignatia amara
Kali bromatum
Lachesis muta
Lycopodium clavatum
Natrum muriaticum
Nux vomica
Oopherinum
Phosphorus
Secale cornutum
Sepia succus
Staphysagria
Sulphur
Thiosinaminum
Zincum metallicum

Section Four

POSSIBLE REMEDIES FOR SPECIFIC CONDITIONS

REMEDIES AND SPECIFIC CONDITIONS

The first and most important rule of homeopathic treatment is that we are t**reating the patient and not the disease.** There is never a time in homeopathic treatment when this basic rule should be relegated to second place. Certainly it should never be ignored altogether at any time.

It is the totality of the person's symptoms—mental, physical, emotional—and the stressors that affect them, that tells us what remedy to give in any circumstance.

We must never be guilty of taking the western medical approach of giving a disease name to a few symptoms and then assuming there is a remedy for that ailment that will be of benefit to every person! Homeopathy doesn't work that way. No healing does!

You have perhaps noticed by now that ailments are rarely listed by the name a medical doctor would use for them. Symptoms, not disease names, are what counts in homeopathy. The newer versions of the repertories and Materia Medicas are beginning to list disease names. This will give you a "starting point" in looking for a remedy. After that you must look at the symptoms and modalities that are unique to this person if you are to find the right remedy.

There will be dozens of remedies that have the basic symptoms of the disease listed in the symptom picture. What will set the case apart and guide you to the remedy that will clear the whole illness in the least amount of time are those symptoms that are different from the symptoms of family members and friends who may be suffering from the same ailment.

That being said, emphatically, we can now discuss groupings of remedies that have been successful for homeopathic physicians around the world in the treatment of specific conditions. ***The basic symptoms of the malady are not discussed.*** What is listed under each remedy are the ***keynotes that set that remedy apart from others on the list.***

These lists are starting points only—just ways to get you thinking and looking and knowing that there is a remedy for everything. A remedy is on a list because its physical characteristics match that of the disease. You will then need to use the mental/emotional, better for/worse for states to match the exactly right remedy to the person. Only then will you be really effective, especially in dealing with some of the really nasty and scary things discussed in the next few chapters.

Most of the time in homeopathic prescribing you have time to clear 40% of the symptoms with the first remedy, rethink the case, and give a second remedy. With epidemics and contagious diseases, time is often a critical factor because the disease will move so rapidly. The first remedy needs to bring the vital force online strongly enough to eradicate the malady almost completely. Any follow-up remedies need to be for the purpose of convalescence, recovery, and the elimination of a few remaining symptoms.

Chapter Twenty - Homeopathy and First Aid

FIRST AID MATERIA MEDICA

The next few pages provide the names of some of the frequently used homeopathic remedies for first aid situations, indications for their use, and some very basic information about each one. Be sure to consult a more in-depth Materia Medica to match the symptoms more perfectly to the person once the initial crisis, which may have required you to act quickly, has passed.

ACONITUM NAPELLUS (MONKSHOOD)
CONDITIONS: Sunstroke; shock; flu; fever, with great thirst; chills; eye injuries and inflammation ; earache; headache; follows exposure to cold, dry wind, too much sun, or fright.
COMMENTS AND INDICATION: For the first stages of an illness; symptoms come on suddenly and dramatically and are accompanied by anxiety and restlessness; particularly suited for anything that is the result of shock or extreme fear and fright.

ALLIUM CEPA (RED ONION)
CONDITIONS: Colds; hay fever, especially with red, watery, burning eyes that have become sensitive to light; also may include dry, ticklish throat and sneezing; follows exposure to pollen, dust, animal dander, molds, or damp cold winds.
COMMENTS AND INDICATION: This remedy covers more symptoms of the common cold than any other and a cold is what the allergy and hay fever symptoms look like, also.

APIS MELLIFICA (HONEY BEE)
CONDITIONS: Hives; insect bites and stings; earache that is worse for heat; allergic swelling of face, eyelids, lips; fever; headache; joint pain; diarrhea.
COMMENTS AND INDICATION: The symptoms of Apis include burning and stinging sensations; thirstless but usually better for a cold drink; symptoms are better for cold worse for heat and touch; red fiery tongue; the person is often irritable and restless (much like a honey bee); tearful; whiny.

ARNICA MONTANA (LEOPARD'S BANE)
CONDITIONS: Bruising; sprains; strains; falls; blows; sports injuries; overexertion; exhaustion; headache; pain; inflammation; bleeding; head injuries; eye injuries; joint pain; post surgery pain; shock; injuries to muscles; sore, bruised feeling all over the body.
COMMENTS AND INDICATION: Arnica is the #1 remedy for any type of injury, even if received years earlier. Keynote: the person often refuses examination, telling you they are just fine when they obviously are not. Arnica promotes healing, controls bleeding, reduces swelling, and prevents infection and the formation of pus—amazing! **It is recommended to use only the homeopathic Arnica on open wounds.**

ARSENICUM ALBUM (ARSENIC)
CONDITIONS: Allergies; diarrhea; fevers; flu; food poisoning; nausea; pneumonia; weakness.
COMMENTS AND INDICATION: A true polycrest remedy and should be used as a first response remedy whenever there is flu, food poisoning, diarrheas, nausea, great weakness, and a host of other symptoms.

BELLIS PERENNIS (ENGLISH DAISY)
CONDITIONS: Bruises; joint pain from getting chilled or drinking cold water after being very hot; headache; pregnancy: pain in groin when walking (trapped nerve).

COMMENTS AND INDICATION: Small but important remedy in first aid; it is indicated for any ailment that follows a plunge into cold water (or even a drink that was too cold) when a person was overheated; a follow-up to Arnica if Arnica fails to act or the action stalls out after a time.

CALCAREA CARBONICA (OYSTER SHELL)
CONDITIONS: Sprains (of ankle, hand or wrist—mostly); stiff neck; backache; earache; eye inflammation; headache; exhaustion.

COMMENTS AND INDICATION: Calcarea carbonica is vital to the health and growth of healthy blood and connective tissue cells as well as bones and teeth. This remedy is indicated during the last phase of healing from an injury or when there is lingering pain from an old injury or sprain. Excellent remedy for weakness or exhaustion during convalescence. Indicated when there is exhaustion with even slight physical or mental exertion.

CALCAREA PHOSPHORICA (CALCIUM PHOSPHATE)
CONDITIONS: Broken bones—is particularly indicated when healing is slow. Phosphorus in the name of a remedy always indicates exhaustion of some sort.

COMMENTS AND INDICATION: Promotes the ossification (knitting together) of bones, especially in the elderly or those whose bones have become thin and brittle.

CALENDULA OFFICINALIS (POT MARIGOLD)
CONDITIONS: Cuts; wounds; abrasions; abscesses; lacerations; fever; surgeries; bleeding from wounds; head injury or concussion; wounds penetrating into joints; burns; sunburns; fever; especially indicated when the pain seems to be excessive for the amount of injury.

COMMENTS AND INDICATION: Calendula may be given internally or applied externally to the area. Given internally, it slows bleeding and helps with exhaustion from loss of blood or excessive pain. Calendula should be given before and after surgery.

CANTHARIS VESICATORIA (SPANISH FLY)
CONDITIONS: Burns; scalds; acute and sudden inflammations; severe cystitis.

COMMENTS AND INDICATION: Pain is raw, smarting, stinging and relieved by cold applications. The face will usually be pale with an expression of extreme suffering.

CARBO VEGETABILIS (VEGETABLE CHARCOAL)
CONDITIONS: Food poisoning; indigestion; acid stomach.

COMMENTS AND INDICATION: Condition may be the result of bad food, overindulgence, or the lingering effects of old illness aggravated by over eating.

COCCULUS INDICUS (INDIAN COCKLE)
CONDITIONS: Motion sickness; nausea; jet lag; sleep deprivation; vertigo.

COMMENTS AND INDICATION: Besides motion sickness and jet lag, this is a remedy for any ailment that has come about because of lack of sleep (when caring for loved ones, for example).

ECHINACEA ANGUSTIFOLIA (CONE FLOWER)
CONDITIONS: Irritation from insect bites and poisonous plants. Headache with dullness of mind. Blood poisoning.
COMMENTS AND INDICATION: Echinacea is a blood purifier and immune system tonic. Modalities include better for lying down, pains come and go suddenly, and worse in the evening.

EUPATORIUM PERFOLIATUM (BONE SET)
CONDITIONS: Chills; bone pains; fever; flu; diarrhea.
COMMENTS AND INDICATION: Conditions where there is a great deal of bone pain and the muscles feel bruised and sore in illness such as flu and fever. Person is restless and is often moaning from the pain. Often there is throbbing pain in the back of the head.

EUPHRASIA OFFICINALIS (EYEBRIGHT)
CONDITIONS: Allergies; hay fever; conjunctivitis.
COMMENTS AND INDICATION: The sensation is that of grit or sand in the eyes and tightness in the chest. Burning and swelling of the eyelids with the eyes watering continuously.

FERRUM PHOSPHORICUM (IRON PHOSPHATE)
CONDITIONS: nosebleeds; bruises; contusions; injuries; inflammation; wounds; weakness; fever; earache.
COMMENTS AND INDICATION: Especially indicated for the first stage of fevers and earaches. Ferrum remedies are indicated for anemia and blood disorders. Ferrum phosphoricum is particular to bright red nosebleeds with the spitting of blood. This remedy also controls soreness and bleeding after surgeries.

GELSEMIUM SEMPERVIRENS (YELLOW JASMINE)
CONDITIONS: Anxiety; chills; chronic fatigue; debility; diarrhea; fatigue; fevers; flu; muscle weakness; sunstroke; vertigo; weakness; often used as a follow-up or convalescent remedy.
COMMENTS AND INDICATION: Symptoms come on gradually and are accompanied by intense weariness and feeling of heaviness in the arms and legs. Person will be trembly from exhaustion and worse for any additional exertion. The mind is unusually sluggish when illness is present.

HAMAMELIS VIRGINIANA (WITCH HAZEL)
CONDITIONS: Bruises; burns; bleeding; open painful wounds; venous congestion of any kind; nosebleeds; hemorrhoids; vertigo.
COMMENTS AND INDICATION: No remedy has a wider range of usefulness with vein and blood disorders. It ranks with Arnica and Calendula as a topical application for burns and wounds.

HEPAR SULPHURIS CALCAREUM (SULPHUR - OYSTER SHELLS)
CONDITIONS: Earache; slow healing of cuts, wounds, and injuries; joint pain; sore throat.
COMMENTS AND INDICATION: Hepar sulph calc is a very chilly remedy. Ailments needing this remedy are often brought on by exposure to cold and are always made worse by cold. The person for whom this remedy is effective almost always lacks internal warmth, which makes them especially susceptible to the cold.

HYPERICUM PERFORATUM (ST. JOHN'S WART)
CONDITIONS: Injuries to nerve-rich parts of the body (fingers, toes, etc.); coccyx injuries; puncture wounds; lacerations; spinal injuries; bites; bruises; hemorrhoids; sciatica; post-operative pain; nerve pain that is tingling, burning, or numb.
COMMENTS AND INDICATION: This remedy is good for backaches after surgeries in which a spinal anesthesia was applied and for old injuries where there is still nerve pain.
Excessive pain and nerve pain is the keynote indications for this remedy.

IPECACUANHA (IPECAC ROOT)
CONDITIONS: Food and drug poisoning; morning sickness; nausea; migraine with vomiting; nosebleeds; fever with nausea; convulsions
COMMENTS AND INDICATION: This remedy is likely to be of great value whenever there is constant nausea and aversion to food. The nausea is not relieved by vomiting—rather there is the desire to vomit again, continuously. Ipecacuanha is useful in pregnancy if the symptom picture fits, but is more often a flu and food poisoning remedy.

KALI PHOSPHORICUM (POTASSIUM PHOSPHATE)
CONDITIONS: Anemia; diarrhea; fatigue; headaches; nosebleeds; pneumonia; nervous prostration; insomnia.
COMMENTS AND INDICATION: Kali phos is the nutrient found in the tissues and fluids of the brain and nervous system. Indicated when there is exhaustion and fatigue following illness or exertion with increased sensitivity to external stimuli such as light and noise.

LEDUM PALUSTRE (WILD ROSEMARY)
CONDITIONS: Bruises; puncture wounds and wounds of all types; insect bites and stings; skin eruptions.
COMMENTS AND INDICATION: Ledum helps prevent tetanus and sepsis in wounds. Most effective for bruising (black eyes or blows from objects) where the affected part feels cold yet pain is relieved by cold applications.

RHUS TOXICODENRON (POISON OAK)
CONDITIONS: Sprains; strains; injuries to ligaments; bruises; sciatica; stiff muscles or joints; swollen glands; cold sores; fever blisters; hives; poison ivy or poison oak rashes—any itchy rash with vesicles.
COMMENTS AND INDICATION: This is a remedy for the straining of muscles and tendons and for dislocated joints. It is good for lameness after a sprain, especially in the wrists or ankles. Rhus toxicodendron pains are aggravated by initial motion, but better upon continuing the activity. Like Arnica, Rhus toxicodendron is a remedy for physical strain that as come about by overdoing some activity.

RUTA GRAVELoENS (GAREN RUE)
CONDITIONS: Severe sprains with damaged tendons, split ligaments, or bruised periosteum—covering of the bones (making it a remedy for bruised shins.) Backache; Carpal tunnel syndrome; Dislocated joints; Eye strain; Joint injuries; Tennis elbow; Tendonitis; Nosebleeds; Fevers.
COMMENTS AND INDICATION: Ruta graveolens may be used for pains due to recent or old injuries, especially to the knees or elbows. Ruta graveolens has an affinity for fibrous tissue, flexor tendons, joints, cartilages, periosteum, skin, and eyes. This remedy is often indicated for any condition of prolapse. A keynote is the slipping out of place of vertebrae and a feeling of coldness in the spine.

SILICA TERRA (PURE FLINT)
CONDITIONS: Splinters and slivers; slow recovery or healing; boils; headache; glandular swelling; whitlow and other nail problems; pus formation; scarring; abscesses.
COMMENTS AND INDICATION: Some of the ailments of Silica seem to be brought about by shock or mental strain. Silica will bring an abscess to a head or cause a sliver or other foreign object to leave the body. The object will work its way to the surface where pus will form from which the object can be removed—rather amazing, actually.

STAPHYSAGRIA (STAVESACRE)
CONDITIONS: Bites; stings; cuts and wounds to nerve rich areas; eye injuries; motion sickness; styes; sciatica
COMMENTS AND INDICATION: Bites, stings, eye injuries, and wounds are very sensitive to touch. Staphysagria is particularly indicated if the injury came with feelings of humiliation, indignation, and anger. This can occur with abuse or even after an operation to a sensitive or embarrassing body part (such as stitching after childbirth). There is usually inflammation of the injured part.

SYMPHYTUM OFFICINALE (COMFREY)
CONDITIONS: Broken bones; fractures that are slow to heal; bone bruises; wounds; injuries to ligaments, tendons, and periosteum; sprains; phantom pain in amputated limbs; eye injuries.
COMMENTS AND INDICATION: This is an herbal remedy that has not been proven extensively by homeopathic researches. (I find this almost impossible to understand.) It is of great value as a first-aid treatment for injuries to the eye, especially for direct blows to the eyeball. Symphytum speeds the healing of broken bones and other injuries.

URTICA URENS (STINGING NETTLE)
CONDITIONS: Burns; bites; stings; sore throat; eczema; itchy blotches; hives with a constant desire to rub—and may actually be better for rubbing; allergic reactions experienced after eating shellfish.
COMMENTS AND INDICATION: Urtica is helpful for diminishing the pain of burns. This remedy is helpful in the passage of accumulated uric acid. Supporting the kidneys and clearing the cells and tissues of uric acid crystals is important to the clearing of hives and itchy patches and to the relieving of pain with burns and bites.

VERATRUM ALBUM (WHITE HELLEBORE)
CONDITIONS: Collapse; dehydration; head injury; diarrhea; flu; shock sunstroke; convulsions.
COMMENTS AND INDICATION: Collapse with extreme coldness, mild blueness of lips usually brought on by severe illness with diarrhea and dehydration or from sunstroke. Usually there is vomiting, cramping, vertigo, delirium and sleepiness.

FIRST AID - CONDITIONS

Emergency first aid treatment should almost always include **RESCUE REMEDY,** a Bach Flower Essence remedy also known as **FIVE FLOWER FORMULA**. If there has been an accident or a trauma of any kind, Arnica or Aconitum, depending on symptoms, should also be given. Arnica is indicated by an insistence from the person that they really are fine, while the Aconitum person will be very anxious, probably hysterical, and often screaming in pain.

This is meant as a collection of remedies that have a reputation for effectiveness for many years and in many places. Your use of them, and when to call for medical assistance, must—as always—be your own responsibility and be based upon your own skill, competence, and confidence. I hope this list is helpful in some way to someone, somewhere, sometime. There are many other remedies that may have deserved a place in this list. Please treat this work as only a beginning in your repertory of emergency remedies.

It is a fine thing to develop the knowledge and skill to cope competently with emergency situations as they arise with yourself and in your families. It is probably best, at least at first, to be under the watchful eye of a more experienced person or a physician.

ABSCESSES
HEPAR SULPHURIS CALCAREUM: Aids in bringing boils to a head and in the clearing of abscesses and suppurating sores.
SILICA TERRA: Brings abscesses to a head quickly and prevents the formation of scar tissue.

ALLERGIES
ALLIUM CEPA: Reactions that look much like a cold.
APIS MELLIFICA: Allergic swelling of the face, eyelids, and/or lips.
ARSENICUM ALBUM: All types of allergic reactions.
EUPHRASIA OFFICINALIS: Reaction centered in the eyes, with a feeling of grit in eye.
RHUS TOXICODENDRON: Predominantly for the relief of hives, fever blisters, cold sores, and eye irritation symptoms from allergic reactions.
PHOSPHORUS: Toxic poisoning or allergic reactions from chemical fumes; panting, gasping for air, vertigo; any strong reaction to odors.

BACK INJURIES
RHUS TOXICODENDRON: Back strains or injuries from over work or heavy lifting. Spinal paralysis of infants; stiffness and lameness in sacrum.
HYPERICUM PERFORATUM: The spinal cord is the major nerve highway of the body. Hypericum is indicated for injury to any nerve-rich area. Spinal or coccyx injury from a fall or surgery. Pinched nerves in back.
RUTA GRAVEOLENS: Herniated, slipped, or ruptured discs from weight lifting or over exertion. Vertebrae slip out of place easily creating chronic back pain.
ARNICA MONTANA: Take immediately after any back injury. Consider alternately with Ruta graveolens

BITES AND STINGS (SEE INSECT BITES AND STINGS)

BROKEN BONES
ARNICA MONTANA: Arnica is always given in an injury situation to treat for shock and to reduce bruising, swelling, and trauma to the surrounding tissues.
CALCAREA PHOSPHORICA: Promotes the knitting together (ossification) of bones.
SYMPHYTUM OFFICINALE: Comfrey has been referred to as knit-bone for many years because it speeds the healing and strength of broken bone.
RUTA GRAVEOLENS: Much like Arnica, Ruta graveolens is for fractures with bruising. The difference is in the emotionals. With Arnica the person is explaining that they are just fine and need to go home or back to work; with Ruta graveolens there is anxiousness and fear that things are worse than they seem to be; broken jaw.

BRUISES
ARNICA MONTANA: To be used externally and internally to relieve pain and reduce bruising and swelling. Use as soon after injury as possible and repeat the dose as needed.
BELLIS PERENNIS: Use predominantly as a follow-up remedy when Arnica has either failed to work or usefulness has ended.
HYPERICUM PERFORATUM: Bruises where there is injury to the nerves.
LEDUM PALUSTRE: Bruise feels cold but is better for cold application.
RHUS TOXICODENDRON: For bruising with strained muscles or dislocated joints.
RUTA GRAVEOLENS: Particularly for bruises to the bones, such as shins, etc.
SYMPHYTUM OFFICINALE: Bruises connected with the bone fractures.

BURNS AND SCALDS
CALENDULA OFFICINALIS: Used mostly as a topical in a gel form. Very good that way.
CANTHARIS VESICATORIA: One of the best remedies for burns; helps the burn heal and lessens the amount of pain felt.
HAMAMELIS VIRGINIANA: Not a common remedy for burns, but very useful if the burns are deep or have become inflamed (pre-infectious).
URTICA URENS: Useful for the minor burns and scalds of every day. Really relieves the stinging and burning sensation.

CUTS AND WOUNDS
CALENDULA OFFICINALIS: Externally, for minor cuts and wounds, along with a remedy that most closely matches the symptoms.
FERRUM PHOSPHORICUM: Ferrum remedies build the blood, correcting anemic conditions. This promotes healing, controls bleeding and fever, and prevents sepsis. The phosphoricum part of this remedy helps with weakness, exhaustion, and debility.
HAMAMELIS VIRGINIANA: Use for open, painful wounds with weakness from blood loss. Also relieves pain following surgery.
HEPAR SULPHURIS CALCAREUM: For wounds with redness and inflammation.
LEDUM PALUSTRE: Puncture wounds, such as to the sole of the foot or palm of the hands. Hypericum is better for extremities, such as fingers and toes. Ledum prevents infection.
STAPHYSAGRIA: Specific mental picture of humiliation or anger with a puncture or stab wound.
SYMPHYTUM OFFICINALE: Speeds the healing of wounds and the reconstruction of tissues.

DENTAL EMERGENCIES AND SURGERIES
MERCURIUS SOLUBILIS (VIVUS) To be taken at the first sign of dental discomfort to prevent further development until a dentist is available (may even fix the problem); pain is worse from cold drinks and from cold air; gum boils; mercury toxicity from dental fillings.
HYPERICUM PERFORATUM: Injuries to dental nerves; trauma to front teeth (try St. John's Wort (Hypericum) Tincture locally at the same time.)
RUTA GRAVEOLENS: Pain from dry socket, infected tooth socket, or tooth that is loose in the socket, or pain from a tooth that has been loosened by traumatic injury; speeds healing of bone and periosteum.
ARNICA MONTANA: Trauma from dental work or surgery; creation of or worsening of TMJ symptoms following dental work; toothache after head injury; alternate Hypericum and Arnica before, during, and after tooth extractions, root canals, and fillings.

DRUGS, ADVERSE REACTIONS
ARSENICUM ALBUM: Deep acting remedy which acts on every organ and tissue; should be the first thing reached for while further determining symptom picture and fine tuning the homeopathic response; side effects of chemotherapy—prophylactic if taken before treatments; anaphylactic shock; exhaustion; collapse.
SULPHUR: Hypersensitive reactions to drugs of any type, but especially antibiotics; cleanses system of previous allopathic drug use; counteracts the drugs suppression of the disease.
CADMIUM SULPHURICUM: Specific to the symptoms of radiation and chemotherapy; quells violent nausea and persistent vomiting, allowing the sufferer to hold down nutritious foods (person may vomit once, violently after first taking the remedy, but then feel much better); lifts the spirits generally.
PHOSPHORUS: Dependency on prescription medications; need for instant gratification; body odor similar to the odor of the drug.
ARNICA MONTANA: For convulsions after drugs.
GELSEMIUM SEMPERVIRENS: Bad reactions to and never-the-same-since symptoms from flu shots and allergy injections.
THUJA OCCIDENTALIS: Number one polycrest remedy for reactions and long-standing symptoms created by vaccinations.
APIS MELLIFICA: Sudden illness or swelling after a vaccination; edema and swelling at the site of administration of a local anesthetic—there will be burning or stinging pains.

EXHAUSTION
ARNICA MONTANA: For the exhaustion that follows overexertion or traumatic accident.
ARSENICUM ALBUM: Deep acting remedy which acts on every organ and tissue. Use when the exhaustion seems out of proportion to the illness.
CALCAREA CARBONICA: Exhaustion with dizziness and breathlessness, especially worse for walking up a hill or up stairs. Often the exhaustion comes on as a result of physical exertion.
CALENDULA OFFICINALIS: Exhaustion from loss of blood or pain, usually following a surgery or traumatic accident.
GELSEMIUM SEMPERVIRENS: is usually great anxiety and trembling.
KALI PHOSPHORICUM: Especially suited to overworked business and professional people and those who are constantly keyed up mentally. Helpful for nervous exhaustion.
SPONGIA TOSTA: Affects the heart valves. Exhaustion with dizziness and heart valve insufficiency. Exhaustion after even slight exertion.
VERATRUM ALBUM: Collapse with extreme coldness.

EYE INJURIES

ARNICA MONTANA: Black eye (bruising); traumatic injury with hemorrhage; absorption of clots following retinal hemorrhage; bruised iris after cataract surgery; floaters in vision after an accident.

ACONITUM NAPELLUS: Acute inflammation after eye injury; inflammation from having had a foreign object in the eye.

LEDUM PALUSTRE: Bloodshot or bruised; black eye from injury; hemorrhage in the eye; drooping of lid from an injury to the eye.

RUTA GRAVEOLENS: Eye injuries where tissue surrounding the eye is also very inflamed.

SYMPHYTUM OFFICINALE: Injuries to the eyes from blunt instruments or a blow to the eyeball, eye socket, or sclera; bleeding inside the eye after injury; traumatic conjunctivitis; long-term pain or soreness in the eye after an injury.

FEVERS

ACONITUM NAPELLUS: Sudden high fevers; fevers with one cheek red and hot and the other pale and cold; worse in the evening.

EUPATORIUM PERFOLIATUM: Fever with great weakness; burning heat; fever with bone pain.

GELSEMIUM SEMPERVIRENS: A remedy for the fever and sweat stages of illness; fever with drowsiness, stupor, dizzyness, faintness, and weakness; fever with nervous restlessness; fever with intense burning; thirstless during fever.

ARSENICUM ALBUM: This is a polycrest remedy for sudden acute illnesses and flu; fever at night with restlessness and anxiety; extremely high fever; septic fevers; feeling as if there is hot water running in the veins.

FERRUM PHOSPHORICUM: Fevers of unknown origin; early stage of illnesses with inflammation and fever; high fever of 102° or higher; fevers with sore throat or lung affliction; red face that feels cool.

IPECACUANHA: Fever with nausea and vomiting; catarrhal or gastric fevers.

FLU

ACONITUM NAPELLUS: First stages of a flu that comes on suddenly. Hot inside and chilly externally. Very thirsty.

ARNICA MONTANA: Flu with sore, bruised feeling in muscles. Body aches as if beaten and joints feel as if sprained.

ARSENICUM ALBUM: This is polycrest, first response remedy. Often all that is needed. Flu will begin with either cold symptoms or upset tummy. Gastric/intestinal flu will usually be accompanied by diarrhea. Usually with headache. Indicated for relapse situations—person got well but then the same illness returned.

EUPATORIUM PERFOLIATUM: Awful flu with characteristic intense pains in bones and lower back (even hips). Skin all over feels dry and sore. Even the eyeballs and scalp feel achy and tender. Fever with chills. Nausea. Vomiting of food and bile. Very thirsty but vomits after drinking anything.

GELSEMIUM SEMPERVIRENS: Flu with deep fatigue and feeling of heaviness. Chilly, can't seem to get warm. Fever with shivering. Headache. Often indicated in the final stages and during convalescence.

IPECACUANHA: Nausea from smell of food. Very weary, as if he has carried a heavy load. Pain in bones and in the back. Fever. Chills are worse in a warm room and better for fresh air. Often accompanied by headache. Belching and much saliva. Often extreme nausea with desire to vomit but unable to.

VERATRUM ALBUM: Sudden and violent with collapse, coldness, blue tinge to skin, great weakness. Diarrhea will be violent. Symptoms often accompanied by fainting. Feels hungry and thirsty, even when eating and drinking causes immediate vomiting. Gastric flu is accompanied by mucus in bronchials.

FOOD POISONING
ARSENICUM ALBUM: For food poisoning with diarrhea and extreme nausea. This is the first remedy I would reach for with any digestive upset, particularly if it was intestinal to any degree. Exhaustion and weakness is a keynote of this remedy.
CARBO VEGETABILIS: Similar to Arsenicum but more specific to food poisoning from bad meat.
COCCULUS INDICUS: Nausea with belching, metallic taste in the mouth, and feeling of faintness.
IPECACUANHA: Nausea, with chilliness and often with pains in the bones.

HAY FEVER
ALLIUM CEPA Symptoms similar to those experienced when peeling onions.
ARSENICUM ALBUM Like a cold with violent sneezing and thin watery discharge.
EUPHRASIA OFFICINALIS Similar to a cold with eye inflammations. Worse evenings.

HEAT EXHAUSTION/HEAT STROKE
The Bach Flower Combination, **RESCUE REMEDY,** is always a good choice.

Heat exhaustion: Loss of fluids and electrolytes can also produce a condition where there is nausea, dizziness, weakness, cramps, headache and fainting. In the instance of heat exhaustion, the person will be dehydrated. Replacing bodily fluids and having the person lie down in a cool room helps with recovery.

Heat stroke: When the body is unable to control its temperature after lengthy exposure to heat and the sun, sometimes a fatal condition known as heat stroke occurs. An early sign is the lack of sweating. The body temperature may rise to 105 degrees Fahrenheit or higher and there will also be dehydration and a loss of electrolytes. Seizures, severe headache, confusion and rapid breathing are also evident. This is an emergency situation and generally calls for immediate medical attention.

GLONOINUM: First remedy for sun stroke. Severe congestive headache after exposure to sun and heat. Hot face with cold extremities. Irritability. Confusion. Pounding pain. (Compare to Belladonna)
GELSEMIUM SEMPERVIRENS: Sun stroke. Headache in the back of the head. Weakness. Possibly comatose. No thirst.
LACHESIS MUTA: Headaches from heat and sun exposure. Faintness. Dizzyness. Mental confusion. Symptoms are worse after sleep. Faintness. Dizzyness.
NATRUM CARBONICUM: Chronically affected by heat and sun stroke. Extreme fatigue that is the result of heat and exposure to the sun. Headache is worse from the slightest mental effort.
BELLADONNA Agonizing sudden shooting headache with intense throbbing. Bright red face. Dilated pupils. Glassy-eyed, fixed stare with no expression. Mouth dry but no sensation of thirst.
BRYONIA ALBA: Severe headache made worse by the slightest motion. Extremely thirsty for large amounts of cold water.
ACONITUM NAPELLUS: Faint and dizzy with headache after prolonged, direct exposure to the sun. Individual will be anxious and restless. May tell you he is dying.
CARBO VEGETABILIS: Collapse from excess heat. Skin feels clammy. Nausea. Better for moving air around him (fanning).

HIVES
APIS MELLIFICA: Much burning and stinging. Rosy red. Very sensitive and sore. Often with fever and sweating. Worse at night.
RHUS TOXICODENDRON: Burning, itchy hives with joint pain
URTICA URENS: Red, raised blotches with constant desire to rub. Rubbing sometimes brings some relief. Always consider when the hives may have been a reaction to eating shellfish.

INJURIES
ARNICA MONTANA: Give Arnica as a routine after any injury to prevent shock, swelling, and bruising.
CALCAREA CARBONICUM: Vital to healthy blood, connective tissue, and bones. For old injuries where there is lingering pain or slow healing.
CALENDULA OFFICINALLIS: Wounds which have extended into or are affecting joints.
FERRUM PHOSPHORICUM: Helps with soreness and bleeding. Phosphoricums are indicated when there is fatigue and weakness.
HYPERICUM PERFORATUM: Damage to nerve-rich areas—fingers, toes, coccyx, spine. Post-operative pain (take as a preventative before surgeries).
HEPAR SULPHURIS CALCAREA: Wounds with inflammation where healing is slow
RHUS TOXICODENDRON: Stiffness remaining after strains and sprains to joints, ligaments or the back. Limbers up with movement.
RUTA GRAVEOLENS Sprains, particularly in ankles or wrists. Bruises to the covering of the bone (periosteum) such as on shins. Pains of Ruta graveolens are constant and worse from movement or pressure.

INSECT BITES AND STINGS
APIS MELLIFICA: Burning and stinging. The person is tearful and whiny.
ECHINACEA ANGUSTIFOLIA: Blood purifier, so speeds recovery and return to normal.
HYPERICUM PERFORATUM: For exceptionally inflamed and painful bites to nerve-rich areas with the pains shooting or tearing up neural pathways.
LEDUM PALUSTRE: Ledum prevents sepsis and infection and should routinely be given when a person is bitten or stung. It may be given, in low potency, along with the remedy that most clearly indicated.
STAPHYSAGRIA: Indicated when the bite or sting stays sensitive to the touch for a longer than the usual period of time.
URTICA URENS: Give internally. Apply locally for the burning and itching

JOINT PAIN
APIS MELLIFICA: Arthritic pains with stinging sensation. Other symptoms must match, of course.
ARNICA MONTANA: Joint pain and stiffness from injury or overexertion. Ache as if beaten.
BELLIS PERENNIS: Use if Arnica has not brought relief.
HEPAR SULPHURIS CALCAREUM Swelling in joints of fingers. Bruised, pulling, tearing pain in hips or shoulders. Better for heat, much worse for cold.
RHUS TOXICODENDRON Polycrest remedy for many types of sciatica and joint pain. There is lameness and stiffness which is worse for rest and much worse when forced to move again after a rest. Continued movement brings relief but pain soon returns with weariness. Pain can be brought about by overexertion.
RUTA GRAVEOLENS Injured joints and bruised bones. Sprains with weakness in joint. Bursitis. Cracking in joints, worse for movement. Parts lain on get very painful. Knees give way. Pain in feet, ankles, wrists, hands. Ganglion of wrists. Nodes in joints of palms.

NAUSEA (SEE FLU AND FOOD POISONING)

NOSEBLEEDS
FERRUM PHOSPHORICUM: Bright red blood, with spitting of blood, especially in children.
HAMAMELIS VIRGINIANA: Profuse nosebleed with failure to coagulate. Typical blood vessel congestion, causing tightness at bridge of nose.
IPECACUANHA: Nosebleed during cough or with headache, bright red.
KALI PHOSPHORICUM: Deficiency of the blood, resulting in nosebleeds, fatigue, and weakness. Profuse flow of blood.
RUTA GRAVEOLENS: Pressure and aching at the root of the nose, like a blunt plug, with nosebleed.

SHOCK
FIVE FLOWER FORMULA (commonly called **RESCUE REMEDY**) should always be given if shock is experienced or pending. Aconitum shock and Arnica shock are exact opposites. Aconitum or Arnica may be used in addition, but Rescue Remedy is essential!
ACONITUM NAPELLUS: Mental and emotional shocks. Panic and great fear. Tingling coldness and numbness. Eyes will be glassy and staring. This is a remedy that is used in childbirth, especially for a fast labor where the mother is shaking with shock (baby may be very still with a fearful look on its face).
ARNICA MONTANA: The first remedy to reach for when there has been an accident or injury accompanied by delayed shock. Person will claim to be fine. Use of Arnica Montana at this time will most likely prevent the person going further into shock.

SPRAINS
ARNICA MONTANA: As immediately after injury as possible to reduce swelling and bruising and to speed healing.
BELLIS PERENNIS: As a follow-up remedy to Arnica, if the action of Arnica was insufficient or has halted.
CALCAREA CARBONICA: Particularly useful for old sprains where there is still pain and weakness.
RHUS TOXICODENDRON: For muscle or tendon strain from over lifting. Use Arnica first. Rhus toxicodendron is then indicated if there is inability to grip or lift after healing should have occurred.
RUTA GRAVEOLENS: Use for old injuries that still stiffen up with changes in the weather.
SYMPHYTUM OFFICINALE: Symphytum aids the body in uptake and distribution of calcium, thus assisting healing of bones and tissues.

SPLINTERS
SILICA TERRA: Silica will encourage any foreign object to work its way to the surface of the body where pus will form from which the object may be ejected or removed.

TOXIC POISONING, CHEMICAL ALLERGIES
APIS MELLIFICA: Anti-inflammatory and antihistamine; multiple chemical sensitivities; hypersensitivity and anaphylactic shock from allergies (foods such as nuts), insect bites and stings; chemicals and chemical fumes, and drugs; swelling of face and throat; difficulty breathing.
PHOSPHORUS: Toxic poisoning or allergic reactions from chemical fumes; panting, gasping for air, vertigo; any strong reaction to odors.
BOVISTA: To be used until medical help arrives to prevent asphyxia and death by suffocation from gas fumes; heart feels enormously large; body, the extremities first, will be puffy and swollen.
CARBO VEGETABILIS: Asphyxia from carbon monoxide poisoning or any other situation where there is lack of oxygen; difficult accelerated breathing; headache; head feels very heavy.

TRAVEL SICKNESS
COCCULUS INDICUS: Travel sickness where there is nausea, diarrhea, headache, dizziness, feeling of faintness, and vomiting. Person must lie down to prevent vomiting. Worse for fresh air, eating, drinking, movement, or sitting up.
STAPHYSAGRIA: Indicated when the traveller is extremely annoyed and difficult and usually complaining loudly about the injustice of this nausea happening to him at a time like this!

NOTES

Emergency first aid treatment should almost always include Rescue Remedy, a Bach Flower Essence remedy also known as Five Flower Formula. If there has been an accident or a trauma of any kind, Arnica or Aconitum, depending on symptoms, should also be given. (Please see Shock on previous page)

This table is meant as a collection of remedies that have a reputation for effectiveness for many years and in many places. Your use of them, and when to call for medical assistance, must—as always—be your own responsibility and be based upon your own skill, competence, and confidence. There are many other remedies that may have deserved a place in this list. It should be only the start of a repertory of emergency remedies.

It is a fine thing to develop the knowledge and skill to cope competently with emergency situations as they arise with yourself and in your families. It is probably best, at least at first, to be under the watchful eye of a more experienced person or a physician.

Chapter Twenty-One - Learning and Behavioral Disorders

We should not make the mistake of thinking that a homeopathic can immediately cope with any behavioral problem. Homeopathic remedies merely punch a hole in the wall that is keeping someone locked into a specific behavior pattern. Homeopathy allows a person to look at the world and see other ways of being in each situation. The person still has to widen the hole and climb through. The use of behavior therapies, energy and allergy work will speed the healing according to how much work the person is willing to put forth.

Where there are bad habits, they will need to be broken and better habits put in their place. The remedy has only made it easier by loosening the chains and letting them see themselves, and their past if necessary, in new lights. Where there is an emotional payoff (such as getting out of certain tasks or getting extra attention) that pattern will need to be recognized and abandonment encouraged. If the patient is a child, they will need considerable help from mom and dad to make the necessary changes.

Homeopathic remedies can change the energetic charge of habits or memories. Wounds can be healed and habits can be recognized and changed.

CHRONIC ANXIETY-BASED DISORDERS

Most of the time demands, challenges, and temporary moments of anxiety are taken in stride. Fear of this or that is part of life in this world. Sometimes the things we fear, or are uncomfortable about, obtain too much power in our lives. The medical world is only too happy to provide us with a drug to take the edge off for us, but all drugs have side effects. Drugs taken for normal, everyday anxiety and depression can become a slippery slope as they interfere with the absorption of nutrients and mess around with hormones.

It is estimated that about 15% of the population suffer from panic attacks and anxiety disorders serious enough to have an impact on their quality of life. (More women than men—really? What do women fear that men do not?) Many times, the right homeopathic treatment at the right time, along with an improvement in nutrition and lifestyle, is all that is needed to take back control of one's life and situation. Other times, medical intervention may be necessary, at least for a time. Once again, the choice and the responsibility belong to the sufferer alone. *Never make the mistake of thinking you have all of the answers for everyone.*

There are over 300 remedies listed in the repertories for anxiety-based problems. In most cases, the appropriate remedy should, of course, be selected using the totality of symptoms. For a full-blown panic attack you will treat using the symptoms of that attack. Life issues will need to be addressed to eliminate the problem long term, but the panic attack is the most dramatically presenting symptom at the moment. Underlying issues and nutritional imbalances will need to be addressed after the attack subsides.

ARSENICUM ALBUM This remedy is recommended for those who are more than usually concerned about their health. Panic attacks occur more frequently in the middle of the night or in the early hours of the morning. There is exhaustion, but it is accompanied by restlessness, fidgeting, pacing, and if they do sit down for a moment they immediately jump back up and move to a new room or chair. Digestive complaints and/or asthmas attacks often accompany the anxiety. There is an underlying concern with order and security and a need to be in control of every detail of their lives. Also an excellent remedy for flu. *(psora miasm)*

CALCAREA CARBONICA This remedy is suited to normally dependable, solid people who have become overwhelmed from physical illness or overwork. Their thoughts have become muddled and confused, especially when tired. Bad news or concern over family, friends, or work may agitate them. They have developed a feeling of dread that some disaster is about to fall on them or on some member of their family. They are, or have become, sensitive to the slightest cold and are having trouble keeping warm. There is a constant craving for sweets. Fear of heights, claustrophobia, and fatigue are also common. Acute attacks consist of increased perspiration, dizziness, nausea, and a pale face. These symptoms, along with night sweats, cold hands and feet, and slow digestion, may occur at any time—not just during an acute attack. *(tubercular miasm)*

GELSEMIUM SEMPERVIRENS Indicated when the panic attack is a feeling of weakness, trembling, and mental dullness—literally being paralyzed by fear. Gelsemium is also useful when there is anxiety about an upcoming event such as a performance, interview, test, or visit to the dentist. There is often a fear of crowds or a fear of falling. A fear that the heart will stop or become impaired is also part of the picture of *Gelsemium*. There is great fatigue, aching of the whole body, limbs and eyelids feel heavy, headache, and dizziness. Unusual-type symptoms, commonly seen with this remedy however, include lack of thirst and the scalp becoming sore to the touch. *Gelsemium* is often a follow-up or a convalescent remedy. **(Sycotic miasm)**

IGNATIA AMARA The primary indication for Ignatia is emotional stress, especially disappointment, loss, criticism by loved ones, or grief. There will be a defensive attitude, mood swings, frequent sighing, sudden bursting into either tears or laughter. Difficult to comfort because they do not want company, especially sympathetic company because of fear of being hurt even further. They are very sad, introspective, and brooding. Insomnia will have become a problem, although they probably won't tell you about it. The picture of *Ignatia* is very similar to the symptoms of the **cancer miasm.**

KALI PHOSPHORICUM Indicated when a person has become exhausted by overwork, illness, bad news, or thinking too much about world conditions. There is a deep anxiety about personal competence and ability to cope with life. Insomnia, an inability to concentrate, jumpiness, over-sensitivity, startling at sounds, and nervous digestive upsets are part of the picture. Although the stomach is upset, eating, warmth, and rest are often all that is needed for temporary relief.

LYCOPODIUM This is a picture of anxiety created by a deep sense of inadequacy that is being covered by pretending to be capable and competent. A lot of mental stress develops and they become self-conscious and intimidated around people they perceive as more powerful or more competent than they consider themselves. There is always a deep sense of anxiety and feelings of failure at the beginning of any task or project; they usually do well once the project is underway. If the problem becomes more serious, there will be a breakdown under stress, bullying tendencies, irritability, claustrophobia, and—eventually—just wanting to be left alone. This is a **psoric** remedy but its picture is of a **very deep version** of this miasm.

NATRUM MURIATICUM The anxiety disorder is brought about by a conflict between a desire to be of service and help others, and an inherent shyness and awkwardness in social situations. Easily hurt or offended, bears grudges, and dwells on unhappy feelings. Anxiety is worse at night, is accompanied by fear of being alone, but consolation or mention of their fear annoys them. Migraines late at night and insomnia are common. *(Alzheimer's miasm)*

PULSATILLA NIGRICANS Pulsatilla personalities express anxiety by becoming discouraged, moody, tearful, whiny, and even emotionally childish. Getting too warm, being in a stuffy room, hormonal changes, and lack of attention and sympathy are some of the triggers for Pulsatilla-type anxiety and fear. Attention and sympathy—really just the opportunity to whine a little without anyone thinking they need to fix it—are just what is needed. **(Sycosis miasm)**

SILICA TERRA Indicated for people who are capable and confident most of the time, but prone to temporary loss of confidence when under stress or embroiled in the criticism common to family disputes. Worry and overwork can bring on headaches, difficulty concentrating, exhaustion, over sensitivity, dread, and just plain panic when faced with public performances that they would normally have taken in stride. Loss of stamina becomes a keynote if the stress is not removed and balance restored. **(predominantly a psora miasm but also sycotic)**

PANIC ATTACKS

ACONITUM NAPELLUS This is the #1 polycrest remedy for panic attacks and shock. An Aconitum panic attack comes on suddenly. There will be a lot of fear—even fear of death. The anxiety may be accompanied by heart palpitations, shortness of breath, gasping, and flushing of the face. (Frightening to observe) There may or may not have been an original fright or fearful situation which triggered the first attack, although these types of attack become more common in the general population after an event like 9/11. **(acute miasm if tend to pass quickly; AIDS if symptoms are more severe or occur constantly)**

ARGENTUM NITRICUM Attacks occuring with claustrophobia, fear of heights in anticipation of doctor or dentist appointments, or giving a performance. This remedy can be given, in low potency, as a preventative when one must go to the dentist or speak in church, etc. The emotional issues of this remedy can be deep, making it possibly indicated for the *Alzheimer's* miasm, with *psora* if symptoms are mild.

KALI ARSENICOSUM Panic attacks related to health worries, particularly concerns for the heart or with asthma. Attacks are a surprise to friends and relative as Kali-anything people are typically conservative, reserved, and not prone to emotional outbursts. This remedy also applies to fairly deep issues.

PHOSPHORUS Nervous, sensitive people in whom anxiety can be triggered just by thinking for a moment about almost anything. The fears are intense and vivid and are often accompanied by palpitations, nausea, and weakness. They are often exhausted from sensitivity to and sympathy for others and they require a lot of company and reassurance for themselves. A Phosphorus personality becomes physically ill from stress, worry, or overwork. A keynote of this remedy is that fears become worse when they are left alone at home. When alone, they often turn on the radio or TV for company. This remedy is characterized by feelings that "something bad is about to happen" to someone. They literally work themselves into a state of panic. They are easily reassured, but the panic returns just as easily when they are alone again. Useful for the tubercular, Alzheimer's, and AIDS miasms. A deep remedy, for issues sliding further down with every passing day.

SPONGIA TOSTA Attacks that occur with a feeling of tightness or strangulation in the throat, accompanied by fear of death from suffocation. Causes may be emotional (freedom or agency issues or fear and anxiety centered around heart health) or physical (glandular or endocrine disorders).

EATING DISORDERS

ANOREXIA

Anorexia is a psychological disorder in which a person, most often female, refuses to eat sufficient calories to maintain health. While there are certainly issues about body size, weight, or attractiveness, anorexia is often about control of one's environment or of oneself. Guilt and self loathing often also play a part. Actual cases of anorexia nervosa have been successfully treated using the following remedies:

NATRUM MURIATICUM This is the most often indicated remedy for anorexia, as well as for head injuries. There is a lot of guilt, fear of being rejected, hurt feelings, self-consciousness, perfectionism, and a driving fear of being fat. *Natrum mur* is a remedy that is often used for head injuries, which is interesting. ***Alzheimer's miasm because it is moving toward destruction.***

ARSENICUM ALBUM Extreme nervousness. Anxiety about the future. Fear that the earth has been poisoned and food supply is contaminated. There is anger at himself and others which alternates with despondency and fear that the world's problems, and her own personal problems, have no workable solution. (rare but interesting)

CARCINOSIN Centers around control issues in the family. Sometimes the result of abuse, either perceived or real. There is an underlying fear of not being good enough that drives perfectionism and the need to succeed and do enough in every aspect of their lives.

CAUSTICUM Overly sympathetic to others and guilt-ridden that they have not done enough for everybody. Feels hungry when there is no food around, but appetite vanishes at the sight and smell of any food at all.

CHINA OFFICINALIS Aversion to most kinds of food, with occasional craving for sweets. Anorexia characterized by feeling full all of the time. There is a marked lack of self-confidence with apathy and indifference.

IGNATIA AMARA Loss of appetite from deep grief. Sadness and sighing with an empty feeling in the pit of the stomach that, when food is taken, becomes great nausea.

PULSATILLA NIGRICANS Feelings of worthlessness and loneliness. Creates ever-expanding lists of food that are bad for health. Great fear of gaining weight (Pulsatilla personalities, or women who have uank back into a Pulsatilla profile, actually do gain weight easily). There is a constant need to weigh themselves.

SEPIA SUCCUS Sepia is a complementary remedy to Pulsatilla nigricans. The anorexia of Sepia often has a hormonal base. There is usually nausea, with a sensitivity to smells, creating a genuine disgust for foods.

STAPHYSAGRIA This remedy is the acute of Carcinosin and is often administered intercurrently with it. Staphysagria alleviates the immediate symptoms of worthlessness and depression created by humiliation or the perception of humiliation (deep enough for suicide to be a concern), while Carcinosin begins to unravel the deep seated abuse, fear, and perfectionist issues.

SULPHUR The keynote of Sulphur is complete loss of appetite followed by ravenous appetite. Expresses the feeling that all foods taste too salty and has an aversion to meat. Milk usually seriously disagrees. A sulphur personality is usually willing to drink liquids but eats very little solid food.

HYOSCYAMUS NIGER This remedy usually indicates a more serious behavioral disorder (or whatever else it might be prescribed for). There is a real fear of being poisoned, along with other suspicions and jealousies.

PHOSPHORICUM ACIDUM Grief with loss of appetite. The debility of the acids is manifest as great emaciation—literally pining away from grief or lost love. The passage of time, instead of bringing healing, brings instead indifference to all emotions and food—a feeling of total deadness inside.

VERATRUM ALBUM The keynote of this remedy is guilt. The anorexia of Veratrum is often driven by fasting, more and more frequently, to appease God and expiate guilt for imagined sin.

VIOLA ODORATA Inclined to weep without knowing why. Childish behavior, being too stubborn to eat just because an issue has been made of it. This type of anorexia is usually not serious and is gotten through quite easily.

BULIMIA

Known also as binge-purge syndrome, bulimia is characterized by an abnormal, constant craving for food and eating binges. The binges are followed by self-induced vomiting and/or laxative use. With bulimia, the list of remedies that have been used successfully narrows dramatically, although there are many other remedies that may fit certain people and certain scenarios.

ARGENTUM NITRICUM The binge eating centers around chocolate or salty foods. The person will eat and eat chocolate long after they know they are getting sick from it. The purge is not so much a deliberate thing at the end of the binge as it is just the natural result of such an overwhelming eating session.

CARCINOSIN Keynote is the need to do everything to absolute perfection. The eating disorder seems to be driven by the need to be the perfect size and weight and to look just right, coupled with insecurity and fear of rejection.

PHOSPHORUS Complete loss of appetite alternating with binge eating and then attempts to purge by vomiting or by the use of laxatives. There is a great deal of fear running all through the mental and emotional symptoms of phosphorus. Very sensitive people in every way.

CINA MARITIMA Characteristic wanting everything but then dissatisfied or mad at themselves for eating it. A keynote of Cina is habitual chewing on the hair, fingernails, lips, or some other part of the body. Children display extreme naughtiness, including kicking and biting. Teens and women become indifferent to touch and caresses. This is a remedy for worms and the possibility of that sort of thing should be considered.

Both of these eating disorders, anorexia and bulimia, appear to be anger/self-hate issues. They are sometimes, but certainly not always, tied to abuse. When they are the result of abuse, the feeling seems to be that since it would be wrong to hate the person who abused them (because it is a parent or sibling or they have been taught that hating others is bad), they turn the hatred inward on themselves. Low self-esteem and dissatisfaction with their physical attributes and appearance, for whatever reason, is a contributing factor.

PICA

Pica is an eating disorder characterized by an appetite for substances that are largely non-nutritive. Common substances eaten are metal, clay, coal, soil, feces, chalk, paper, soap, hair, wool, urine, wood ash, and gum. Pica can also be an abnormal appetite for some things that are considered foods when not eaten to excess—flour, raw rice, starch, noodles, ice cubes, and salt, to name just a few. Of course, the consumption of everything they can get their little hands on by crawling babies is not an indication of pica.

Suspected causes are many and varied. Causes include: mineral deficiencies—with iron being the most common, parental separation or neglect, child abuse, disorganized family structure, and poor parent-child interaction. Parasite infestation of the colon is often seen with pica. The question is, "Was the pica caused by a nutritional deficiency set up by the parasite infestation, or did the parasites gain a foothold or be introduced to the body because of the ingestion of indigestible things?"

Constipation, chronic abdominal pain, nausea, vomiting, and loss of appetite for normal foods are some of the physical symptoms and results of pica.

ANTIMONIUM CRUDUM Characterized by cravings for nothing but raw food and vegetables. This almost sounds good except for there is bloating of the abdomen and other signs of inability to digest what is being eaten and a tendency to put on weight from this diet. Eventually there will be a craving for acids, pickles, and bread. The person becomes peevish, irritable, and cannot bear to be touched or even looked at.

ALUMEN CRUDUM This remedy is usually suited best to thin, delicate children who are exhausted physically and mentally. Averse to potatoes, they crave other starches, chalk, charcoal, cloves, coffee or tea grounds, raw rice, and acidic foods. This remedy is a polycrest antidote for lead poisoning, which is frequently a complication of pica. Emotionally, the symptom picture of Alumen is of a mild, cheerful disposition.

CALCAREA CARBONICA The cravings are for chalk, charcoal, coal, and pencils (also crave eggs, which is good). The person is usually pale, weak, tires easily, fearful, shy, and is very susceptible to cold. There is also a marked restlessness and a need to wander about.

CALCAREA PHOSPHORICA Desires lime, slate, pencils, earth, chalk, clay, and other things. Usually the child was slow in learning to walk and had digestive problems that included colicky pains and a distended abdomen. Symptoms are aggravated by damp, cold weather. Picture also includes restlessness.

CICUTA VIROSA Abnormal appetite for chalk, charcoal, coal, and—interestingly—cabbage, which is really enjoyed. Unusual keynotes include grinding of the teeth and a tendency toward convulsions in which the body bends backwards.

IGNATIA AMARA Characterized by great grief and cravings for acidic fruits, sour things, raw or indigestible things, cheese, bread, sweets, and chocolate. Food must be eaten cold because warm food causes indigestion. Deep sadness with continual sighing are keynotes of Ignatia.

NATRUM MURIATICUM Keynotes are a craving for salt and an aversion to bread and anything fatty. Usually poorly nourished and emaciated, even when eating fairly well. The skin of the face has an oily feel.

NITRICUM ACIDUM Desires lime, slate, pencils, papers, charcoal, fats, and salt. There will be cracks at the corners of the mouth and fissures at the anus with strong smelling urine and frequent diarrhea. Emotionally head-strong, irritable, vindictive, and fearful with a great sensitivity to noise and light.

NUX VOMICA Cravings for charcoal, chalk, fats, spicy foods, and pepper. Usually the person is thin and chilly with a nervous disposition that includes great sensitivity to noise, odors, lights, and music. The person needing this remedy is characteristically quick, active, impatient, irritable, spiteful, and even violent.

SILICA TERRA Cravings are for lime, sand, and raw foods. Extremely chilly and all symptoms are made worse by cold except for stomach complaints which are made better by cold. Glandular disturbances and a tendency to sweat profusely, especially on the feet. Children were usually slow in learning to walk and complain of weak ankles into adulthood. Emotionally obstinate, irritable, and headstrong, there is also nervousness, apprehension, and over-sensitivity to criticism. They often cry when spoken kindly to.

GRIEF ISSUES

Please note that many of the same remedies listed for anxiety and panic and for eating disorders are the same ones we will be listing here for grief. Grief, in one form or another, seems to be a factor in many negative behavior patterns. The following is a list of remedies that are useful for various stages of grief and the various ways in which people become stuck in one stage or another of the grieving process.

IGNATIA AMARA Used when the grief or disappointment is still fresh. This does not necessarily mean that whatever it was happened yesterday in the literal sense (although it is of the most benefit right at the time of the grief). This remedy is especially effective when the grief, disappointment, or fear is still as present and as painful to the person as it was when it first occurred.

NATRUM MURIATICUM People who have never been the same since (NSS) a grief or a series of griefs and disappointments. An "Eeyore" quality to the grief—it's not so bad but will probably never be any better.

PHOSPHORICUM ACIDUM In whatever combination an acid is contained, there will be an association with extreme physical fatigue and flat, listless emotions—feeling dead inside. The person seems more collapsed than grieving and is often slow to answer when spoken to. Serious illness or hopeless situations can also produce these feelings and will often respond well to this treatment.

CAUSTICUM This remedy has been found to be very effective against grief that has been buried. There has been a wall built up to protect against similar circumstances and the risk of similar grief in the future. Unresolved emotional wounds caused by loss are still holding the person in their grip.

CARCINOSIN is discussed in detail in the section on miasms and nosodes. Note that this remedy is used for people who suppress emotions, usually either grief or guilt. As a result the buried emotions are, quite literally, eating at them and producing the pathologies associated with Carcinosin.

NATRUM SULPHURICUM The grief of Natrum sulphuricum is usually tied to unsuccessful relationships. May also follow a head injury from which the person has never been the same since.

PULSATILLA NIGRICANS Pulsatilla is for warm, caring people that are very sensitive emotionally. Their giving nature sets them up in relationships where they feel resentful because they are constantly giving and giving but often feel disappointed in the emotional response of those closest to them. Typically, they suppress these disappointments for long periods of time, so there is a pattern of buildup of repetitive small griefs rather than one big thing that causes their deep resentment.

Pulsatilla people often blame other people for not listening to them or caring about what they said when, in reality, they prefer to keep their resentment inside, rather than speak up and possibly provoke an argument. Unfortunately, the resentment which they do not speak festers. They often think they have expressed themselves clearly when, in reality, they have not. Pulsatilla nigricans promotes the release of this toxic buildup, puts things in perspective, and allows the person to relate to others more openly and without the resentment and disappointment characteristic of this remedy. They often act as though the other person in their close relationships is more important than they are.

STAPHYSAGRIA (See notes on violence disorders.) Staphysagria has a history of suppression, usually of anger, insults, and humiliation. There are usually physical ailments that have already manifested from the suppression of multiple small griefs over the years. Check closely to see if the person matches the overall symptom picture of Staphysagria; if so, this can be a wonderful remedy to help them process the anger and grief. It will also have an impact on their physical issues if followed up on.

SUICIDAL DEPRESSION

Suicidal depression is sometimes another self-hate issue—again often tied to abuse. For one reason or another, hatred has turned inward on themselves. Depression this deep can also be a nutritional or chemical imbalance, or the certainty that another way out of a situation is not feasible. Of course, there is always another option, but sometimes perception becomes narrow and desperate, and courage and resilience become lost for a time.

AURUM METALLICUM The picture of Aurum metallicum depression is a very specific and particular one. This remedy is for people who set very high standards for themselves and feel that they have failed to meet them. There is always a fear of failure in people needing Aurum. Consider this remedy for depression brought on by business reversals, a lower grade than usual on a report card, or not the expected A grade. Consider Aurum also for someone who has lost or fallen from a perceived social position. *miasm: syphilis.*

This type of suicidal intent or talk is not a cry for attention; suicide is seen as the only way to gain relief from the pain they feel as the result of their perceived failure! The person is often experiencing chronic insomnia. Aurum metallicum is not a cure-all for depression. It is essential that the basic Aurum symptoms be present in other aspects of the person's life. *miasm: syphilis.*

NATRUM SULPHURICUM All Natrum remedies share a tendency for depression, but Natrum sulphuricum is famous for suicidal thoughts that have resulted from or follow a head injury. Another cause of this type of depression is grief from an unsuccessful or failed relationship or the death of a spouse.

The desire for suicide can be very strong, but the Natrum sulphuricum person will usually not follow through on the thought because of his concern about the effect his death would have on his family (no one is capable of doing his job or things would fall apart without him). Even though they are in misery, Natrum sulphuricum people usually do not take the remedy as prescribed, even when the first dose or two makes them feel considerably better. *miasm: sycosis.*

NATRUM MURIATICUM is very similar to Natrum sulphuricum. The depression often comes after grief from divorce or the death of a loved one. People who will benefit from Natrum muriaticum may contemplate suicide. More often, however, they will hold grudges and dwell on past unhappy memories. They cannot cry in front of others and do not like to be consoled. They are quite likely to develop a chronic physical problem as a result of their grief. Compare: Causticum and Phosphoricum acidum. *miasm: Alzheimer's.*

CAPSICUM ANNUUM This remedy is for people who have deep depression with nostalgia for another time or place. For homesickness that becomes suicidal depression. The person wants to be left alone and is peevish, irritable, and easily offended. Capsicum people have a tendency for weight gain and usually crave stimulants and peppers. *miasm: malaria.*

ANACARDIUM ORIENTALE Anacardium always has an undercurrent of feeling humiliated. Feelings of estrangement from society or family can lead to deep depression. Anacardium people have two sides to their personalities—one side compliant and wishing to please others, the other side seeking power and authority over others. It is this conflict—not approving of either part of themselves—that creates the suicidal tendencies. *miasms: cancer, leprosy, AIDS, Alzheimer's—all rather deep and desperate.*

ARSENICUM ALBUM This remedy is for anxiety about things that cannot be controlled. There is an overwhelming sense of vulnerability and depression, even to the point of suicide, because of fears concerning health and material security. Arsenicum album is marked by compulsiveness, fastidiousness, need for control, obsession with planning, and sometimes avarice. *miasms: psora, vaccinosis, Alzheimer's.*

KALI BROMATUM Keynote of all Kalis is duty, keynote of Bromatums is guilt. Hence, overwhelming feelings of guilt about failure to do their duty. The person feels that he will never, ever achieve salvation, so may as well end it all now. You should look for restlessness with fidgety fingers and frequent wringing of their hands. The person usually experiences terrifying dreams at night. *miasm: Alzheimer's.*

MERCURIUS SOLUBILIS As the Mercurius personality becomes more and more out of balance energetically, suicidal impulses are sometimes seen. Use a remedy guide or other discussions in this text to refresh your memory about the Mercurius solubilis picture (jab, poke, kick, etc.). *miasms: syphilis, vaccinosis.*

LACHESIS MUTA Many of the major polycrest remedies have dual natures—an ***active, upbeat side and a passive, insecure side.*** Most of the time we see the characteristic intensity, passion, jealousy, and verbosity of this remedy. The insecure side can manifest extreme anxiety, addictive behaviors with feelings of guilt, and deep depression, even to the point of suicide. *miasms: psora, vaccinosis.*

ZINCUM METALLICUM Most often used in people with over-excited nervous systems that are manifested by great restlessness, twitches, and constant mental activity. The over-stimulated state is followed by dullness, depression, and occasionally, suicidal thoughts. There are keynotes of irritable disposition, constant complaining, and feeling that nothing in their life is any good at all. *miasms: psora, Alzheimer's*. Interesting since psora and Alzheimer's are opposite ends of the desperation spectrum as well as, typically, opposite ends of the life cycle—in an energetic sense if not in life. Many symptom pictures and ailments begin gently but spin downward into ever-increasing desperation.

SELF-MUTILATION

Whenever we see people who harm themselves in ways such as cutting themselves, burning themselves, or biting themselves, we turn to a very short list of remedies used in a deep regimen to correct this problem. Start at the 1M level and continue treatment clear through the 50M, with possible follow-up regimens every year or so if the need arises.

Behaviors such as body piercing, nail biting, constant picking of scabs, and multiple tattoos can, sometimes, be early warning signals of this problem. Self-destructive behaviors of this type can signal the early stages of a depression deep enough to become suicidal. Be sure other aspects of the symptom picture of the remedy you choose fits before prescribing at the higher potencies. The person is already on an emotional roller coaster ride and doesn't need a hastily chosen remedy to make them feel even worse.

SYPHILINUM This remedy is the nosode for the syphilis miasm which is, as you know by now, one of the most desperate and destructive of the miasms. Both the Syphilinum remedy and the syphilis miasm are marked by hopelessness with despair of recovery. This despair may not be expressed directly—most likely it will be expressed in a jocular manner. Responses to offers to help may be met with such statements as, "You are not qualified in that department," meaning, usually, psychiatric help—their way of indicating that they are broken beyond repairing.

HYOSCYAMUS NIGER The Hyoscyamus picture includes the desire to strike, bite, fight, insult, scold, and even kill. This pattern is seen in teens and even in children and can worsen into actions taken against themselves as they age. Under certain conditions of despair or self-anger, these impulses do turn inward.

ARSENICUM ALBUM The Arsenicum picture is one of extreme nervousness and anxiety with fear of death, fear of disease, and fear of being left alone being a large part of the things they are anxious about. There is sometimes a desire to commit suicide to avoid current or future suffering. In milder forms the self-mutilation may take the form of extreme nail biting, piercings, or tattoos.

STAPHYSAGRIA The Staphysagria pattern is one of very low self-esteem and feelings of utter worthlessness. This remedy is for persons who are easily offended and take insults entirely to heart and have great difficulty letting go of them. They have a perception of being humiliated or sad—often based on incidents in the past, but just as likely to be misperceptions they have formed based on very little, and quite different from actual reality. Staphysagria people are often overly nice, hiding their anger and then hating themselves for not having defended themselves. It is this anger at self that results in self-abuse. There is also an undercurrent of trying to make the people whom they feel are humiliating them understand how badly they are hurting as the result of the insults they feel they are suffering.

TUBERCULINUM BOVINUM Part of the Tuberculinum picture is deep feelings of being unfulfilled by life as they are currently living it. This dissatisfaction manifests as restlessness and destructiveness. Contradictory behavior and changing moods are also keynotes of this remedy as well as violent outbursts of temper. When in a temper, a Tuberculinum person will pick fights or throw things. It isn't often that the destructiveness turns on oneself, but if the tuberculosis miasm seems to fit, this is the remedy to reach for.

Since you will probably be working with high potency remedies, be sure that you refer to a homeopathic repertory to help you sort the symptom pictures until you are sure that you have chosen the correct one. Pay particular attention to the mental/emotional and better for/worse for symptoms.

The depression may have been triggered by many things and part of the picture for many depressed people, especially suffering from the Tuberculinum pattern, is to do their best to hide it from those around them. Bad things, hidden, usually refuse to stay out of sight. The desire to have everything in their lives appear to be perfect can create sufficient stress that may manifest in some other way such as anorexia, bulimia, temper tantrums, self-mutilation, maliciousness, and foul language. Bad behavior is bad behavior and needs to be contained and changed, but sometimes it helps to know what the bad behavior is trying to communicate to the outside world.

VIOLENCE DISORDER (AND POST-TRAUMATIC STRESS)

The experience of violence against oneself, the witnessing of violence, and the constant exposure to violence in the media and movies, can create feelings *of fear and a deep sense of vulnerability* to personal danger, especially in children. Deep and continual inner fear often becomes rage. In adults, the anger may be controlled and kept within acceptable bounds, but a child may lack sufficient self-control and act out his fear and anger. Below is a list of the more common remedies and some of their indications for dealing with PTSD and other violence disorders.

STRAMONIUM This is the first remedy considered when violence and extreme fear of violence are seen in a child. Stramonium children act out violently *to keep the perceived and feared threat at a distance.* Their attitude is one of, "I'll be so mean and tough that no one will ever dare mess with me." The extreme inner terror can lead to wild rages, and even homicidal impulses. The rage is impulsive (an outburst), and not the cold, planned variety. There is usually an extreme fear of the dark, of being alone, of violence, or of death which accompanies these tendencies. Stuttering, stammering, epilepsy, attention deficit disorders, and sleep disorders are common symptoms. Often, there is clustering together into gangs.

TUBERCULINUM BOVINUM The fear of violence runs through this remedy. Differs from Stramonium in that the child is coldly and deliberately destructive and malicious. There is indifference to punishment, except that the child will later break a favorite object of his parent's as retribution for any punishment or any other happening that he/she disliked. (See ADHD and Learning Disabilities section, next.)

MEDORRHINUM (Described in ADHD/Learning Disabilities section beginning on the next page) Medorrhinum children are sometimes aggressive—kicking and striking parents or other children, but this remedy is one of many contradictions. Sometimes Medorrhinum children are pale, almost sickly and appear sensitive and withdrawn when they are not in a violent and aggressive mode. There is often exce,ssive attachment to animals, with the inner rage erupting into violence toward their well-loved pets.

HYOSCYAMUS NIGER (More details in ADHD section.) These children live with fear—real or perceived. What is perceived is reality to all of us, and what they perceive is what they will act upon. As children they will probably lack the self-control not to act on the impulses to strike, hit, kick or poke that are part of this picture.

ANACARDIUM ORIENTALE (Also in ADHD/Learning Disabilities section, next.) Keynote: split personality. Two contradictory natures—one wishing to please, the other obstinate and disobedient.

TARENTULA HISPANICA (also in ADHD/Learning Disabilities section.) Keynote is hurry, hurry, hurry, and deep annoyance at the slower pace of others. They are always wound up tight.

Every remedy listed above is also listed for ADHD and hyperactivity
Does this tell us something about the role of fear and anxiety in any negative behavior patterns of children?

STAPHYSAGRIA: *Keynote here is a history of humiliation (real or perceived) and suppression of anger. Children are sweet and gentle most of the time, suppressing anger until it boils over.* The anger is expressed by throwing things or hitting someone. Staphysagria people suffer from low self-esteem and, often, depression. One useful keynote that helps distinguish this remedy from the others is the tendency to be sleepy in the day, but sleepless at night.

CAUSTICUM A person needing this remedy exhibits great emotional sensitivity and tends to build protective walls around their heart. May have great anger towards perceived injustice or the abuse of authority by others. Resent any turn-the-other-cheek teachings. Grief issues have been scarred over. With Causticum, there is usually the need for another remedy also. Extreme adult Causticum cases are anarchists.

LEARNING DISABILITIES

A whole book could be written on the subject of learning disabilities and ADHD syndrome. I am reasonably certain that there are very few of us who have not known or had occasion to work with a child or adult who has struggles with one educational/learning skill or another and/or has trouble being still in school-type situations. In addition, most of us seem to have stress issues left over from our own school days.

Many times little boys—who probably ought to be out-of-doors with Daddy for a least a few more years before being stuffed into a school desk—seem to be the hardest hit by learning disabilities of any type. They are also the most likely to have their futures negatively impacted by mind-altering prescription drugs.

Dana Ullman, who is probably America's best known homeopath, says, "It deeply saddens me that so many parents and doctors give powerful drugs to infants and children. They unknowingly are committing what I *call medical child abuse.* Homeopathic medicines provide a viable alternative to the powerful conventional drugs of our day, and I sincerely hope that parents and doctors learn about them soon. Although these may be harsh words today, I believe that history will show them to be accurate."

I can only agree. Statistics and research are, more and more, supporting these conclusions.

Children who have been labeled as *learning disabled* often hear (and their parents are told) something similar to one or more of the following statements—and, too often, these statements are made with the child listening and taking it all to heart.

"He has the ability, if he just tried harder, he could do it. He chooses not to do the work."
"If she would just pay attention like the other children, she would get it."
"He sits there and stares at his paper. He is just not motivated." (Or say that he is lazy.)
"He is completely out of control/undisciplined, etc.. He obviously needs medication."

WHAT IS A LEARNING DISABILITY?

If you are the parent of a child who has been diagnosed with a learning disability you have probably heard a great many explanations and definitions. In short, learning disabled means that there is some type of difficulty in processing sensory information. **You are not learning disabled just because your mind (and energy system) sees, hears, and understand things differently from most people.** That last sentence is my personal bias and not what you will hear from a school counselor, social worker, or prescriber of medications.

Let's use the analogy of a telephone system to define real learning disabilities. Faulty wiring with static on the line disrupts normal functioning. The phone company responds by rewiring the connections and then protecting the new connections from further damage in the future. Under the right educational conditions, and with the help of herbal medicines, homeopathic remedies, essential oils, and nutritional therapies, the brain also has the ability to rewire itself—to form new neural connections. This is done when there has been serious brain injury, and it can be done for children who struggle with basic learning tasks. These new connections, or the clearing of static along the old connections, make skills like reading and writing easier, and even enjoyable, for many children.

TO PARENTS

Whether or not your child has a learning disability, the fact is that the way you behave and what you do will have a huge impact on your child. Everyone faces obstacles and difficulties. As a parent, you can help your child learn how to deal with obstacles and come out victorious. A good attitude won't immediately solve a problem with some phase of education, but it can give your child enough confidence to avoid becoming discouraged and feeling sure that he is broken and not worth fixing!

A FEW SUGGESTIONS FOR YOU, AS A PARENT:

Keep things in perspective. All people learn differently, and some of us just do not learn best in the left-brained format of America's school system. Your most important job is to keep your child's self-esteem intact. Challenges are meant to be overcome. Don't get distracted from your most important job of providing your child with emotional, moral, and educational support.

Do your own homework. You may, out of fear or instinct, look to others for solutions at first if your child is struggling but, ultimately, you need to take charge when it comes to finding the tools your child needs to succeed.

Remember that your influence on your child outweighs that of all others. If you approach his learning challenges with optimism, hard work, a sense of humor, and no embarrassment or apology to your friends, he will likely pick up on your attitude. He will come to view the situation as an obstacle and not a roadblock. Trying to change the school or his teachers is usually futile. Focus on finding solutions and what works for your child, and implement it the best you can. Allowing other people (teachers and school officials) to be imperfect underscores your message that imperfection is a challenge and not a terminal illness.

Give your child many chances for success in other areas. This cannot be overemphasized. Even though they may require extra time for school work, make time for them to work at, and succeed, in other areas. They need to grow up knowing that while so-and-so is better than they are at math or reading, they are particularly good at art, throwing a ball, tending their baby sister, or being depended on. This is very important!

SOCIAL AND EMOTIONAL DIFFICULTIES

Social and emotional difficulties are an area where you, as a parent, can make a huge difference. Challenges with learning may lead to low self-esteem, anger, withdrawal, and other behavioral problems. In fact, *social and emotional skills are the most consistent indicator of overall success in school and in life.* Confidence and emotional stability outweigh, many times over, all academic factors. Give your child a strong support system. Help him learn to express himself appropriately and deal with frustration properly. Your focus on his growth as a person will help him develop the right tools for lifelong success.

HOMEOPATHIC REMEDIES AND LEARNING DISABILITIES

Can a homeopathic remedy really affect a learning disability? This has certainly been my experience time after time. Of course, I am also using essential oils (the Butterfly Express blend, ^{Le}Millenia, being the most important) along with better nutritional habits and allergy work, using energy modalities. I know that when the appropriate homeopathic remedy begins to smooth out dysfunctional energy patterns, true healing begins. This healing often changes the way sensory input is perceived, and when that has been accomplished, the work of rewiring the neural pathways in the brain proceeds very quickly.

I suppose that nearly all homeopathic remedies are potential remedies for ADHD, hyperactivity, autism, or any learning disability. These learning disabilities often match quite closely the description of one miasm or another. It is my personal belief that we could put a great many learning disabilities under the label "vaccinosis" or "drug" or "environmental pollution" miasms and be quite accurate. The fact that there are so many more children suffering from learning disabilities needs some serious explaining. Let's try to deal with causes, instead of effects, whenever we can.

It is something to think about that every remedy listed for PTSD is also listed for ADHD and hyperactivity.

As always, when using homeopathy, the procedure is to match the symptoms—and **not just the ones pertaining to learning**—to a remedy and start with that remedy. There are a few remedies whose symptom pictures include problems with the processing of sensory information. I will list them, along with a few key symptoms, to get you started on your task of sorting through them.

Remember as you go along, that the symptoms will change. The remedy you give next month will need to change to fit the new picture. Do not become discouraged. This is progress—real and measurable progress—even though, sometimes, it looks for a time like things are getting worse.

LABELS

I really hate labels, especially when applied to children. And the descriptions of the various learning disabilities tend to make me very angry. I am going to give you just one example. Here are some of the official symptoms of Asperger's Syndrome. (I have been working with children and their parents for quite a few years—and I had children of my own with various learning styles—and I had never heard of this one until recently. Now I get at least two calls a week from distraught mothers. What is going on here?)

I will be quoting directly from WebMD and the Autism Spectrum Disorders Health Center for the next few paragraphs. Indented paragraphs are direct quotes from this site. Italics are comments I simply couldn't resist making. If you are the parent of a child who has been diagnosed with Asperger's syndrome, I assure you I do not mean offend—only to encourage you to think about which of your child's behaviors are a real concern and which are not.

Although there are many possible symptoms of Asperger's syndrome, the main symptom is trouble with social situations. Your child may have mild to severe symptoms or have a few or many of these symptoms. Because of the wide variety of symptoms, no two children with Asperger's are alike. *(I should hope not, since no two children anywhere are alike!)*

Parents often first notice the symptoms of Asperger's syndrome when their child starts **preschool** and begins to interact with other children. Children with Asperger's syndrome may:

Not pick up on social cues, such as being able to read others' body language, cannot start or maintain a conversation, or take turns talking. *(Remember, we are talking about preschoolers, here!)*

Dislike any changes in routines. *(Sounds like a normal preschooler to me.)*

Appears to lack empathy. *(I think they mean that this child has not learned a very adult skill yet.)*

Your child may not understand a joke or may take a sarcastic comment literally. *(Again, please remember that we are talking about a preschooler here.)*

Have a formal style of speaking that is advanced for his or her age. For example, the child may use the word "beckon" instead of "call" or the word "return" instead of "come back." *(When my mother was a parent, having a child behave in this way was an indication that the parent was spending some time with the child and not talking down to them while they were doing it. It was considered a good thing—a mark of both the child's intelligence and the parent's good parenting.)*

Have unusual facial expressions or postures. *(Imagine that! A preschooler pulling faces and pretending to be something he is not, like a dinosaur, maybe.)*

Talks a lot, usually about a favorite subject. One-sided conversations are common. Internal thoughts are often verbalized. *(I thought one-sided conversations were part of immaturity, another word for childhood, and I would have given quite a bit to get my children to verbalize their internal thoughts in any manner!)*

Have delayed motor development. Your child may be late in learning to use a fork or spoon, ride a bike, or catch a ball. He or she may have an awkward walk. Handwriting is often poor. *(This is the only set of symptoms that make any sense at all to me. And even then, what would be in the best interest of the child? Take him to a specialist, label him as broken, point out his problems—often to everyone who will listen—and make sure he knows he is broken and a problem, or to work with him as a loving parent and maximize his abilities in every way possible?)*

Please do not misunderstand. I believe that learning disabilities and behavioral disorders are real and that children often struggle with learning and the school environment. I raised seven children, and at this moment, have 30 grandchildren. Many of them could have (and would have been, if it had been allowed) labeled with one learning disability or another.

What I question is how much that is labeled *learning disabilities* is childhood stuffed into a classroom, differences in learning and personality styles, reactions to some type of chemical toxicity, allergies, or development at different rates. After all, in the typical first grade classroom there are kids nearly a year apart in age. This matters in childhood. If a slower developer is also one of the youngest in his group, or if his learning style is differentfrom that valued in the classroom, he will likely be having problems of one sort or another. Is it in his best interest to label him *learning disabled*?

I know, very dearly and personally, a young man who would have fit into several learning disability categories as a child. He did OK in his home school, but he certainly learned in his own obsessional way (one subject at a time, mostly). He served a mission for the Mormon church, and was a couple of years into college when he called his mother because his roommates thought he might have ADHD and he wanted to know what she thought. His mother asked him where he was, usually, when doing his math as a child. He responded that he was most often to be found upside down, spinning in circles, in the big family rocking chair while doing the math in his head. They concluded together that maybe this was as good a definition of ADHD as they had ever heard, but wondered what difference the definition really made.

My question is, "Would it have helped him to know that he had ADHD and couldn't possibly be expected to sit still, behave, pay attention, and get his school work done?" This young man completed his master's degree, with high honors, and is in the final weeks of his doctoral program. I think it is quite fortunate that he avoided drugs and his professors didn't know that he was one of the "broken children" when they were evaluating him for awards and programs.

HOMEOPATHIC REMEDIES
FOR ADHD, LEARNING AND BEHAVIOR DISORDERS

At the beginning of this section on behavioral disorders, it was stressed that homeopathic remedies are not magic pills. They do not make a problem simply disappear. Children, especially, will need considerable help from mom and dad to make changes in their behavior. Homeopathic remedies remove inherited or acquired energy malfunctions that are contributing to the problem. They do not immediately alter *learned* behavior patterns, bad manners, selfishness, or being allowed to get away with things. Sometimes it is tricky to tell what is what—whether, as a parent, you should apply patience or discipline in each particular instance of misbehavior. If you recognize your child in one of the following descriptions, the homeopathic remedy will likely be an aid to you in your search for answers but it will certainly not absolve you of all further responsibility.

Many homeopathic medicines are potential remedies for both hyperactivity and learning disabilities. *I have recently been studying butterfly remedies and their use with learning problems and ADHD. I think they will be an amazing addition to protocols for children who are struggling.*

In my limited experience, but wide range of study of butterfly remedies, I have concluded (at the moment) that these remedies probably belong predominantly in the *sycosis miasm with psora underpinnings*. They must because butterflies are creatures of the sky and because one of their main themes is transformation, they must be strong remedies for all aspects of the *AIDS miasm.*

One small study of 43 children with ADHD observed that Stramonium was the most prescribed remedy—35% of the cases fit the Stramonium pattern. Cina maritima and Hyoscyamus niger were each given in 19% of the cases, Tarentula hispanica and Veratrum album were also used. It would be very educational to stop for a moment and note the wide variety of very different symptoms described by these 3 remedies.

When you are working homeopathically, the symptoms you should give the most attention to are those that are different from the *normal* pattern of the problem. The pattern of the ailment needs to be there, but it is the things that are unique to that individual that determine your choice.

Homeopathic remedies function as a catalyst to send the body's own inner healing mechanisms and resources into action to correct imbalances. If the homeopathic being taken is not necessary, then nothing much happens! If not used excessively, there are no harmful side effects to worry about such as are encountered with most prescription drugs.

STRAMONIUM With stramonium, the mind is very active and the speech is rapid, usually with a lot of gesturing. There is often great anger (rage) and violent behavior (see Violence Disorder information given previously). The violence is the result of fear and they will explain it with phrases such as, "They started it," or "They were about to hit me," or even, "They were looking at me funny." It is as if they must keep threats away by striking first or being so mean and tough that no one dares mess with them. The anger, and most other actions, are impulsive. There is not usually a pattern of vindictive revenge or cool planning, just an uncontrolled impulse of the moment. Clustering together into gangs or clubs with other children (for the feeling of protection) is common.

HYOSCYMUS NIGER This is one of the most important remedies in childhood behavioral problems. These children may be clinging to a parent one moment and doing silly annoying things the next moment. **There is poor control over impulses.** The child wants it now and may throw a tantrum if he doesn't get his way. There may be violence toward other children, and eventually towards the parent of the opposite sex. In most cases there is an early sexual awareness and precocious behavior. There may also be cursing or lewd talk.

If Hyoscyamus seems to be indicated this might be one of the few times you would consider giving the 50M remedy more than once. Indication for this would be good progress during the regimen but some returning problems 5 or 6 months after the 50M remedy was given. The 50M may be given 3-4 times at 6 month intervals, if needed. During the intervening months it may be necessary for someone to **help the child develop new habits. Some of the negative behaviors have become just that, habits,** and are no longer part of the underlying emotional or mental problem. These behaviors **need to be dealt with as simple bad behavior.**

CINA MARITIMA A keynote of Cina is habitual chewing on the hair, fingernails, lips, or some other part of the body. Children display extreme naughtiness, including kicking and biting. Want to be carried, held, or rocked, but are not comforted by these actions or anything else. Teens and women become indifferent or annoyed by touches or caresses. There is often a history of periodic bed-wetting, more often at the time of the full moon. Cina is considered a remedy for parasites and I have often wondered how much a part parasites play in behavior and learning difficulties.

TARENTULA HISPANICA There is a piece of dance music called The TarantelLa, meaning the Tarantula, that is descriptive of this remedy. Tarentula types have a tremendous love of music and dancing. This remedy is indicated when there is over-stimulation of the nervous system. The outstanding characteristic of this remedy is hurry—it is the most hurried of the remedies—and in children this translates, of course, to hyperactivity. The child simply cannot stand to be sitting still and is even annoyed, almost unbearably, by the slowness of those around him. In a few cases there may be cunning and deceit or a destructive desire to break things or tear them up. This is, after all, a spider remedy and may fit that part of the spider picture very clearly.

VERATRUM ALBUM This remedy is a little different in that the very young child is often very well behaved. The pathology of this remedy in children begins with **excessive, early mental development.** The child is curious and almost adult-like in ability to understand abstract concepts. This over-stimulation of the mental faculties eventually seems to lead to frustration which manifests as restlessness, disobedience and behavior problems. The doing of meaningless, repetitive tasks such as cutting paper into smaller and smaller bits is often seen. A keynote symptom of this remedy is a **detachment when punished or reprimanded**—the child shows no emotion or turns away. You will know what I mean by this if you have ever seen it. The child's eyes just get a vacant look and they look away from you. This is a very important signal that you may be dealing with something more than just a very intelligent child. Use of this remedy may prevent problems later on. In adults there is a manifestation of religious mania, the beginnings of which can be glimpsed in the child.

ARSENICUM IODATUM This is another frequently used remedy for hyperactive children. In these cases the child simply tears apart a room, not from maliciousness, but rather from restlessness and constant motion. This is generally considered a hot remedy. The *Iodine in the remedy is indicated by the tendency to be on the move* and by the fact that the person feels better for being allowed to get out and run.

ARSENICUM ALBUM There is extreme anxiety; the child is usually clinging to mother's hand. The child is constantly changing position, wanting to move from desk to desk and even teacher to teacher and room to room. A *keynote* is that the child is continually climbing on things, usually from a very young age. These children have active imaginations and are quite fragile emotionally, with over sensitivity to disorder and confusion. They experience difficulty concentrating, especially when tired, are inclined to selfishness, and their desires greatly exceed reasonable needs. Lycopodium personalities frequently have difficulties with milk, wheat, and sugar. Ice cream is often a particular problem for them with its combination of milk and sugar. Symptoms often disappear when these foods are eliminated or allergy work (using alternative therapies) has been done. *Using this remedy (or any other remedy) throughout early childhood for flu and digestive disorders, whenever indicated, may prevent this pattern from developing as the child reaches school age*

ANACARDIUM ORIENTALE This remedy is strongly indicated for past *sexual abuse*. *The child needing this remedy shows a distinct split in their personality—two contradictory natures*. On the one hand they have feelings of inferiority, are eager to please, and are a bit timid, while at other times they can be cruel and obstinate. The opposing nature of this inner conflict makes Anacardium a leading remedy for bipolar disorders, also. This child seems to delight in cursing and swearing. There is a definite display of feelings of worthlessness and inferiority. *There are remedies among the butterflies that have this dual nature.*

LACHESIS MUTA Lachesis personalities are very creative and their minds become crowded with thoughts and ideas that need expression. Whether an adult or a child, they have overly strong emotions, particularly *feelings of jealousy*. In the child this often manifests as a *need for the spotlight*, or resentment if they are not in the spotlight. Jealousy can often be seen toward siblings, especially a new baby in the house. At school, this jealousy focuses on a student that seems to be getting extra attention from the teacher (see also Hyoscyamus niger, Anacardium orientale, Veratrum album for this characteristic). A child may be possessive of his friends and demand that they pay attention to only him (or her) and not play with other friends at all. These children are often sarcastic and aggressive, with an uncanny ability to find a vulnerable spot and strike at it.

NATRUM MURIATICUM A child who would benefit from this remedy is usually a loner, indifferent to other children, and actually seems to enjoy being alone. Quiet and melancholic with a dislike of answering questions and being made to talk and play with other children. She cries easily but wants to be left alone rather than consoled. Often there is delayed development and smallness for their age. Displays anxiety and agitation alternately with indifference. The child is usually quite adept at academic skills but reacts poorly to criticism and instructions about how to accomplish a task. Reaction to criticism is anger, followed by poor memory and muddled thought patterns. A *keynote* is anger at self when even the slightest mistake is made.

NATRUM SULPHURICUM A keynote of this remedy is mental troubles arising from head injury, or concussion from falls and blows (sounds like a playground environment to me). Other symptoms are inability to concentrate, with the symptoms getting worse from extended mental exertion. They feel a great need to defend other children if they are being picked on in any way.

TUBERCULINUM BOVINUM This is one of the principal remedies for hyperactive children. The child is unable to remain long in any one place, can be loud and obnoxious. We often think of this remedy when children are deliberately destructive to other children's or parent's things and indifferent to punishment.

MEDORRHINUM In this case the child may express violent or aggressive tendencies. He may have a strong passionate nature, with temper outbursts, or fights with other children. He may have strong attachments to animals, or alternatively, be cruel to them. He may also be sensitive and withdrawn from parents, siblings and the world in general.

LYCOPODIUM When under stress, these children experience periods of time when thoughts vanish and concentration is nearly impossible. They have difficulty with reading comprehension and difficulty expressing their thoughts in writing. School work is frustrating to them because they misplace words, use the wrong words, or spell words wrongly by omitting letters or syllables. Emotionally, Lycopodium displays a contradictory nature. The child lacks confidence so is sometimes shy, submissive, and melancholic; at other times they compensate by being dictatorial and self-righteous—demanding that everyone do everything their way all the time.

ARGENTUM NITRICUM Hurry and worry are keynotes of this remedy. These children are always in a hurry and always in a state of anxiety about upcoming tests, book reports, or projects. They are always in motion, moving impulsively and suddenly. All symptoms get worse if the room becomes too warm or they have been allowed to consume sugary treats. A keynote is creative rationalization about why they may not do well on the upcoming test, etc. These children often complain that their stomach is upset before tests or performances.

ZINCUM METALLICUM Anemia, poor nutrition, or poor assimilation of nutrients is part of the Zincum symptom picture. These children are easily startled or distracted by noise. They are often fidgety, especially their feet, and symptoms improve—for a time—if they are allowed to run about for a few moments.

SILICA TERRA Sand—gritty but not stable. Silica children are sure they have an inner weakness or inadequacy. They compensate for this by being defiant and obstinate and pushing themselves too hard. These children need others to think well of them and appreciate their abilities. They suffer extreme anxiety before tests and performances. Occasionally, the flip-side of yielding will be seen, but not often.

NUX VOMICA These children are competitive and independent. They have a desire for freedom so that they can move forward on their own agendas and personal goals (and they always have agendas and goals!). They are optimistic, sometimes unrealistically so, about their goals and feel great satisfaction at their own accomplishments. These children are always on the move, must have everything in order, and are irritable if anyone else's disorganization slows them down in the slightest degree. They are not patient, ever, and they crave stimulants. The Nux child tends to have had colic and stomach problems since birth.

Nux vomica balances and detoxifies the liver and other digestive organs and is a remedy for adrenal stress. Adrenal fatigue leads to the opposite set of symptoms which out-of-balance Nux people show as they get older—a pattern of extreme fatigue, often chronic fatigue syndrome. They have simply worn themselves out. Like the nut from which this remedy is made, Nux people have a hard outer shell but are sensitive, passionate, and compassionate on the inside, most particularly with people closest to them.

CALCAREA CARBONICA It is estimated that almost 40% of children fit the Calcarea carbonica picture at birth. As a midwife I think this is a nutritional deficiency or calcium absorption problem on the part of the mother during pregnancy. These children are slightly slower in learning to walk, have weaker bones, and often have trouble teething. They may have many cavities in their baby teeth. They can be stubborn and insistent on doing things their own way and in their own time. They really do not like to take breaks in the middle of a task and do not like changes in their daily routines. They almost always object to new ways of doing things. They have strong cravings for sugar and milk, and often have nutrient absorption problems of their own.

CHAMOMILLA VULGARIS These children are highly emotional, temperamental, irritable, and over-sensitive. They want to be held and can only be quieted when rocked. Chamomilla children are excessively irritable and are known for their tantrums. They want instant relief from pain or annoyance and are often quarrelsome with little regard for the opinions or needs of others.

BELLADONNA This is not a common remedy for learning and behavior disorders, but unique enough to be essential, nothing else will work if the symptom picture fits. **Keynotes** are fear of both real and imaginary animals, swollen glands and tonsils, sudden rages that include tearing things and destroying things, and throwing the body forwards and backwards.

CARCINOSIN The behavioral problems connected with Carcinosin have to do with the need to do everything to the absolute best of their ability. The child is enraged with himself over even the slightest mistakes and then becomes discouraged and refuses to work at all.

SULPHUR Sulphur is a remedy for the vaccinosis and Alzheimer's miasms. This tells you a lot about the symptoms of children needing this remedy. Some keynotes are that they hate to bathe, like to wear their clothes until they are disgustingly worn and dirty, think rules are made to be broken, and want to do everything themselves. They need little sleep, are careless with their possessions, and have no sense of time as far as turning in assignments or showing up where they should be on time. These children hate standing and will always be looking for a place to sit down.

HEPAR SULPHURIS CALCAREUM These children are very hurried, especially in speech, they're quarrelsome, and very dissatisfied. Nothing ever seems to please the Hepar sulph personality. This type of personality often feels that the people they should be depending on for support treat them badly, put them down, and say things just to humiliate them. In children, these feelings often translate into violence and making threats of violence towards other children. They may try to carry a knife or some such thing to school. A keynote is feeling better when the weather is cold, but feeling very much worse if the weather is wet, even wet and cold.

CHINA OFFICINALIS These children are delicate (like a beautiful china cup) and artistic with a sense of beauty and connection to spiritual realms. They often lack self-confidence and suffer from mental exhaustion. The mind of a China child is most clear at night. In fact, they often have an abundance of ideas and clearness of mind in the evening. They may stay up late at night because of an overactive mind, or because they want to get their ideas into production. These late nights contribute to the exhaustion and fuzziness that they feel the next day. The exhaustion will likely manifest as inability to concentrate, inability to arrange thoughts, reluctance to express themselves because their thoughts are muddled, and mistakes in writing. Eventually, these children display apathy, indifference, despondency, or disobedience (they simply won't do the things that they don't feel they can do well enough). China is a remedy of extreme exhaustion.

IGNATIA AMARA This homeopathic remedy is almost always associated with grief or a bad fright of some kind. Often employed for adults and children alike when there are ailments that seem to stem from grief or fear. The basis is often the death, or near death, of a parent or sibling, or the recent divorce of the child's parents. The child is grieving, but their grief is compounded by the fear that nothing and no one in their lives can be counted on to stay with them. These children are oversensitive and nervous. Their moods undergo rapid alterations and they are often quarrelsome. They are intolerant of contradiction or reprimands. A reprimand will cause them to immediately show anger, followed by the return and intensifying of their grief and sorrow. *A keynote is the volatility of emotion—laughter turns suddenly to tears.*

MERCURIUS SOLUBILIS is an extreme remedy and indicates a personality that is in fairly serious trouble. These children really dislike the school environment because they feel completely suppressed and closed in by authority. They consider any person in authority to be the enemy, but they are themselves often dictatorial with other children and with their younger siblings.

Like the mercury from which it is made, these children are as changeable as the weather. They are extremely restless and act in a hurry, without thinking things through. Sometimes, on the other hand, they have been in so much trouble with authority that, although still moving a million miles an hour *inside,* their actual movements are extremely slow and careful. They may even avoid other people and seclude themselves from social situations.

Mercurius children are often very talented and highly intelligent. It is not unusual for them to skip a grade, or be leaders among their peers. There is a deep conflict between desire for law and order and almost violent impulses to do something to upset the status quo. These patterns are considered behavioral disorders but do not usually come under the heading of ADHD.

SUMMARY

There are many remedies listed in the foregoing pages. Perhaps I should have broken the different learning disorders and behavioral difficulties of children down into more detailed groups. That would have required listing many of these remedies more than once in category after category and would, of necessity, have contained a lot of redundancy. Homeopathic treatment of emotional patterns is, as always in homeopathy, based on the symptom picture. These descriptions are brief. If one seems to fit your child, be sure to look it up in a more complete reference. *Be sure to remember the butterfly remedies as possible solutions.*

CONCLUSION—AN INTERESTING STUDY

A carefully controlled clinical trial conducted in Switzerland has shown that homeopathy does significantly improve ADHD. This study was published in the July 27, 2005, online edition of the European Journal of Pediatrics. *One interesting aspect of this study was that no other treatments or medications of any kind were allowed during the course of the study.*

The Conners Global Index rating system was used to assess the children's response to treatment. The Conners Global Index is an 11 item rating scale containing the most important ADHD symptoms. These symptoms are:

1. temper outbursts
2. excitability
3. impulsivity
4. over-activity
5. crying often
6. inattentive
7. fidgeting,
8. disturbing other children
9. easily frustrated
10. failure to finish things
11. quickly changing moods

RATING SCALE
0—never   2—often   3—very often.

As you can see, the higher the score is, the more prominent and severe the symptoms. Other assessment instruments included standardized achievement and intelligence tests.

The study was set up in three phases. In phase one, the children were given a remedy closely determined to match their symptom pictures (an example of proper homeopathic treatment). Only children showing at least 50% improvement after 6 weeks of homeopathic treatment became part of phase two of this study.

Phase two involved continuing to give half of the children the homeopathic remedy and giving the other half of the children a placebo—a double blind study. The children and their parents did not know whether or not the child was taking a homeopathic remedy or a placebo. In the middle of this phase a crossover was implemented; the groups were switched—those who had been given a placebo were put back on homeopathic treatment and the others were then given a placebo.

In phase three each child was put back on the remedy that had been specifically matched to their original symptoms.

The median Conners rating of the children at the beginning of the study was 19. Remember, the higher the number, the deeper the pathology. At the end of phase one the median rating of the children as an entire group was 8—a substantial improvement having been accomplished with every child!

Both group's ratings went up to a median range of 12 at the conclusion of their 6 weeks on the placebo. The group that had the placebo first and then returned to homeopathic treatment had a median range of 9 at the conclusion of phase two. In other words, both groups, at the conclusion of the placebo stage, had lost ground measurably but improvement was reestablished when the homeopathic regimen was begun again.

Does this mean that the children will need to take their remedies for the rest of their lives to maintain improvement? No! It means that follow-up work with higher potency, deeper acting remedies needed to be done. These children were taking very low potency remedies and taking them every day with no interruptions to allow their body's own vital force to implement the new energy patterns.

In addition, a different remedy was not given as the symptoms changed. In properly done homeopathy, the children would have been given a different remedy as some symptoms were eliminated and the over-all picture changed. Although it is one of the better tests for following *some* of the basic principles of homeopathy, these children improved *in spite* of the violation of several basic rules of homeopathy.

This was homeopathy poorly done, and still the results, especially at first when the remedies were given somewhat properly, were very impressive.

In this study, the remedies which proved most effective were Calcarea carbonica, Sulphur, Chamomilla vulgaris, Lycopodium, Silica terra, Hepar sulphuris calcareum, Nux vomica, China officinalis, Ignatia amara, and Mercurius solubilis.

Chapter Twenty-Two - Chronic Fatigue Syndrome (CFS)

Chronic fatigue syndrome has become so widespread in the United States that it qualifies as an epidemic. The cause, or causes, of chronic fatigue syndrome are still not well understood, even after years of research. The Epstein-Barr virus is often seen in people who suffer from this syndrome. However, just as many people test positive for this virus without exhibiting CFS symptoms. This has led some experts to conclude that the condition may be triggered by *any* viral attack that the body did not handle well.

Another claimed, or suspected, cause is chemical poisoning from one source or another, including dental fillings and prescription drug use. Other experts suspect an unidentified immune system dysfunction, or a defect in the mechanisms that regulate blood sugar or blood pressure. Other proposed causes include anemia, diabetes or hypoglycemia, hypothyroidism, a *Candida albicans* overgrowth, food or chemical allergies, or intestinal parasites. Fatigue in muscles or tissues is <u>always</u> the result of an overly acidic condition, and an acidic condition is perfect for the growth of virus and bacteria. Stomach and intestinal difficulties are always a part of chronic fatigue syndrome.

SYMPTOMS:

Determining if CFS Could Be What's Wrong With You
Like any true chronic condition, **chronic fatigue syndrome does not manifest the same way in every person**. It is more a matter of having a number of symptoms from a list of possible symptoms. A family history of mononucleosis or hepatitis is considered an indicator of exposure to whatever is the cause. A family history of other infectious diseases, multiple allergies, asthma, and certain cancers may indicate an underlying immunological predisposition. Recurring sore throats and/or swollen glands, frequent colds or other infections, and various hormonal imbalances are also considered pre-indicators.

Dietary habits are extremely important to recovery, as is the need to eliminate as many chemical poisons as possible (alcohol, tobacco, recreational drugs). "Current medications, or medications taken in the past, may also be significant. For example, prolonged and multiple antibiotic use, steroids, birth control pills, chemotherapy (just about any drug, really) can have a suppressive effect on the immune system." <u>Chronic Fatigue Syndrome, The Hidden Epidemic</u>, Jesse A. Stoff, M.D. and Charles R. Pellegrino, Ph.D.

Symptoms include abdominal bloating, migratory aching muscles and joints with increasing stiffness and loss of motion, marked irritability or personality changes, anxiety, depression, difficulty concentrating, a significant loss of stamina an hour or so after meals, cravings for sugar or caffeine, sudden episodes of dizziness, rapid onset of fatigue at odd times, fever, headaches, digestive and/or intestinal problems, mood swings, muscle spasms, recurrent upper respiratory infections, sensitivity to light and temperature, onset of food and environment sensitivities, sleep disturbances, temporary memory loss, and finally, extreme and often disabling fatigue.

Chronic fatigue syndrome (CFS) affects the entire person (every organ and system is a potential target). The entire person must be considered in looking for symptoms and finding a treatment modality that will be effective. It is not the presence of any one symptom that indicates CFS. It is the presence of a constellation of symptoms, including any combination of the above list. CFS is difficult to diagnose.

An unusual phenomenon is that from time to time, in the midst of the disabling fatigue, a CFS sufferer will hit upon an idea (they were often very creative and dynamic people before the overwhelming fatigue of CFS) and suddenly the energy just flows for a time—until the project is completed, or nearly so. This is remarked on time and time again in the literature and is not understood. I can only tell you that it is not that the person is lazy the rest of the time, and it does not necessarily indicate that they are suddenly on the road to recovery.

The best description of CFS I have ever found is in the chapter entitled Footprints: The Diagnostic Dilemma in the book <u>Chronic Fatigue Syndrome, The Hidden Epidemic,</u> referred to above. This book is a wealth of excellent information and is written in a very readable and entertaining style. The information in this book was the basis for the creation of the first four of the CFS homeopathics listed in this book.

HOMEOPATHY AND THE TREATMENT OF CFS

To treat homeopathically is always to treat following the **law of similars.** The specific name of the disease is **not relevant;** what matters is that your symptom picture and the symptom pictures of the remedies you choose match!! A struggling adrenal cortex always manifests in certain ways, as does a clogged liver or colon. ***Symptoms are what matter*** and symptom-picture methodology is where homeopathic remedies shine!!

Since CFS is a syndrome and is diagnosed from any combination of symptoms (do not have to display all of the symptoms) nearly all of the remedies with fatigue in their picture are candidates for use with CFS. There are a lot of these remedies listed in the repertories.

STRESS AND CFS

The following is a quote from Norman Cousins in *Anatomy of an Illness*, and re-quoted in *Chronic Fatigue Syndrome, The Hidden Epidemic* by Stoff and Peligrino

Adrenal exhaustion could be caused by emotional tension, such as frustration or suppressed rage. . . the negative effects of negative emotions on body chemistry. The inevitable question arose in my mind: what about the positive emotions? If negative emotions produce negative chemical changes in the body, wouldn't positive emotions produce positive chemical changes? Is it possible that love, hope, faith, laughter, confidence, and the will to live have therapeutic value? Do chemical changes occur only on the downside?

Stress and its relationship to physical and mental health is an elusive subject to study or to treat. It is not so much a matter of what stresses are in our lives, but it matters very much how we handle the stresses under which we live. Our responses to stress should be very carefully considered—and chosen.

There are 4 main ways of responding to daily stresses of living and to major disasters in our lives. They are:

1. *We surrender* to the flow of circumstances in our lives *fatalistically*, as though we have no control, and therefore, cannot possibly have any say in the direction our lives are going in. This makes us either victims or martyrs and is one of the most destructive things that we can do to ourselves.

2. *We ignore* the struggles of life as we pass through them, **pretending** that all is well and there is nothing to be concerned about or dealt with. This inevitably leads to an accident or an illness as our body tries to make us consciously aware of our own needs.

3. *We attempt to resist,* which often wastes energy, adds fuel to the destructive processes of stress, and usually gets us nowhere very fast. Rather than simply resist, we need to actively seek ways to make changes or learn to cope with stress in a better way.

4. *We learn* from our circumstances and use them as stepping stones and catalysts for our growth and for the achievement of our goals. Needless to say, this last one is the only appropriate response to stress.

In order to discover a possible psychological underpinning for any chronic illness, there are several difficult questions that need to be asked—and thought about deeply. Some examples are:

1. Am I using my illness to get the care and attention that I feel I deserve or need and am not getting?

2. Do I enjoy not having to deal with people and situations I dislike or find overwhelming?

3. Am I using my illness to avoid the possibility of failure, or even of success?

4. Do I feel sorry for myself and see myself as either a victim or a martyr?

HIGH OR LOW POTENCY REMEDIES

A few years ago—back before the dawn of time—when I first heard the term *Chronic Fatigue Syndrome* and then came across Jesse Stoff's book (referred to previously), I felt like a great light had dawned. My husband was very sick. He had a great many of the symptoms listed for this syndrome and nothing we were doing seemed to help much. This book, *Chronic Fatigue Syndrome: The Hidden Epidemic*, not only explained the disease but it provided nutritional counseling, advice on depression, and a section titled "For the Physician." I didn't know any homeopathic physicians at the time. The United States was not, at that time, a friendly environment for homeopathic remedies or homeopathic physicians.

I had read quite extensively about homeopathy and I had used a few basic remedies. I took what Jesse Stoff had to say, went online to homeopathic sites in England and began to gather up the remedies that he recommended. When I couldn't find a particular one I repertorised, looking for a similar remedy that matched my husband's symptoms.

The remedies I ended up using were the low potency variety. Higher potency ones were not available in the United States at that time. I knew very little about their use and Dr. Stoff's notes didn't make much sense to me at the time. Nevertheless, the combinations I made began to make a difference for my husband.

Looking back at it now, I find the whole thing rather amazing. I have learned a lot about homeopathic remedies over the years. I now know that chronic, deep maladies like chronic fatigue syndrome usually **require a gentle and long-term approach,** using lower potency remedies in the early stages.

Step one of effective treatment is low potency remedies and changes in nutritional patterns. The person's system is too debilitated to be hit by a high potency remedy right at first, and a body cannot heal until it has the proper nutritional building blocks.

Gentle nudges, and the support of all of the organs and systems at the same time, is the best way. Low potency remedies get the energy system moving, there is less likelihood of healing reactions that the very debilitated person would have trouble coping with, and you can target more organs and systems by using the remedies simultaneously. I stumbled into doing all of this pretty much correctly with too little knowledge and no help (except from Heaven!).

I believe, however, that low potency remedies, even with good nutrition, will take you only so far toward complete wellness. If you wish to avoid a repeat of CFS, a bout later on with mononucleosis, or a never the same since chronic fatigue scenario, you must continue on with the appropriate deeper acting, higher potency remedies. The protocols will be very much like any constitutional or chronic program.

COMBINATION HOMEOPATHIC REMEDIES FOR CFS

The first four remedies discussed below are the ones I made up years ago based loosely on Dr. Jesse Stoff's recommendations. The next two are other combinations, made later, that have proven helpful over the years. These remedies are described in this book. Other combination remedies are described in the companion book to this book, _Butterfly Miracles with Homeopathic Remedies, II_.

Energetic remedies similar to these original homeopathic formulas have been available from Butterfly Express llc (208-747-3021). You can, with effort, purchase each of the ingredients listed and create your own combination remedies if Butterfly Express, llc no longer has them available. The descriptions below are, of necessity, brief and are included to help you see what is available in the homeopathic world and how they might be combined to assist the healing process.

CFS #1 (12X)

HOMEOPATHIC INGREDIENTS:
Echinacea angustifolia/purpurea (purple cone-flower), Argentum nitricum (silver nitrate), Ferrum phosphoricum (iron phosphate)

ECHINACEA stimulates the immune response and is a tonic for the blood. The symptom picture includes many of the physical and mental symptoms of CFS and supports liver function. Great fatigue and prostration are keynotes of this remedy. Taking Echinacea as an herbal supplement should be considered. Echinacea protects against bacterias, viruses, and chemical toxins and supports the immune system.

ARGENTUM NITRICUM has listed in its symptom picture fears, phobias, and anxiety—especially about upcoming events or performances. There is fear of failure (or success), impulsiveness—wants to do things in a hurry. Physically, the symptoms include colic with much gas and distention, lassitude, and weariness. Keynotes are craving for sweets and fear of something bad happening.

FERRUM PHOSPHORICUM is the great polycrest for debility, exhaustion, and anemia. It is said to increase hemoglobin in the blood and is indicated for the first stage of all inflammatory disorders.

CFS#1 is an outstanding example of synergy, the combining of remedies so that the sum is greater than the total of the parts, in a healing sense. In this case, the *Argentum nitricum* and the *Ferrum phosphoricum* greatly enhance the immune strengthening properties of the Echinacea. This remedy helps the regenerative process of the individual cells of organs, tissues, and nerves

CFS #2 (6X)
Targets the Nervous System and Brain

HOMEOPATHIC INGREDIENTS:
Apis mellifica (honey bee), Belladonna (deadly nightshade)

APIS MELLIFICA In research studies a few years ago, the sting of the honey bee was being used experimentally in the treatment of nerve and immune disorders such as multiple sclerosis. Being stung by bees brought temporary relief from the symptoms of multiple sclerosis. Apis, at this potency, has a slow action and must not be discontinued too soon. Increased flow of urine will indicate that it is detoxifying the body, as intended. A keynote is the hot, stinging, burning sensation, the location of which may be anywhere in the body. Other keynotes are extreme tenderness in the abdominal region, nervousness, and restlessness.

BELLADONNA acts on the brain, nerve centers, glandular, and lymphatic systems. It is noted for the suddenness of the onset of symptoms. Abdominal symptoms include extreme sensitivity to touch, with tenderness, and swelling. These abdominal symptoms are common in all stages of CFS. Belladonna is also useful for several kinds of insomnia and other sleep disorders.

CFS #3 (6X)
Targets Liver, Pancreas, Adrenal Cortex, Digestive Function

HOMEOPATHIC INGREDIENTS:
Hepar sulphuris calcareum (calcium sulphide), Mercurius solubilis/vivus (mercury vivus), Spongia tosta (roasted sponge), Taraxacum officinale (dandelion)

HEPAR SULPHURIS CALCAREUM The mentals of this remedy include oversensitiveness to people and places, extreme irritability, and impulsiveness. Hepar has a definitive action on the liver and action on the lymphatic and glandular systems. Other symptoms include depression, desire for death, and a ferocious temper.

MERCURIUS SOLUBILIS/VIVUS People needing Mercurius are often described as human thermometers. Their moods and energy levels go up and down, all over the scale, in a constantly changing pattern. Mercurius clears the lymphatic system and increases glandular activity. Like all remedies for CFS, this is a remedy for pervasive exhaustion. Mercurius is one of a very small number of remedies whose symptom picture also includes the days when the fatigue backs off and the person is, for a short time, able to move quite freely and energetically. Like the mercury in a thermometer, however, the weather will soon change and the person will return to exhaustion, discouragement, pancreas dysfunction, liver enlargement, and stiffness in the joints.

SPONGIA TOSTA is specific to the adrenal glands. With improved adrenal gland function comes more energy, and more ability to accomplish the day's tasks. Some of the symptoms for which Spongia tosta is effective are: clothes feel uncomfortable, especially at the waist, stiffness in muscles, constipation, and fear of the future. Spongia tosta acts as a stimulant to the liver.

TARAXACUM OFFICINALE Debility, liver clogging, headache, gastric distress, impatience, irritability, grumbling, deficiency of liver and bladder, and feelings of bubbles bursting in abdomen.

CFS #3 seems to stimulate the anabolic metabolism of the liver. Doing so supports the immune system, takes stress off the pancreas and adrenal glands, and improves digestive function. *The abdominal pains and bloating often noted by CFS sufferers should subside with the use of this combination.*

CFS #4 (6X)

HOMEOPATHIC INGREDIENTS:
Sepia succus (cuttlefish ink), Ignatia amara (St. Ignatius bean), Calcarea carbonica (calcium carbonate)

With this compound you should notice, over several weeks, *a lessening of both fatigue and irritability* and a *clearing of the dark circles under the eyes.*

SEPIA SUCCUS The picture of Sepia is that of a person mentally and physically worn out, with laxness of tissues and organs. There is irritability with family and a feeling of being just too tired to cope with even one more demand. The liver is sluggish and there is the sensation of something twisting in the stomach and intestines. I have heard it described as a knife twisting in the guts at the slightest movement.

IGNATIA AMARA The symptoms of Ignatia always have to do with grief, worry, and fear. The debility of CFS often leads to a grief for plans made and goals set aside because of poor health. As the health deteriorates, there is always worry and fear of what the future holds. The symptoms of Ignatia may or may not be part of the original bacterial invasion, but certainly are part of the development of the malady.

Physical symptoms include spasms and cramps in the back and other muscles, sciatic pain in back and hips, and joints that feel as if they have been dislocated. Ignatia can help with insomnia that is due to the mind focusing on griefs, disappointments, or worries.

CALCAREA CARBONICA Constantly worrying about all their responsibilities and duties and the things that their poor health is not letting them accomplish deepens the fatigue. Periods of mental and physical effort that end in great fatigue are also part of this remedy. The person suffers from nightmares and poor sleep. There is frequent sourness and nausea in the stomach. Ignatia is considered the polycrest of antipsoric remedies and CFS is certainly a manifestation of psora in many ways.

CFS #5 (6X)

HOMEOPATHIC INGREDIENTS:
Calcarea muriatica (calcium chloride), Kali phosphoricum (potassium phosphate), Reserpinum (alkaloid of Rauwolfia serpentina), Zincum muriaticum (zinc chloride)

CALCAREA MURIATICA The focus of Calcarea muriatica in this combination is the relief of glandular swelling and gastric pain. This remedy also relieves anxiety and should help lessen periods of weakness and trembling.

KALI PHOSPHORICUM All phosphoricum remedies have fatigue, nervous prostration, and a weakened state from mental or physical stresses in their symptom picture. The Kalis are related to duty and feelings of not having done one's duty. Whether the negative emotion of guilt made them susceptible to chronic fatigue, or the chronic fatigue brought about the feelings of guilt because of the things they aren't accomplishing, is not relative to relief. If there are these feelings, the addition of this remedy to the regimen is very helpful.

RESERPINUM The most interesting symptom of reserpinum from a CFS standpoint is alarming fatigue in normally hyperactive and aggressive persons. Almost all CFS sufferers were dynamic individuals before the CFS slowed them down so drastically.

Reserpinum's symptoms include the slowing down of mind and body, fatigue and the inability to work in the evening, the need for sleep or a period of rest after meals, and nervous depression. Physically there are spasmodic attacks of pain in colon; constipation followed by diarrhea, and gastric and duodenal ulcers. All of these symptoms are common among many CFS sufferers.

ZINCUM MURIATICUM is for brain and nerve fatigue and changeable moods. There is an unusual symptom of craving for some particular food in an attempt to relieve irritation and nausea of the stomach. With CFS, this craving is often for potatoes or other starches, which also stabilize the blood sugar.

Glandular #3 (9X)
Supports Organs, Glands, and Nerves

HOMEOPATHIC INGREDIENTS:
Chelidonium majus (greater celandine), Crataegus oxyacantha (hawthorn berries), Avena sativa (oatstraw), Lobelia inflata (indian tobacco), Equisetum hyemale (horse-tail)

CHELIDONIUM MAJUS Symptoms of this remedy include liver disorders, gallbladder pains, nausea, and vomiting. An overloaded or poorly functioning liver creates headaches. These headaches are frontal and usually centered over the right eye—it feels like a sharp object is being driven into the head above the eye.

CRATAEGUS OXYACANTHA is added to this combination because it is a heart tonic and blood pressure stabilizer. It is also useful for insomnia and certain types of nausea.

AVENA SATIVA is useful during the recovery period from illness and is added to this combination in hopes that the periods of energy and well-being can be encouraged to last a little longer each time. The picture also includes chronic insomnia with nervous exhaustion and weakness.

LOBELIA INFLATA is specific for conditions that drag on and on with the person never quite returning to full health and vigor. There is the unusual symptom of prickling sensations and itching all over the body.

EQUISETUM HYEMALE Support of the urinary tract and other eliminative organs.

Detox #1 (6X)
Detox from Chemical and Environmental Poisons.

Clay foot soaks and herbal and essential oil support during the detox period are recommended. Take this one slowly—take the remedy for a few days, then rest from it until cleanse symptoms have subsided. Making yourself sicker is not a good idea.

HOMEOPATHIC INGREDIENTS:
Arsenicum album (white oxide of arsenic), Berberis vulgaris (barberry), Glycyrrhiza glabra (licorice root), Lycopodium clavatum (club moss), Natrum muriaticum (sodium iodide), Nux Vomica (poison nut), Phytolacca decandra (poke root), Stillingia sylvatica (queen's root), Thyroidinum (thyroid gland extract), Trifolium pratense (red clover)

ARSENICUM ALBUM is the great, deep-acting, polycrest remedy for any type of influenzas or poisonings. Particularly useful for CFS because the picture includes sudden great weakness and shortness of breath. Arsenicum album is a restorative for all systems of the body (digestive, urinary, circulatory, lymphatic, glandular, all of them), and has a particular affinity for the liver.

BERBERIS VULGARIS is useful in arthritic and hepatic (liver) disorders. The main function of Berberis in this case is to support the urinary tract and protect against kidney inflammation as the body sends the poisons being pulled out of the tissues through them. Poisonous chemicals can only leave the body safely by attaching to mineral compounds such as calcium and passing through the kidneys.

GLYCYRRHIZA GLABRA is a liver remedy, useful in both detoxifying and protecting the liver and hepatic ducts. It is a powerful anti-inflammatory. Glycyrrhiza's frequent use with chronic fatigue syndrome illustrates its viral fighting and restorative properties.

LYCOPODIUM CLAVATUM is best suited to gradually developing ailments with functional weakness. This is a very good description of chronic fatigue syndrome. Lycopodium targets digestive problems and liver dysfunction. It is used in other ***deep-seated, progressive chronic illnesses*** and is a true polycrest for these illnesses.

NATRUM MURIATICUM is one of the cell salts. It encourages the uptake and proper distribution of minerals and salts throughout the body and has a positive effect on the heart, kidneys, spleen, and immune response. Natrum remedies are about gloom—nothing will get any better and they have to do all the hard work all alone.

NUX VOMICA is pre-eminently for men who have been under stress and strain for a lengthy period of time. Included in the symptom picture is disorders of the stomach and bladder, sleep disorders, irritability, nervous tension, and fiery displays of temper.

PHYTOLACCA DECANDRA acts powerfully on the muscles of the back and neck, all fibrous tissues, all tendons, and joints, and has a strengthening effect on the glandular system.

STILLINGIA SYLVATICA has an effect on the respiratory, lymphatic, eliminative, and glandular systems. Removes toxins from the body by forcing the poison to a pustular head somewhere. Perfect for chronic fatigue because it alleviates cramping and the pressure of gas from the abdomen and relieves pain and stiffness in joints.

THYROIDINUM is a sarcode, and as such is useful for stimulating, strengthening, and regulating the thyroid. Sarcodes are excellent in combinations since they are most effective when taken with a symptomatic remedy.

TRIFOLIUM PRATENSE The herb is useful as a blood purifier and is indicated for anyone with predisposing factors for any type of cancer. As a homeopathic, Trifolium is a powerful detoxifying agent and useful for the deep respiratory illnesses that people with chronic illnesses are prone to.

HOW TO TAKE THE REMEDIES

The remedies discussed so far are low potency combination remedies. They are designed to very gently start strengthening and cleansing the various organs of the body. Almost every remedy in them works on various aspects of emotional health. Like all low potency homeopathics, take the remedy several times a day for 4 or 5 days, followed by a break of 2 or 3 days. This protocol brings both the negative patterns that need eliminating and the positive patterns that need supporting to the attention of the vital force.

There are several reasons for the 2 or 3 day break with no remedies taken. The first of these is to guarantee that there is not even the slightest possibility of taking any remedy long enough to set up a symptom picture of any symptoms of a remedy that you do not already have.

The second, and very important, reason is that a homeopathic remedy is meant to be a catalyst to the healing abilities of the person's own body. The break allows the immune system to take over the healing process. It also allows you to assess how well the vital force (immune system) is doing at that task.

It is vitally important that as the symptom picture changes, the remedies taken also change. At times, it will be important to give extra support to the glandular system. At other times the keynote symptoms may be in the joints or in the digestive system. Symptoms *always* guide the prescribing. Muscle testing is very effective, although intuition and intellect make a very powerful combination in homeopathic health care.

Fresh air, sunlight, good nutrition, *mild* exercise, family support and patience, and a program for spiritual growth are also essential to healing from chronic illness.

SINGLE HOMEOPATHIC REMEDIES FOR CFS

The following are single remedies, listed with a few keynotes appropriate to chronic fatigue. These remedies are appropriate for use in higher potency later on in the treatment. Only rarely will you use a higher potency remedy at the same time as you are taking lower potency combinations. I have listed, mainly, the symptoms that apply to chronic fatigue here. PLEASE, always make sure that the symptom picture of the remedy fits the person as a whole. They, of course, need not have every symptom listed in the Materia Medica. The symptoms listed there are the whole gamut, right up until the person is very debilitated and almost dead. The basic pattern of the destructiveness and out-of-balance state should be there, however.

AMMONIUM CARBONICUM One keynote of this remedy is that lack of endurance, rather than pain or fatigue, is the main complaint of the person. This is a cold remedy; the person may suffer from thyroid problems and chilliness after eating. There is absentmindedness and bitterness toward the world.

ARSENICUM ALBUM is a picture of a collapsed state. It is keynoted by a sense of restlessness. The person is too exhausted to move. The restlessness is expressed more in discontent than in motion. Anxiety and control issues are also common with this remedy.

CALCAREA CARBONICA is for overworked, overwhelmed, overburdened patients who constantly worry about what other people are thinking of their performance and abilities. There are pronounced feelings of vulnerability and deep needs for security and safety.

CAMPHORA is the universal antidote for homeopathic remedies—but also a remedy in its own right. Serious cases of chronic fatigue with almost total collapse, extreme coldness, and little vitality at all often require a round or two of Camphora before any other regimens can take effect. Keynote: person is chilly but does not like to be covered up.

CARBO VEGETABILIS This remedy, while containing symptoms of exhaustion, indigestion, and intestinal problems common to CFS, is often most useful for a person who has been doing so much better for a period of time but is not quite back to normal. The complete picture is of a person who has not quite fully recovered from a chronic or serious illness. Their vitality is low, they are exhausted by the slightest activity, and they often lie down and sleep for a bit one or more times during the day. Sleep is un-refreshing however. They lie down because they are exhausted, then fall asleep. They often wake with cold legs, especially cold knees.

CARCINOSIN is a nosode of particular value where the chronic fatigue is the result of allopathic cancer treatment. Whenever possible, give this remedy before the chemotherapy as a preventative for some of the worst side effects. A regimen of this remedy may also be undertaken where cancer or diabetes is prevalent in the immediate family of any person.

CAUSTICUM is indicated for neurological problems. Causticum is a grief remedy and usually applies best where there has been a history of repeated griefs. Causticum people feel other people's pain, as well as their own, with unusual intensity. This constant bombardment of pain often results in a pervading sadness that may settle in to depression.

CHINA OFFICINALIS (also called CINCHONA) The personality picture of China officinalis makes this remedy especially appropriate for teenage boys and idealistic men who may spend time fantasizing about situations where they can shine. Frequently, the person is sensitive to noise and smells and has become introverted and touchy. This is the first remedy that is considered for hormone imbalance in men (a polycrest for men much like Sepia succus is for women).

COCCULUS INDICUS Cocculus indicus works on *progressive* nervous disorders, so the symptom picture runs from mild restlessness through deeper patterns like vertigo, and literally, being extremely sick from stress and grief. There is sensitivity to light and noise and the person is always made worse from loss of sleep. Motion sickness is often extreme, making any kind of travel difficult.

GELSEMIUM SEMPERVIRENS Great fatigue, trembling, dullness of thought, worsening of symptoms when anticipating an event (stage fright or performance anxiety) are keynotes of Gelsemium. The fatigue of Gelsemium is intense. The whole body feels very heavy, as if the arms and legs have been weighted down with lead. Gelsemium strengthens the nerves, with the symptoms more likely to clear first on the left side of the body.

Oddly, Gelsemium is likely to be needed when the weather changes from cold to warm as winter passes away. This is a common remedy for people who spend their time in overly warm houses or work places.

IGNATIA AMARA The complaints and problems of Ignatia amara often come on or get worse after an emotional upset of some kind. The physical symptoms cover a wide range because they develop, following the emotional upheaval, in areas of weakness unique to each person. Some people manifest their stresses in their hearts, others in their digestive processes. Someone else may get a headache. A sore throat is common in people who cannot, or are not allowed to, express themselves openly.

KALI PHOSPHORICUM Phosphorus is an essential nutrient for healthy nervous systems; phosphorus remedies are pictures of neurological stress. Kali phos is used for mental or physical exhaustion after periods of high stress or exertion. The person felt like it was their duty to see it through no matter how worn out or sick they were getting. Kali people insist on doing their duty and feel guilty if they don't do enough.

MAGNESIA CARBONICA People who would benefit from Magnesia carb have an overwhelming need for peace and harmony and an aversion to conflicts or quarrels of any kind. (An aversion to conflict that can be an indication of a weak liver, generally.) They typically have a tired and long-suffering look and attitude. Symptoms get worse at night, preventing sleep. They often wake more tired in the morning than they were when they went to bed the night before. There is usually diarrhea, flatulence, and various forms of indigestion.

MURIATICUM ACIDUM All acid remedies are associated with fatigue and collapse in one way or another. Muriaticum acidum is a picture of profound physical weakness. It may be the entire body, or a specific organ or system. The body is sore and achy all over and the muscles feel completely exhausted. The person appears restless because they are constantly seeking a position that is more comfortable to them.

NATRUM MURIATICUM Chronic fatigue which has developed in individuals who are very driven emotionally to achieve success in their profession. There are grief issues—either a serious loss or two or a series of repetitive small losses. These people drive themselves at top speed and then crash. At any sign of recovery or with the slightest improvement in energy levels, they are off and running until they have exhausted themselves again.

NUX VOMICA Nux has a very definite remedy picture and is easily recognized by homeopaths and the people who live with this type of personality. Nux vomica is the typical Type A personality who consistently runs faster than he has strength and is competitive, ambitious, and impatient with the normal pace of life. These are strongly aggressive personalities. Nux vomica is excellent for alleviating collapsed states and will also help temper the personality to avoid the excesses that led to the collapse in the first place.

PHOSPHORICUM ACIDUM This is a very powerful chronic fatigue remedy. In one remedy we have the Phosphorus neurological picture of sympathy and dread and the fatigue of all acids. This produces a remedy of great potency for emotional burnout, especially when tied to the needs of family and friends. One keynote of this remedy is the intense craving for chocolate. There is often expressed a fear of running out of chocolate. (Chocolate contains phosphorus. Is there a connection?)

SCUTELLARIA LATERIFOLIA The keynotes are fatigue, anxiety, cloudy thinking (slow to answer), flu-like symptoms and vertigo. A symptom that sets Scutellaria apart from other fatigue remedies is that the tiredness is usually associated with the suppression of sinus problems by repeated antibiotics. This remedy is made from skullcap which, in the herbal world, is renowned as a nervine and heart tonic.

SULPHUR This is a deep psora miasmic remedy. The symptoms always worsen in warm, stuffy rooms and are better for fresh air. Any type of hot flush or symptom as the result of getting over heated will respond to Sulphur. A Sulphur personality is always very intelligent with a mind that questions the why of everything.

They are full of ideas, but in an-out-of balance state, they have difficulty implementing their visions. Sulphur types are often self centered, impatient, irritable, and critical of how others are running their lives. They manage this, somehow, in the face of their own almost total lack of organization and cleanliness. They will frequently tell you how they could do whatever you are doing better than you are doing it.

COMMENTS

The single remedy you choose will depend—very much—on your constitutional type and which miasm is at play in your life currently. The homeopathic remedy should be chosen to support and strengthen the various organs and systems of the body, according to which ones are in trouble with each person.

It is always beneficial, even necessary, to include herbal remedies and nutritional supplementation to the regimen. The body cannot rebuild, no matter how badly the vital force wants it to and understands the correct pattern, if it lacks the basic building materials to do so. These building materials are vitamins, minerals, fat, and proteins, and they must be ingested in order to be utilized.

A FINAL WARNING

The Epstein-Barr virus is almost always present in people who have been diagnosed with chronic fatigue syndrome. The really alarming statistic, however, is that it is estimated by the medical community that at least 85% of Americans have the Epstein-Barr virus in their bloodstreams.

According to Jesse Stoff, MD (previously quoted on the topic of CFS), the Epstein-Barr virus not only weakens the surveillance system that guards against deviant cells, but is itself oncogenic, meaning that, under the right circumstances, it can create deviants and can cause several different varieties of cancer.

The research indicates that the Epstein-Barr virus acts as an initiator when potentiated by a promoter of some sort. Research into what constitutes a promoter continues. Some of this research is very much focused on emotional triggers which weaken the immune system. This research makes a connection, scientifically, between how we handle mental and emotional stress and how well our immune systems handle physical stressors.

The list of EBV-associated cancers grows every day. The common denominator seems to be confusion of the immune system as to what is and what is not an invader. In other words, the same thing that is causing such an increase in allergies may also be causing an increase in EBV-related cancers. The first thing that comes to my mind is the immune-suppressant drugs added to medically required and publicly accepted vaccinations and given so freely to our infants and children. The second link seems to be the vast array of chemicals that we ingest or take into our bodies in other ways every day.

According to some studies, EBV attacks the antibody producing B-cells. Once inside, the virus causes the B-cells to reproduce the virus along with any new B-cells that are produced. The very cells that are usually our defenders have become hosts for the virus. As the T-cells set about destroying the virus, B-cells are also destroyed. This causes an immune deficiency because, as B-cells are destroyed, there are too few remaining to build a strong immune response. Just like soldiers in battle, some T-cells are destroyed in the battle against the virus filled B-cells. The thymus, where T-cells are produced, then goes into overdrive to make up the losses. This overproduction of T-cells, over an extended period of time, results in thymus gland fatigue. The fatigued thymus then produces immature and atypical T-cells, thus deepening the immune system compromise and opening the body to disease, including cancers.

Is this going on in the bodies of the 85% of us who have Epstein-Barr in our systems? Probably, but do not despair. The best defense is often a good offense. Strengthen your immune system every day and use homeopathy to communicate with your immune system. A strong B-cell does not succumb to the attack. It does not let the virus inside. When it reproduces itself, it reproduces healthy, resistant B-cells like itself. The immune system remains (or becomes) strong and active.

If you are reasonably healthy, do not wait until you are fighting something nasty to support your immune system. If you are already in trouble, get to work right now, today!

Chapter Twenty-Three - Heart Problems

Defects in the structure or function of the heart seem to be part of an inherited syphilitic miasm, while congestive heart tendencies are more often part of the sycosis miasm.

Congestive heart failure means that the heart is no longer able to pump enough oxygen-rich blood out to the rest of the body, especially during exercise. As the heart's pumping action is lost, blood may back up in other areas of the body. Fluid then builds up in the lungs, the liver, the gastrointestinal tract, and the arms and legs. As a result, there is a lack of oxygen and nutrition to organs, which become damaged and fail to work properly. This is a long-term, chronic condition although the realization that you have it may occur quite suddenly.

CAUSES OF CONGESTIVE HEART FAILURE:

Narrowing of the small blood vessels that supply blood and oxygen to the heart (coronary heart disease).

A heart attack

Heart valve disease or damage

Severe anemia

An infection has weakened the heart (cardiomyopathy)

Some types of abnormal heart rhythms (arrhythmias and murmurs)

Hyper- or hypothyroidism

COMMON SYMPTOMS:

- Shortness of breath with activity or after lying down for awhile
- Cough
- Swelling of feet and ankles
- Swelling of the abdomen
- Weight gain
- Irregular or rapid pulse
- Sensation of feeling the heart beat (palpitations)
- Difficulty sleeping
- Low oxygen levels, especially at night
- Fatigue, weakness, faintness
- Loss of appetite, indigestion
- Decreased alertness/difficulty concentrating
- Decreased urine production
- Nausea and vomiting
- Need to urinate at night
- Fluid around the lungs
- Distended neck veins
- Swelling of the liver

Homeopathic Remedies

The following homeopathic remedies are included because their symptom pictures contain many of the symptoms listed for congestive heart failure and they are specific to heart damage and overall heart function.

APOCYNUM CANNABINUM The specifics of this remedy are congestive heart problems that are accompanied by renal (kidney) failure. There is swelling and edema (water retention in the tissues—usually lower extremities) that is characteristic of kidney problems and poor circulation.

ACONITUM NAPELLUS Aconitum is used as a shock remedy for good reasons, and that characteristic should carry over into your choice of this remedy for heart issues. Aconitum is effective for palpitations brought on by shock or fear, angina, and acute myocardial infarctions. An infarction is usually defined as the blockage of an artery, etc. and the term acute means something that has come on suddenly or become dangerous quickly. A keynote symptom here is severe, radiating chest pain, with numbness down the left arm. Aconitum is a heart attack remedy, but congestive hearts, under stress, are at risk and should be prepared.

ARSENICUM ALBUM Congestive heart failure with irregular rhythm, cyanosis (blue tinge to skin from lack of oxygen), dyspnea (labored breathing), weakness, feeling of cold, restlessness, and anxiety

CRATAEGUS OXYACANTHA Acts on the muscles of the heart, smoothing out irregular heartbeats and reducing high blood pressure. Is reputed to have a solvent action on the calcareous deposits in arteries without creating clumps that might produce a stroke. Particularly suited to the symptoms associated with congestive heart failure.

DIGITALIS PURPUREA Digitalis is used when there is an abnormally slow pulse (bradycardia), or (tachycardia) rapid pulse with inadequate conduction of oxygen, etc. Indicated for rheumatic heart disease or heart problems that are the result of other serious illness.

GELSEMIUM SEMPERVIRENS The keynote of Gelsemium is an empty feeling in the chest that is worse for being still. The person feels as if his heart will stop beating if he is not constantly in motion. There is hoarseness and loss of voice, which are also indicators for this remedy.

GLONOINUM Glonoinum is made from nitroglycerine which, when used allopathically stimulates the heart to beat faster, but sometimes produces pulsating headaches as a side effect. These indications of the remedy's symptom picture make it the obvious choice to treat intense pulsation of the heart, heart murmurs, pulsating bursting headaches, and many other congestive heart issues.

KALI CARBONICUM is a polycrest remedy but has a very specific symptom picture. If a person has the keynote symptoms of this remedy it can be very effective when used to treat both angina and congestive heart failure. Kali people are duty and principle people. They are responsible, optimistic in the sense that they are always sure situations and people will be better tomorrow than they are today. They often hang on to negative situations while waiting for a better tomorrow. They also tend to ignore symptoms because they are sure that things will be better tomorrow.

KALMIA LATIFOLIA The suppression of rheumatic or arthritic heart conditions with drug therapies frequently shows up later as rheumatic heart, valvular diseases, arrhythmia, cardiac hypertrophy (enlargement) or congestive heart failure. This remedy is for those situations and is most effective where there is both neuralgia and rheumatic conditions. It has been proven effective even in advanced stages.

LACHESIS MUTA Being a snake remedy, Lachesis is indicated for circulatory problems, particularly blockages and/or hemorrhages. Lachesis should be used for angina and congestive heart failure if the basic personality symptoms match. Some of the symptom picture is a perfect description of a myocardial infarction. I would consider this one to give quickly as you rush a heart attack victim to the hospital.

LAUROCERASUS OFFICINALIS The keynote of this remedy for cardiac or respiratory problems is **great coldness and total collapse**. The person has no energy or strength and does not seem to be recovering at all in response to other therapies.

MEDORRHINUM This is the *surprise heart attack remedy because patients show few if any symptoms before the actual heart attack occurs.* Consider giving as a preventative to people with a history of heart attacks in their close family background or angina (chest pain) beginning when quite young.

NAJA TRIPUDIANS Another snake remedy (circulation) and similar in many ways to Lachesis. Some of the differences between Lachesis and Naja are: Naja is not as effective for hemorrhages but the cardiac symptoms are more pronounced. This is a specific remedy for valvular diseases (James Tyler Kent Materia Medica) even in advanced cases. Also, if indicated, for cardiac murmurs, cardiac asthma, and angina. Naja is particularly suited to heart people who are nervous, excited, and tremulous and who brood over imaginary troubles and other people's problems.

PHOSPHORUS *A Phosphorus personality is soft, sensitive and has a gentle nature.* This should be reflected when this remedy is chosen. Phosphorus has been used successfully on congestive heart failure, heart murmurs, and angina. The hemorrhagic indicators are strong enough that this one is even recommended for hemophilia.

Chapter Twenty-Four - Contagious and Epidemic Diseases

GENERAL INFORMATION

The right homeopathic remedy at the right moment—which is at the first indication that you are not feeling as well as usual—can make the impact on your body and energy system from any disease much less than it otherwise might have been. If enough people responded homeopathically at the onset (outbreak stage) of an epidemic, perhaps the epidemic could be averted altogether.

Epidemics have ravaged our planet for many thousands of years. A study of history reveals that the rise and fall of nations is frequently connected with the weakening of a culture as the result of successive years of debilitating and deadly epidemics.

Greece, for example, gave us many great thinkers, statesmen, and even conquerors. Among them were the philosopher Plato, the mathematician Pythagorus, Hippocrates (considered the father of medicine), and Alexander the Great, who expanded the borders of Greece through conquest but died under the age of thirty as the result of a malaria epidemic. There is no doubt that malaria played a role in the history of Greece and also in the conditions which eventually led to the fall of the Roman empire. Wars, famines, and pestilences like the Black Plague ruled Europe for nearly a thousand years.

In statistics compiled by Stanford University, it is claimed that the pandemic of 1918-1919 killed more people than the Great War (World War I) with death tolls calculated as between 20 to 40 million people and is considered the most devastating epidemic in recorded world history. This influenza had the unusual characteristic of an unusually high mortality rate among younger persons. The death rate from influenza and accompanying respiratory pneumonia for 15 to 34 year old individuals was 20 times higher in the 1918 flu than in previous years. The effect of the influenza epidemic was so severe in the United States that the average life span was depressed by a full 10 years. More people died of influenza in a single year that in four years of the Black Death Bubonic Plague (1347 to 1351). Bubonic plague in its heyday affected nearly 100% of the population and sometimes killed anywhere from 40% to 80% of the residents of a city or village, and in places wiped out entire populations leaving few, if any, survivors. It is incredible to me to think of a flu epidemic as even worse than this.

In our times we have learned to control some of these epidemics through improved sanitation, better nutrition, quarantine, and isolation. But the enemy is not so very far off. Partially because transportation has improved dramatically and people travel all over the world continually now, we are able to carry any local germs or potential epidemics with us wherever we go.

As always, the first rule of homeopathic treatment is to treat according to the totality of symptoms and not by the name of the disease.

However, there are specific remedies that have been found by some to be effective against some of the epidemic diseases that currently abound in the world. There are also remedies whose symptom pictures match closely some of the more modern threats to health. The remedies listed in these pages are meant for your consideration. They are not meant as an exhaustive list. Nor do they give you all of the information available about any disease or the individual homeopathic remedies. They are meant to give you a place to start should you need one. They should also provide you an opportunity to see clearly how one remedy differs from another, according to the characteristics of the person, even in the treatment of a specific epidemic disease. This book is meant to be an educational tool.

A nosode of the appropriate disease, if available, should always be considered in an epidemic situation.

Remember that a nosode should always be used in conjunction with a remedy that is specific to the person and supportive of the organs and tissues that are under attack.

SOME THINGS TO CONSIDER
WHEN TREATING CONTAGIOUS AND/OR EPIDEMIC DISEASES

MIASMS
Inherited conditions and miasms—which are the major focus of constitutional treatment philosophies—are not a factor in contagious epidemics, except to the degree that a person's inherited constitution makes him susceptible to a particular epidemic. Many of the rules and protocols of constitutional homeopathy do not apply, or need to be modified somewhat, to be effective in the treatment of epidemic diseases.

The non-inherited miasms (those created by drugs, pollution, toxins, vaccines, and chemicals) may have weakened the person and made them more susceptible to the current epidemic's bacteria or virus. There isn't much you can do about it in the time frame you will be working with once an epidemic has begun, but constitutional aspects must be factored in if the most effective and quickest acting remedy is to be found and utilized.

The compromised eliminative organs must be supported as the therapies you use for the epidemic situation cause dead and dying bacteria to leave the body through the kidneys and the intestinal tract.

ACUTE AILMENTS
Acute ailment homeopathic treatment is aimed at those conditions which are 1) short-lived; 2) non life-threatening at present; and, 3) would clear up by themselves through the normal functioning of the body's energy system. Acute prescribing is meant to relieve the suffering of the person and speed the healing process. Homeopathic treatment is also meant to prevent an acute ailment from becoming a more chronic situation.

CONTAGIOUS EPIDEMIC DISEASES
Contagious diseases impact the vital force of the body to such a dramatic degree that, generally, the body cannot throw off the disease without intervention. In fact, many—if not most—of these diseases so seriously impact the vital force of the body that collapse of one organ system or another can come about quite rapidly, resulting in death. The treatment of these diseases, then, is acute prescribing but with a time factor and a seriousness missing in most treatment protocols.

POTENCY
Because the energetic displacement is so deep and the time factor is so pressing, it is essential that a very high potency remedy be used immediately. It is critically important that a remedy matching both the current symptoms and the person overall be used. You must stop the disease in its tracks and you must also support the organs and systems of the body which have come under attack. This is done best by a remedy that matches their needs closely.

HERBAL REMEDIES AND DRUG THERAPIES
Epidemic diseases are usually bacterial or viral in nature. They move very quickly, and many times, they kill quickly. You might think that antibiotics will be your best bet. This is a decision for the person to make, if they are able. There are some things that should be factored into the decision, however.

First, allopathic medicine has a terrible record with epidemic diseases.

Second, a drug must be tailored very closely to the virus or bacteria causing the problems to be effective, and the little critters mutate very rapidly. What has worked on last year's flu strain may not touch this one.

Third, antibiotics are not effective immediately. The first dying bacteria as a result of antibiotic treatment may be 48 hours away, and with a viral epidemic strain, you may not have that kind of time.

Fourth, all drugs have side effects and weaken the vital force of the body and add to the stress of the organs and systems. In addition, some drugs antidote homeopathic remedies. There is not enough literature or testing on this but it seems to be surprisingly rare. There is, however, a possibility that by using the drug you might stop the action of the very remedy that might have saved a life.

Fifth, the right homeopathic works very rapidly—far more rapidly than drugs. If you do not see immediate results, a change in and a lessening of the symptoms, you will know you are on the wrong track and need to try something else.

An allopathic physician often must wait for a disease to progress far enough that the disease can be identified and named before he can make a diagnosis and prescribe the appropriate drug. With the homeopathic method, we treat the very first symptoms of energy displacement and illness. For example, the early stages of polio resemble a summer cold. Treatment of summer colds with Lathyrus sativus resulted in homeopathic physicians speculating that because they had treated a very high incidence of summer colds throughout the epidemic (and a lower than average number—in some cases, none at all—of polio cases), they had many times, in fact, been treating incipient polio.

The above paragraphs may sound like I am saying that the only right choice is homeopathy. That is not my intention! Although homeopathic remedies have been used successfully the world over in the treatment of these contagious diseases, you must use every bit of knowledge, intuition, skill, and treatments available in whatever proportions you see fit. Your skill and previous experience with homeopathic remedies and how they work will be of critical importance! It will be important that you get it pretty much right the first time, although remedies like Arsenicum album fit the initial symptoms of many contagious/epidemic diseases. Hopefully, you will have a support group and some help at the time. Sometimes, the allopathic route buys a little time while someone figures out what is the best thing to do.

Try to avoid letting fear rule either your choices or your actions. Fear will cloud your thinking, make situations look more dismal than they really are, slow your response time, and make you less effective. Good muscle testing skills, developed earlier and good enough to be relied on, would be very helpful.

ONE FINAL NOTE:

When the body is under attack by hostile disease agents it reacts in one of two ways. The first is to fight back, ferociously, and eradicate the disease in its entirety. This results in a complete cure and subsequent immunity to the disease and anything similar to it. The other reaction is to attempt to seal up the disease by encapsulating it in some way. This is often the case with viral attacks, particularly when the vital force is not sufficiently strong to fight the disease off altogether at this time, or a problem has been suppressed by allopathic (treating with opposites/antidotes—in other words, drugs). The disease is known to be present, but is considered to be dormant. It may, of course, resurface at a later date and continue its attack upon the person, especially if the overall system becomes weakened by disease, allopathic drug use, stress, or the normal processes of aging. At this time, the body may be even less able to fight off the disease.

With homeopathic treatment, the vital force is stimulated to throw off the disease altogether. Homeopathic treatment may even bring online other suppressed or encapsulated diseases to be handled. This is often experienced with old, encapsulated maladies. Some examples would be cold sores, herpetic lesions, shingles, or asthma. (The list is quite endless, actually.) It is quite common, when a homeopathic treatment has been used, to find that other suppressed diseases have been cleared at the same time.

Always remember, homeopathy stimulates the vital force to cure the disease and strengthen the entire system; it does not merely hide or cover over the disease.

STATISTICS
HOMEOPATHY IN EPIDEMICS

As you will see from the article quoted below, and from my accompanying commentary, homeopathy has repeatedly proven itself to be an effective method of treatment during epidemics of some of the worst diseases this world has to offer. You will also see that homeopathy has just as often been ruthlessly suppressed when the statistics have proven embarrassing to the medical communities of the day. The same is true of herbal remedies and treatments.

The following is an article showing the research done, and statistics gathered, on various diseases in history. I have quoted it exactly, in its entirety. I have, however, emphasized the statistics by repeating them in bold and centering them below the paragraph which contains them. Please pay attention to the bolding! **The statistics are amazing.** *I have also added an occasional comment of my own, or a comment from another source. These comments that were not part of the original article are in italics.*

Some History of the Treatment of Epidemics with Homeopathy
Adapted from an article by Julian Winston

(I just looked Julian Winston up on the web. He is deceased, but his autobiographical sketch was impressive and amusing. I love brilliant people who don't take themselves too seriously and have a sense of humor.)

From its earliest days, homeopathy has been able to treat epidemic diseases with a substantial rate of success, especially when compared to conventional treatments of the day. It was these successes that placed the practice of homeopathy so firmly in the consciousness of people world-wide *(and seems to have led to the resentment displayed by the medical community over the years)*.

There is a story told about Joseph Pulte, one of the earliest homeopaths in Cincinnati. When he began his practice, many people were so angered by a homeopath being in town that they pelted his house with eggs. He was becoming discouraged enough to think of leaving. His wife said, "Joseph, do you believe in the truth of homeopathy?" He replied in the affirmative. "Then," she said, "you will stay in Cincinnati." Shortly after, when the cholera epidemic swept through the area, Pulte was able to boast of not having lost a single patient—and he was accepted enthusiastically into the community. In the epidemic of 1849, people crowded to his door and stood in the street because the waiting room was full.

Cholera - not a single patient lost!!

In 1900, Thomas Lindsley Bradford, MD, wrote a book called "The Logic of Figures" in which he collected all of the statistics he could find that would compare the conventional therapeutics with homeopathic ones. Many of the figures cited below are derived from Bradford's work.

One of the earliest tests of the homeopathic system was in the treatment of typhus fever (spread by lice) in an 1813 epidemic which followed the devastation of Napoleon's army marching through Germany to attack Russia, followed by their retreat. When the epidemic came through Leipzig, as the army pulled back from the east, Samuel Hahnemann, the founder of homeopathy, was able to treat 180 cases of typhus-- losing but two. This, at a time when the conventional treatments were having a mortality rate of over 30%.

1813 - Typhus Fever - mortality rates
Hahnemann   1%
Conventional   30% +

In 1830 as the cholera epidemic was reported coming from the east, Hahnemann was able to identify the stages of the illness, and predict what remedies would be needed for which stages. When cholera finally struck Europe in 1831 the mortality rate (under conventional treatment) was between 40% (Imperial Council of Russia) to 80% (Osler's Practice of Medicine). Out of five people who contracted cholera, two to four of them died under regular treatment. Dr. Quin, in London, reported the mortality in the ten homeopathic hospitals in 1831-32 as 9%; Dr. Roth, physician to the king of Bavaria, reported that under homeopathic care the mortality was 7%; Admiral Mordoinow of the Imperial Russian Council reported 10% mortality under homeopathy; and Dr. Wild, allopathic editor of Dublin Quarterly Journal, reported in Austria, the allopathic mortality was 66% and the homeopathic mortality was 33% "and on account of this extraordinary result, the law interdicting the practice of homeopathy in Austria was repealed."

Cholera through most of Europe 1830 - 1831
Homeopathy   7% - 9%
Conventional   40% - 80%
Austria - as reported by the allopathic editor
Homeopathy   33%
Conventional   66%

Homeopathy continued to be effective in the treatment of epidemic cholera. In 1854 a cholera epidemic struck London. This was an historically important epidemic in that it was the first time the medical community was able to trace the outbreak to a source (a public water pump), and when the pump was closed, the epidemic soon ceased. The House of Commons asked for a report about the various methods of treating the epidemic. When the report was issued, the homeopathic figures were not included. The House of Lords asked for an explanation, and it was admitted that if the homeopathic figures were to be included in the report, it would "skew the results." The suppressed report revealed that under allopathic care the mortality was 59.2% while under homeopathic care the mortality was only 9%.

Cholera, London, 1854 (Note paragraph above, suppression of results.)
Homeopathy   9%
Conventional   59.2%

It is hard today to comprehend what kind of scourge such an epidemic was. As was seen in the later flu epidemic of 1918, **one could be healthy in the morning and be dead by evening-- it moved that rapidly.** Many books were written about the homeopathic treatment of cholera during these times, among them: _Cholera and its Homeopathic Treatment_, F. Humphreys (1849); _Homeopathic Treatment of Cholera_ B.F. Joslin (1854); _Homeopathic Domestic Treatment of Cholera_, Biegler (1858); _Epidemic Cholera_, B. F. Joslin (1865); _Asiatic Cholera_, Jabez Dake (1886).

The success of homeopathic treatment continued with the later cholera epidemics. In the Hamburg epidemic of 1892, allopathic mortality was 42%, homeopathic mortality was 15.5% During the 1850s, there were several epidemics of yellow fever in the southern states. This disease was eventually found to be transmitted by mosquito. Osler says that the allopathic mortality from yellow fever was between 15-85%. Holcome, a homeopath, reported in 1853 a mortality of 6.43% in Natchez, and Dr. Davis, another homeopath in Natchez, reported 5.73%. In 1878 the mortality in New Orleans was 50% under allopathic care, and 5.6% (in 1,945 cases in the same epidemic) with homeopathic care. The two best books on this topic were: _Yellow Fever and its Homeopathic Treatment_, Holcome, (1856), and _The Efficacy of Crotalus Horridus in Yellow Fever_, C. Neidhard, (1860).

Cholera, 1892
Homeopathic   15.5%
Conventional   42%
Yellow Fever - 1850's - Southern States
Homeopathic   5.6% - 6.43%
Conventional   lowest reported, 15%; highest 85%

Another epidemic disease which was treatable with homeopathy was diphtheria. Since the advent of widespread vaccination, it is a disease not often seen in our modern world. Diphtheria appeared periodically, and rarely had the same presentation. It was, therefore, very important for the practitioner to individualize the treatment in each specific case or generalized epidemic. A remedy which had been effective in treating it one year might not be the same remedy needed the next year. _(Is this because, as homeopaths and many medical people believe, the little "critters" mutate under allopathic drug programs?)_

In the records of three years of diphtheria in Broome County, NY from 1862 to 1864, there was a report of an 83.6% mortality rate among the allopaths and a 16.4% mortality rate among the homeopaths. (Bradford)

Broome County, NY, Health Record 1862 - 1864
Homeopathic   16.4%
Allopathic   83.6%

Perhaps the most recent use of homeopathy in a major epidemic was during the influenza pandemic of 1918. The Journal of the American Institute for Homeopathy, May, 1921, had a long article about the use of homeopathy in the flu epidemic. Dr. T A McCann, from Dayton, Ohio, reported that 24,000 cases of flu treated allopathically had a mortality rate of 28.2% while 26,000 cases of flu treated homeopathically had a mortality rate of 1.05%. This last figure was supported by Dean W.A. Pearson of Philadelphia (Hahnemann College) who collected 26,795 cases of flu treated with homeopathy with these results:

Influenza 1918 24,000 - 26,000 cases reported
Homeopathic   1.05%
Allopathic   28.2%

The most common remedy used was Gelsemium sempervirens, with occasional cases needing Bryonia alba and Eupatorium perfoliatum reported. Dr. Herbert A. Roberts from Derby, CT, said that 30 homeopathic physicians in Connecticut responded to his request for data. They reported 6,602 cases with 55 deaths, which is less than 1%. Dr. Roberts was working as a physician on a troop ship during WWI. He had 81 cases of flu on the way over to Europe. He reported, "All recovered and were landed. Every man received homeopathic treatment. One other ship, however, lost 31 men on the way."

Influenza on Troop Ships 1918
Homeopathic 0% - 1%
Conventional very high

Closer to our present time, there were the polio epidemics in the mid-1950s. Dr. Alonzo Shadman, a homeopath in the Boston area, emphasized that until "actual paralysis" was observed, it was hard to distinguish the prodromal symptoms of polio from those of the common cold -- and he treated many "summer colds" during the time. Were they incipient polio? No one can tell. (When treating homeopathically, remember, you treat what is presenting by giving the remedy that is most "similar." The treatment used would be unaffected by the "name" of the ailment)

Dr. Francisco Eizayaga of Argentina tells of a polio epidemic in Buenos Aires in 1957, where the symptoms of the epidemic resembled, in the very early stages, those of an oncoming cold. Lathyrus sativus appeared to be the remedy that most closely resembled those early symptoms.

The homeopathic doctors and pharmacies prescribed Lathyrus sativus 30c as a prophylactic, and "thousands of doses" were distributed. "Nobody (given the homeopathic remedy) registered a case of contagion." Eizayaga points out that in other epidemics of polio, Gelsemium sempervirens was the indicated remedy—emphasizing, again, the need for individualization in matching a remedy to the emerging symptoms. By treating the earliest symptoms properly, much suffering was avoided altogether.

Homeopathy was very effective in treating many of the epidemics during the 19th and early 20th centuries. Why the successes are not better known is a subject for conjecture. It could be that, like the physician quoted below, some people would rather not acknowledge the ineffectiveness of the conventional therapeutics in certain circumstances nor do they like, for reasons of their own, to accept the efficacy and effectiveness of homeopathic remedies.

One physician in a Pittsburgh hospital asked a nurse if she knew anything better than what he was doing, because he was losing many cases. "Yes, Doctor, stop aspirin and go down to a homeopathic pharmacy, and get homeopathic remedies." The Doctor replied: "But that is homeopathy." She replied, "I know it, but the homeopathic doctors for whom I have nursed have not lost a single case."

The quote at the bottom of the preceding page was found in an article in the Journal of the American Institute of Homeopathy, May 1921, and was cited in *Homeopathy In Influenza—A Chorus Of Fifty In Harmony* by W. A. Dewey, M.D. He attributed the quote to W. F. Edmundson, M.D., a Pittsburgh doctor.

STATISTICS FOR THE LAST 100 YEARS

As you can see for yourself from the statistics compiled by Julian Winston in the article on the previous 3 pages, there are not many reliable statistics quoted from the last 100 years. Why is that? To my mind there are several factors at play here:

Homeopathy was driven out of the United States by the American Medical Association; the practice of homeopathy was declared illegal and homeopathic hospitals and colleges were closed. Where would a statistician get homeopathic results? I'm sure that for a long time there was probably a strong grass-roots homeopathic movement, but they certainly wouldn't be publishing their results, would they?

- As is always the case, when allopathic medicine "fails" it is assumed that "they did their very best and nobody else could have done better anyway." Repeatedly in the herbal, homeopathic and midwife communities you see the medical profession losing the patient with very little, if any, accountability—except to a closed panel of their peers; but if an herbalist or midwife "loses" a patient, or even fails to make a miraculous "cure", it is big news and there is a great likelihood that some one will be fined or jailed!

- If you look honestly at world history over the last 50+ years, you will see that where the World Health Organization— a very allopathic organization—has been, statistics on mortality rates for epidemic diseases are dreadful! In Africa alone, whole tribes have been wiped out by one disease or another, in spite of vaccination and health care programs.

- In the rest of the world, particularly throughout Europe where homeopathy was never illegal and remained in good standing, statistics for the treatment of disease still show that homeopathy is "doing its job' and doing it without major side effects and drug reactions.

- In India, where homeopathy has been an accepted and well-utilized form of medicine for more than 150 years, government intervention has now restricted its practice to graduates of a very limited number of schools. The cost of treatment is out of the reach of the common man in India as a result, and it is becoming difficult to get an appointment.

- Homeopathy is making an amazing come-back in the United States and, I believe, we are seeing the "pushing back" of the A.M.A. as new legislation is being proposed. As in India, these regulations are being promoted as "for the safety of the public" when, in reality, they will only keep these healers out of the hands of ordinary people and protect the interests of "conventional" physicians and the drug industry. Recently, Remedia Homeopathics of England and Scotland has established a policy of not shipping remedies to the U. S.

The great homeopathic physicians of the past spent years observing people, studying remedies and health issues to become good at their profession. In the years that I have been teaching homeopathic philosophy, I have seen an amazing phenomenon. Mothers (and fathers), tired of the standard medical model and the drugging of their children, are turning to homeopathy and other alternative modalities. They back up their knowledge with intuition and muscle testing skills. The results are an excellent, in-the-home, use of homeopathic remedies in improving the health of their families.

PREVENTION AND PROPHYLAXIS

Using homeopathic remedies as prevention or as vaccinations violates at least one basic tenet of homeopathic prescribing. Classical homeopathic philosophy insists that a remedy be given based on the totality of the symptoms that the person is experiencing. With prevention (prophylaxis), the remedy is given to *prevent* the occurrence of disease—*the disease and its symptoms are, supposedly, not presenting*.

When working preventively—since there are no symptoms to make go away—it can always be argued that the people treated would not have developed the disease whether or not they had taken any remedies. Perhaps, this is true. When you are standing at a fork in the road, there is no way to travel down both of those roads and see what is there. The beauty of homeopathics as a preventative measure is that, unlike vaccinations, antibiotics, and other allopathic drugs, the homeopathic remedy has no side effects and does not compromise the immune response in any way. No harm has been done, and statistics indicate that homeopathic remedies have, in past epidemics, prevented people from contracting the disease and have a strong place as preventative medicines.

STATISTICS

Dr. Dorothy Shepherd (1871-1952), an orthodox physician in England who converted to homeopathy, gives many interesting statistics in her book <u>Homeopathy in Epidemic Diseases</u>. I will share a couple of her stories here.

Dr. Taylor Smith (a colleague of Dr Shepherd's) used Lathyrus sativus as a prophylactic during a polio epidemic in Johannesburg, South Africa. Eighty-two people, ranging in age from six months to twenty years, were given the remedy *when not showing any symptoms of polio*. All of them lived in the area of the epidemic—twelve of the children were in direct contact with a person with the disease—*and yet not a single one in this group developed polio*. This is an impressive statistic, indeed.

Pertussis, or whooping cough, was a common (and major) problem in Dr. Shepherd's day. Her description of it is absolutely frightening. Children almost always took weeks to recover from this disease and were often weakened for many months after the so-called recovery.

During an outbreak of pertussis near her clinic, Dr. Shepherd gave the pertussin nosode remedy to every child she encountered, whether or not they were showing any symptoms. She described the results as "so striking that (she) soon used it as both the prophylactic and as the curative remedy after the disease had started."

During a polio epidemic in Buenos Aires in 1975, 40,000 people were given Lathyrus sativus and not one of them developed polio. A homeopathic researcher gave Lathyrus to over 6,000 children during an epidemic with the same 100% no cases of polio results.

PROPHYLAXIS AND CURATIVE—AT THE SAME TIME

Dr. Shepherd reported that if Pertussinum was given within the first day or two of emerging symptoms, the disease was often aborted in under a week. Even when the remedy was not given until the disease was at its height (3 or 4 days after the first symptoms), the disease ran its course in ten to fourteen days, was much less severe, and the children developed none of the usual long-term complications.

Dr. Shepherd used the story of a five-year-old girl to illustrate, not prophylaxis, but cure. The child began with respiratory difficulties a week before Christmas and was deep into the whooping cough pattern before Christmas. A doctor was called, his prescription for a sedative did little good. By January 2nd the child was having 25 to 30 coughing and vomiting attacks a day and was exhausted and weak. Pertussinum 30C was given three times a day. A week later the child was vomiting—only slightly—once a day, and showed no signs of weakness or anemia. Recovery from this point was rapid and complete. In fact, the mother reported that the child was in better health, ate better, and had more energy than before the disease.

Dr. Smith in Johannesburg (previous page) also used Lathyrus sativus on people who had already developed early symptoms of polio. Meticulous records were kept with one group of 34. The symptoms varied. There was muscle tenderness, neck rigidity with high temperatures, pain and resentment when touched anywhere. One little girl, two years old, appeared to be gravely ill. After 2 doses of Lathyrus sativus 30C given a half hour apart, she fell asleep. Twelve hours later, the symptoms had disappeared and she was completely well. Of the 34 people that Dr. Smith treated, only 4 were sent to the hospital for further treatment.

THE PSYCHOLOGY OF FEAR

Another factor that should not be overlooked in an epidemic situation is the effects of anticipation and fear. Fear and panic nearly always affect the morale and immune response of people. Gelsemium sempervirens is the great remedy for fear and nervous anticipation. Gelsemium's description also includes many of the early symptoms of the major epidemic diseases. Its use would not only allay the fear, but could be all that is needed to prevent—or cope with—the epidemic disease itself. In an epidemic, it doesn't really matter whether you are preventing the occurrence of the disease or curing the disease in its early stages as long as the person does not become a statistic of the epidemic.

POTENCY AND PREVENTION

Dr. Dorothy Shepherd speculated that remedies in the 1M potency provide approximately 2 1/2 years of protection. Lower potencies, she believed, proved to be protection for only a few months.

Personally, I would be leery of high potency remedies prescribed when no symptoms of the disease are present and the risk of exposure to the disease is very limited. Deep level homeopathic remedies, given when matching symptoms are not present, occasionally set up a proving, creating temporary but unpleasant symptoms. If an epidemic of something really nasty was going on in my area, however, I would not be reluctant to risk a few "energy" symptoms if it meant not contracting the contagion.

SUGGESTIONS FOR TREATMENT

POTENCY

Many of the contagious, epidemic diseases come on very suddenly and reach crisis proportions almost immediately. The disturbance to the energy system is happening at a very deep level and the destruction to organs and tissues begins very rapidly. Not only must the vital force (immune) response be immediate, it must be to the depth of the energetic and physical displacements that are going on.

The use of 1M levels at the opening stages of disease is appropriate. A 10M may be required and well tolerated if, prior to this crisis, the person was exhibiting a reasonable degree of health.

Being in a state of generally good health—because of lifestyle choices and the use of herbal remedies, homeopathics, and other treatments which do not compromise the immune system instead of allopathic drugs—will enable you to use stronger potency remedies safely should the need arise. Overall good health is also the best preventative possible.

The treatment of non-crisis stages of even serious diseases can frequently and effectively be done using 200C levels of a well chosen remedy. Dr. Shepherd (cited in previous pages) worked almost exclusively with 30C remedies, given more frequently.

FREQUENCY OF DOSAGE

This is a difficult thing to pin down and make an organized description for. Frequency of dose depends so much on the severity of the problem and the overall vitality of the individual. Both factors will need to be considered in making a decision.

A 200C remedy, in classical homeopathic literature, is used every 5-7 days for a chronic problem and may only be needed once or twice for many common ailments. Following the muscle test seems to lead in a different direction, with more frequent usage and for longer periods of time. In a serious contagious disease, a 200C remedy may need to be used 2-3 times a day for several days. Other times, one dose every other day may be sufficient.

If the person's overall vitality—before this illness—was quite good, the use of a 1M level as close together as every other day may be the best solution. It may even be necessary to use the 1M remedy more often than that in certain circumstances. A 10M remedy might also be considered. Muscle testing—as long as you don't let your fears or prejudices interfere—will be your best guide.

Each situation will be unique and will require knowledge and judgement on your part. As a general rule, people with weakened overall vitality will respond best to frequent doses of a lower potency remedy, and because it is exactly what is needed, it will be enough for them if done frequently.

POLYMORPHIC OR "MUTATING" DISEASE ORGANISMS

As long ago as 1931, it was discovered that disease organisms could mutate into differing versions of themselves. We have had many examples of this brought to our attention in recent years, some of them quite terrifying.

Most disease agents have developed several strains already, from simple to more complex ones with more serious manifestations. For the homeopathic practitioner this means that the remedy indicated by the symptoms at the beginning of the disease may not eliminate every strain of the organism, or be the remedy you will need if the disease returns in an altered or more virulent form. You will need to watch the symptoms carefully and follow up with another remedy which matches the new symptoms more closely. This is reflected in the homeopathic literature by such references as "follows well" or "is followed well by." Pay attention to these references. Use them to guide your prescribing and your muscle testing.

REMEMBER THE BASIC PRINCIPLES

Use the most similar remedy as long as it is working well.

When the organism changes or you have eradicated one strain, the symptom picture will change in smaller or larger degrees; your remedy needs to change accordingly.

Remedies are usually given only until improvement begins. Once the vital force has taken over, the remedy should be discontinued to avoid the risk of "proving the remedy" and setting up a symptom picture. In dramatic contagious disease you must watch closely for signs that the vital force is weakening and needs further support. Thank heaven for the additional help that muscle testing gives us, but never stop thinking and analyzing, especially in these serious situations.

LIST OF DISEASE STATES

CONTAGIOUS AND EPIDEMIC

Common Colds
Measles
Mumps
Chicken Pox
Sars
Influenza
Whooping Cough
Diphtheria
Tuberculosis
Strep A
Hepatitis A, B, C, D
Small Pox
Malaria
Typhoid
Cholera
Q Fever
Dengue Fever
Cytomegalovirus
Arboviral Encephalitis
Aids/HIV
Gonorrhea
Syphilis
Polio

ENVIRONMENTAL

Lyme Disease
Legionaires
Hanta Virus
West Nile

BIOLOGICAL WEAPONS

Anthrax
Plague
Botulism

COMMON COLDS, ORDINARY FLU AND HEADACHES

Instead of a flu shot, antibiotics, and cold remedies, perhaps you should consider homeopathic remedies. Homeopathics have no side effects, and will probably be cheaper. For best results, start taking a remedy the very moment you suspect you are not feeling your best or even when someone close to you becomes ill.

POLYCREST FLU REMEDIES

ACONITUM NAPELLUS Aconitum is especially useful and effective if taken very early on in the illness. It is best taken right after you have been caught in a draft or gotten chilled in some way, or at the first sign of fever or headache, or even if you are just feeling particularly tired. If you missed these initial symptoms, you will think that the Aconitum ailment, whatever it may be, has come on suddenly. There is often agitation and great restlessness. Fever may alternate with chills and all symptoms are generally worse around midnight.

ARSENICUM ALBUM A leading remedy for intestinal, stomach, or chest type influenza. Symptoms are exhaustion with great restlessness, shortness of breath when not sitting up, catarrh, abdomen swollen and painful, enlarged spleen and liver, headache which is relieved by cold, nausea and vomiting, craves cold water but vomits it immediately, high fever, and vertigo during coughing or retching spells.

EUPATORIUM PERFOLIATUM This is one of the premier remedies that saved lives in the epidemic of 1918. Achy bone pain, intense back pain, heavy feeling headache with soreness of the eyeballs, high fever with chills, hoarseness and dry cough with soreness in the chest, and thirst for very cold drinks even during the chills that are a hallmark of this remedy. Hiccups often accompany other symptoms.

VERATRUM ALBUM Veratrum album is a picture of collapse which includes extreme coldness, blueness and weakness. Other symptoms include extreme vomiting and diarrhea, cramping in the legs and feet, tip of nose very cold, cold sweat on forehead, heart palpitations, and large hard stools followed by diarrhea. All symptoms are worse for the slightest motion.

BAPTISIA TINCTORIA Very swift onset with mental confusion deteriorating into an almost coma-like stupor, offensive perspiration and breath, reddish congestion of the face, ulcerated throat that is pain-free, slurred speech are some of the keynote symptoms.

GELSEMIUM SEMPERVIRENS Gelsemium colds and flus come on gradually with 2 or 3 days of feeling more tired and out of sorts than usual. Other symptoms include: chills running up and down the back, aching and stiffness in the neck, heaviness and trembling of the legs, and soreness of the scalp with the feeling of a tight band around the head. With Gelsemium, there is never a feeling of thirst. This remedy was also used during the great flu epidemic of 1918 with amazing results and some really interesting statistics. I use Gelsemium both when something is first coming on and as a remedy for the convalescent stage. Headaches of nervous origin are a keynote of this remedy.

HEADACHES
(ALONE OR AS A FORERUNNER OF A COLD OR FLU)

ARNICA MONTANA A concussion, injury, and shock remedy. The headache pain of Arnica is a bruised feeling. The headache is worse for bending over, and the person will wince and draw away if you reach out to touch their head. With movement, the pain sometimes becomes sharp, almost stabbing. Arnica should be taken whenever there has been a blow to the head, especially when there is an accompanying headache.

BELLADONNA Belladonna is for cluster headaches and migraines that come on with suddenness and intensity. Throbbing pain like hammers pounding from the inside. The face will become red and flushed and the pupils will be dilated. The headache always gets worse from direct light.

BRYONIA ALBA Headaches accompanied by nausea. Just want to be left alone, preferably in the dark and where it is very quiet. They will try not to move, or even open their eyes, as this will increase the feeling of hammers pounding in the skull. Bryonia often follows Aconitum.

CHAMOMILLA VULGARIS Similar to Bryonia with the additional symptom of extreme irritableness and whining. The person will be demanding and discontented with whatever is being done for them.

COFFEA CRUDA This is for a headache where the scalp and head are supersensitive. Feels like a nail is being driven through the skull. Hyperactive with dozens of thoughts running around and around in the brain.

GLONOINUM Headache associated with heatstroke or sunstroke. This headache throbs in tandem with the heart beat; the pulse may be felt in the head. The pain is made worse by stooping or shaking the head.

IGNATIA AMARA Headaches that have been brought on by grief or loss.

PULSATILLA NIGRICANS This type of headache is often the result of eating too much rich food. The headache is accompanied by emotions that are like a roller coaster. The person will often feel like crying and will want pampering and sympathy.

RUTA GRAVEOLENS These headaches are the result of eye-strain, overwork, or anxiety of some kind. The pain feels much like a nail is being driven in and is centered in the forehead, often over only one eyebrow.

COMMON COLD

ACONITUM NAPELLUS To be taken when a cold is first suspected because of a tired, rundown feeling.

ALLIUM CEPA Symptoms resemble those you have when cutting onions (from which this remedy is made). The eyes are watery and the nose runs profusely. The nose becomes raw and sore very quickly.

FERRUM PHOSPHORICUM Mild cold, mild cough, mild fever, mild sneezing. The face will be very pale, but flushes easily with red spots appearing on the cheeks. Nosebleed. Physical and mental fatigue.

HEPAR SULPHURIS CALCAREUM Mucus moving from throat to ears or from ears to throat. Sinus involvement, greenish-yellow discharge, and heavy mucus that must be coughed up or blown out. The hoarse, dry cough moves into the chest where it becomes loose and rattling. There will be pain in the ears on swallowing.

NATRUM MURIATICUM For early stages of a cold. Sneezing is worse in the morning and the nasal discharge looks like runny raw egg whites. Sores develop in the nostrils and the person wants to be left alone.

PULSATILLA NIGRICANS Wonderful children's remedy, especially if the child wants extra attention and doesn't want to be left alone. During the day the nose runs profusely but at night both nostrils stuff up and breathing becomes very difficult. Pulsatilla patients, no matter how sick, are better for fresh air and distraction.

CONTAGIOUS DISEASES

GENERAL INFORMATION

Traditional medicine, at the present time, is treating childhood diseases such as measles, mumps, and chicken pox as horrendous, life-threatening problems. Except for rubella and pregnant women, this is a gross exaggeration. In fact, many researchers and physicians (both orthodox and alternative) have come to the conclusion that passing through these illnesses, in the natural order of things, actually strengthens the immune system. The immunity that is created as the body musters its forces and develops antibodies specific to that illness results in life-long immunity *and* increases the immune response to illness in general. There is no need to keep taking controversial booster shots, with their built-in immune suppressants.

No attempt is being made here to provide a detailed description of these remedies; a few distinctive symptoms, so that you can tell one remedy from another, are all that is listed with each one.

MEASLES

The early symptoms of measles are much like the common cold (as are the early symptoms of polio and rubella). It is remarkable how many of the same remedies have been employed around the world against both types of measles and against polio with good results. Although the Morbillinum variety of measles is well-known for the skin rash and the fever, it should be remembered that it is really a respiratory ailment. Often, with measles, the eyes also become sensitive to light.

Rubella (German measles) and the more common Morbillinum (measles) virus are not the same thing. Rubella and Morbillinum are not even found on the same basic viral family tree. Rubella, while the milder of the two diseases when contracted by children, can seriously compromise a fetus if the pregnant woman contracts this disease during the first 20 weeks of a pregnancy.

The MMR (measles-mumps-rubella) is a mixture of both measles strains, with mumps thrown in at the same time. The CDC (Center for Disease Control) says that pregnant women should NOT be vaccinated, nor should a woman get pregnant for at least 4 weeks after vaccination. While they admit that the slight fever and rash which often occurs after a child is vaccinated is a mild case of measles or rubella, they claim that this is no risk to pregnant women and their babies. These two claims—do not vaccinate or expose pregnant women to the MMR vaccine, and that the rubella illness created by the vaccine is not harmful—seem like contradictions to me. I advise women to err on the side of caution and avoid all children who have recently been immunized.

SUGGESTED REMEDIES

PULSATILLA NIGRICANS is often the first remedy selected because of its close match to the symptoms. Pulsatilla was also used for generations in some parts of the world as a preventative following exposure. The recommended dosage was once daily from the 3rd to the 7th day after known exposure.

ACONITUM NAPELLUS is also often given at the time of exposure. Distinctive symptoms include fever with chills, or coldness alternating with heat. The child will be thirsty for cold drinks and very restless.

ARSENICUM ALBUM The keynote with Arsenicum album is the unusual fatigue (described as a collapse state). The person will express restlessness but will be simply too tired to move. Arsenicum can also be given as a preventative.

BELLADONNA As always with Belladonna, the symptoms come on suddenly and develop rapidly. High fever and great sensitivity to movement, noise, temperature, and light is also part of a Belladonna picture.

BRYONIA ALBA The keynotes of Bryonia are a hard bounding pulse, dry cough, and such a deep chill that piles of blankets are desired. The child is worse for motion and just wants to be left alone.

EUPHRASIA OFFICINALIS Euphrasia is specific for measles with burning, itching, streaming eyes.

SULPHUR The important thing to remember about Sulphur is that it is a remedy for those times when a carefully selected remedy (that matched the symptoms well) has failed to produce the desired results. Use it to "kick start" things if progress has stalled out. Sulphur is also a first choice remedy for relapses of illnesses and symptoms.

MORBILLINUM NOSODE Morbillinum should be considered both for prophylaxis and treatment. Nosodes are especially indicated for never the same since situations.

MUMPS

Mumps is viral illness. Typically mumps strikes children between the ages of three and sixteen. When it occurs after puberty, it can cause complications in the ovaries, testes, or pancreas. The mumps patient is contagious up to 48 hours before the symptoms appear. Mumps is characterized by fever, followed by pain below the ear and swelling of the parotid, and sometimes, the salivary glands.

SUGGESTED REMEDIES

ABROTANUM ARTEMISIA This is an important remedy if, during the course of the mumps illness, any swelling develops in the testes of a male or in the breasts of a female. Either Abrotanum, Carbo vegetabilis, Pilocarpinum, or Pulsatilla nigricans should be given if this situation develops.

ACONITUM NAPELLUS is a remedy for the onset of the illness. A keynote is extreme restlessness and constant motion, in spite of being very ill.

BELLADONNA Patients, as always with Belladonna, experience very sudden onset of their illnesses. The child's face will be red, the pupils dilated, and there will be a great sensitivity to movement or touch. The left side will be more affected than the right and there will be intense, shooting pains. The child will be burning hot to the touch and extremely sensitive to cold.

BROMIUM ailments come on slowly—the exact opposite of Belladonna. The swelling will be worse on the left side and the child will be very irritable.

CARBO VEGETABILIS The keynote of Carbo veg is that the face is unusually pale and cold.

LACHESIS MUTA The pain is so severe that the child can hardly swallow liquids or food and jerks away if anyone approaches with the intention of touching them.

LYCOPODIUM The illness will begin in the right parotid gland, then move to the left. The person desires warm drinks.

MERCURIUS SOLUBILIS The person needing this remedy is extremely sensitive to both hot and cold.

PAROTIDINUM is a nosode. Used if recovery is not complete and there are symptoms of continued exhaustion and listlessness. Nosodes invite the body to complete the disease cycle and throw off the last vestiges of illness. Gelsemium sempervirens should be tried if the Parotidinum fails to produce the needed results.

PHYTOLACCA DECANDRA The indications for Phytolacca are swelling that is worse on the right side that extends to the region below the jaw (submaxillary region) and not just in the parotid. The glands will be rock hard with shooting pains on swallowing. There will also be an abnormal amount of swelling in the neck.

PILOCARPINUM Pilocarpinum is another remedy for occasions when the swelling drops into the testes or breasts. An early indication for this remedy is copious saliva.

PULSATILLA NIGRICANS Use Pulsatilla (or Abrotanum, Carbo veg, or Pilocarpinum) if there is swelling in testes or breasts. There will be pain in both ears, the child will chill easily, and be very whiney.

RHUS TOXICODENDRON With this remedy the swelling is abnormally huge and the glands beneath the jaw become highly involved. There is often painful stiffness in the joints, especially in the neck.

CHICKEN POX

Chicken pox is caused by the varicella-zoster virus. It is said that this virus may lie dormant for years and then reappear as shingles in adults. Chicken pox is the virus replicating throughout the cells of the body. With shingles, the virus appears to have lain dormant along a particular section of nerve cells and reactivates there at some future time when immune function is lowered for some reason. Persons with open shingles sores may infect others, but the newly infected person will get chicken pox, not shingles. Prevention, by maintaining a strong immune system, is the best plan.

SUGGESTED REMEDIES

ANTIMONIUM CRUDUM This remedy always includes a white coated tongue, irritability, and the sores get more itchy after a bath. The children are extremely sensitive to touch and usually have upset tummies.

APIS MELLIFICA The keynote symptoms are itching (of course, this is chicken pox) but with a stinging quality that is worse for the application of heat or if the person must be in a warm room.

ANTIMONIUM TARTARICUM The pox sores typically needing this remedy will appear slowly and be unusually large. The child will most likely have a dry cough.

BELLADONNA Belladonna symptoms come on suddenly and include a high fever with red cheeks, skin that is hot and dry to the touch, and a violent headache.

CARBO VEGETABILIS For low vitality and exhaustion, especially in the weeks after a bout of chicken pox.

DULCAMARA should be considered for rashes that are especially thick on the face and scalp with no fever.

MERCURIUS SOLUBILIS Useful if the abnormally large sores become infected. The child will be sweaty and thirsty and will feel worse at night.

RHUS TOXICODENDRON This is the most common remedy for chicken pox. Rhus toxicodendron is for the relief of intense itching and extreme restlessness, especially at night. If Rhus fails, try Urtica urens.

SULPHUR The child will be experiencing extremely itchy sores which they continuously scratch until they bleed. Sulphur is indicated if other remedies fail to work effectively and if the person is drowsy during the afternoon and restless and hot at night.

VARICELLA is chicken pox nosode. Variolinum and Malandrinum should be considered if a nosode is needed. Remember to use the nosode with an intercurrent remedy.

WHOOPING COUGH (PERTUSSIS)

Whooping cough is an acute infectious disease marked by fever and sticky mucus building up in the throat and lungs. There will be frequent attacks of spasmodic coughing as the body tries to rid the lungs and throat of the gelatinous, ropy phlegm. The coughing spasm lasts until the lungs are completely emptied of air; there is a whooping sound as the person finally takes in a large, gasping breath. Whooping cough often leads to pneumonia or enteritis, and was, in the past, often fatal to very small children and very dangerous even to older persons. Often whooping cough leaves its victims exhausted and weak and recovery is very slow.

There has been a resurgence of whooping cough type illnesses recently. Some researchers believe the beginning of this small resurgence has been brought about by vaccination programs. In spite of what is being published in the media, this is a few isolate incidences and not an epidemic caused by unvaccinated people. We have seen this and defeated it using alternative remedies, but it was a long and nasty fight!

SUGGESTED REMEDIES

Antimonium tartaricum, Arsenicum album, Belladonna, Carbo vegetabilis, Causticum, Cuprum metallicum, Coccus cacti, Corallium rubrum, Drosera rotundifolia, Ipecacuanha, Kali phosphoricum, Kali sulphuricum, Magnesia phosphorica, Natrum muriaticum, Phosphorus, Rumex crispus, Sanguinaria canadensis, and Spongia tosta. A few of these remedies are discussed here.

PERTUSSINUM is the whooping cough nosode. According to the Materia Medicas, this remedy can be used as a preventive or to treat the disease and is equally effective if the cough is from some other cause. Being a nosode, this remedy should probably be taken with an intercurrent remedy.

CARBO VEGETABILIS Spasmodic cough with burning the chest; bluish face; body may become blue and icy-cold; this remedy may be very effective during the recovery stage of this disease; alternate chills and fever; cold from the knees down.

KALI SULPHURICUM Rattling of mucus in the chest; post-influenza cough; a remedy for the last stages of whooping cough; engorgement of the pharyngeal mucus membrane.

DROSERA ROTUNDIFOLIA was praised by Hahnemann as a cure for nearly every case of whooping cough he ever encountered. A keynote is vomiting in an attempt to, or as a result of efforts to, clear the phlegm. Attacks follow each other very rapidly, giving the patient little rest night or day.

CUPRUM METALLICUM is for coughs accompanied by convulsions. The cough is so violent that suffocation threatens and the face and lips become bluish. Keynotes are rattling in the chest and relief from a swallow of cold water.

CORALLIUM RUBRUM is characterized by a smothering feeling and lack of air before the cough begins. The cough is short and quick. The child is utterly exhausted after each attack. Corallium is usually called for in the later stages of this illness.

COCCUS CACTI The mucus is long and stringy and comes from both the mouth and the nose, causing the child to strangle. Coccus is especially useful for bronchial catarrh after the whooping cough has passed.

BELLADONNA is for sudden violent paroxysms without mucus. Although the symptoms are not quite whooping cough, Belladonna is believed to shorten the disease when given early and symptoms match.

IPECACUANHA is for the child that becomes blue or pale with the loss of breath. There is great nausea; Ipec provides relief from the vomiting.

MAGNESIUM PHOSPHORICUM is a Schussler tissue salt that has been known to provide almost miraculous relief of whooping cough symptoms and is credited by some practitioners as saving lives.

PHOSPHORUS always great fatigue and debility; whole body trembles with the cough; larynx very painful; worse when lying on the left side; heat between the shoulder blades; worse from any motion; short naps ameliorate; enjoys sympathy.

SANGUINARIA This is an important remedy for whooping cough; most important action is on the spasmodic cough of whooping cough that often returns with every fresh cold; severe constriction of the chest with shortness of breath.

With alternative medicine, beginning treatment early—at the first sign that something is not quite right—is the secret to success. Following one remedy with another as the symptom picture changes also improves the outcome and shortens the illness. The beauty of homeopathy in contagious diseases is that, so often, the disease that was treated properly in the early stages never fully develops. The case does not even make it into the literature and statistics.

Whooping cough is not a disease of the past. Channel 10 news in Los Angeles reported in September of 2010 that the state had at least 4,000 confirmed cases of this highly contagious illness. The CDC reported 11,466 cases nationwide for 2010. In New Jersey, which has stringent vaccine policies, it was determined that 99% of the kids who came down with pertussis had been properly vaccinated. In the winter of 2010-2011 and again this last winter(2014-2015) there has been an illness going around whose picture looks very much like Pertussis (whooping cough). This illness has been miserable for adults and dangerous to little ones but does not seem to be very contagious.

RSV / SARS

The lungs are the most common organ of the body in which to come down with an infection. Illnesses that target the lungs may be either bacterial or viral in nature. Lower respiratory tract infections, especially viral ones, can pose a serious threat to the very young, the very old, and any person with a chronic or debilitating health problem. It is estimated that 35-50% of lower respiratory infections are viral. They are a major worldwide health concern.

I have lumped these two, RSV(respiratory syncytial virus) and SARS (severe acute respiratory syndrome), together on this page and probably should have included all other respiratory influenzas and hantavirus as well. When treating homeopathically, as has been stated before, the name of the disease is not relevant. Nor does it matter much whether the cause is viral, bacterial, chemical, or allergenic. It is the symptom picture and the response of the person to the first remedies given that guide treatment.

RSV, SARS, the wide variety of respiratory influenzas, and hantavirus exhibit many of the same symptoms. There are variations, of course, and variations among persons with even the same virus creating the problem. You should, as always, let the symptoms—with a heavy emphasis on the unusual and unique aspects of each case—guide your remedy choices.

Technically, SARS is a viral respiratory illness that is caused by a coronavirus that has been given only a provisional name, so far. In 2003 the United States reported only 192 cases of coronavirus-related illness and most of these cases were travelers returning from foreign countries. The appellation SARS, since it applies to a syndrome, is sometimes given to a variety of severe lower respiratory illness, especially in infants. More often, however, a lower respiratory illness will be diagnosed as RSV if the infant has been sick for more than a few days. This diagnosis will often be made long before any lab results have come back because RSV is the leading cause of respiratory infections in small children and is likely to be the cause of the problems.

To the physician, correct diagnosis is important. He needs to know if he is dealing with a bacteria which will likely respond to an antibiotic or one of the more dreaded viral illnesses. To the homeopath, there is no need to wait for lab work. The initial symptoms are all the guide that is needed.

Symptoms of SARS include sudden, high fever with chills or convulsions, rapid respiration, difficulty breathing, weariness, fatigue, mental confusion, muscle pain, swelling of the air spaces in the lungs which then fill with fluid creating viral pneumonia, rapid heart beat or—alternately—a slow heart beat with chest pain, and dizziness, sore throat or intense nausea with vomiting and diarrhea. Eventually there will be paralysis of the lungs, respiratory failure or failure of organs such as the heart, liver, or kidneys, with death resulting.

Frequently, with SARS, there is a relapse two or three days after the person seems to be on the way to recovery. There should be no slacking off in attention paid and remedies given—herbal and homeopathic—when improvement begins to be seen.

Symptoms of RSV include fever, breathing difficulties, bluish skin color due to lack of oxygen, cough, nasal flaring, stuffy nose, and wheezing. It should be noted that RSV usually begins with mild upper respiratory involvement and symptoms and then progresses to a more serious lower respiratory infection. Sick children should be watched closely for the retractile breathing that indicates lower respiratory compromise. In retractile breathing, the child's abdomen caves in under the ribs and sternum with each breath. This is a sign of serious lower respiratory problems. The child may be—probably is—in serious trouble. Oxygen deprivation and damage to organs is very near, if not already happening.

There is not a lot of literature yet published by homeopathic physicians outlining what they have learned and what remedies to use in SARS or RSV cases. Mostly that is the case because homeopathic physicians treat on symptoms, not on specific disease names. There are plenty of remedies identified for pneumonia, asthma, and other lower respiratory infections, however. The best thing to do is to repertorize the symptoms and make a list of possible homeopathic remedy choices, then narrow it to the one that most closely matches your observations.

SUGGESTED REMEDIES

Aconitum napellus, Antimonium tartaricum, Arsenicum album, Bromium, Carbo vegetabilis, Crotalus horridus, Ipecacuanha, Kali carbonicum, Kreosotum, Lachesis muta, Mercurius solubilis, Naphthalinum, Natrum sulphuricum, Phosphorus, Pulsatilla nigricans, Rhus toxicodendron, Sepia succus, Sulphur, the Veratrums and, of course, the RSV and SARS nosodes. This list of remedies would be effective against lower respiratory infections. Be sure to match the symptom pictures closely.

Aconitum napellus seems to hold the key to the first stages of these illnesses, followed by Natrum sulphuricum, Carbo vegetabilis, Ipecacuanha, or Chelidonium. If symptoms persist after these treatments, Crotalus horridus might be considered.

As always, the remedy should match the totality of the person's symptoms. As the case progresses, remedies will need to change to match the new symptom pictures. Please remember this in every situation!

One homeopath from New Jersey says that possible SARS remedies need to include all of the remedies that are for severe asthma. He also found remedies that are usually associated with recovery from vaccinations to be useful. These remedies would include Carbo vegetabilis, Spongia tosta, and Thuja—to name just a few. His reasoning is that SARS originated with a live-virus Corona virus vaccine used in Asia on animals.

Common first-response remedies such as Arsenicum album, Carbo vegetabilis, Lachesis, Phosphorus, Sulphur, and the Veratrums are mentioned on this list. My personal opinion is that, when dealing with a contagious epidemic disease you do something—anything—and do it quickly at a high potency and then, while the body is balancing as far as it is able with that remedy, study the symptom picture and the possible remedies for a really close match. As always, change the remedy as the symptom picture changes.

The nosode, **Tuberculinum aviaire**, seems to be the most closely matching nosode remedy. **SARS and RSV nosodes**, when obtainable, might also be helpful.

INFLUENZA

In 1918 a flu outbreak in the United States took more human lives than were lost by America altogether in Word War I. Over 500,000 people died in one two year period alone. Influenza viruses produces enough toxins to cause organ failure and death. Most strains of the flu virus attack the body rapidly and serious organ failures follow very quickly. The scariest statistic that I found with the 1918 flu epidemic was the number of younger adults that died in this pandemic. Nearly half of the people who lost their lives to this virus were between 20 and 40 years old.

SUGGESTED REMEDIES

The principle remedy used in homeopathic hospitals that were having far greater success rates than traditional hospitals was Gelsemium sempervirens. Arsenicum album and Veratrum album were also being used as follow-up remedies. The remedies suggested for SARS/RSV should also be considered.

ARSENICUM ALBUM *This is the first remedy I would reach for if I suspected the flu—intestinal or respiratory.* In fact, I have used it in both intestinal and respiratory flu. Arsenicum's picture is one of exhaustion, but with anxiety and restlessness. There is marked lack of vitality. There is often great nausea with retching and vomiting, that if not corrected will lead to emaciation and weight loss. The abdomen will be swollen and painful with an enlarged spleen and liver. The person will crave cold water but even a small sip will be vomited immediately.

If there is respiratory tract involvement, there will be shortness of breath with suffocative catarrh, especially when not sitting up. Often there will be darting pain through the upper, predominantly right, lung. Arsenicum patients usually experience high fever, a throat that is so swollen that swallowing is difficult to impossible. There is usually vertigo—almost a loss of consciousness—during coughing or retching spells.

Arsenicum album is especially useful for cases where the person recovered well but later has a relapse of the same bacteria or virus.

CROTALUS HORRIDUS being a snake remedy, has hemorrhagic symptoms. This is the remedy that most closely matched the symptoms of the 1918 flu because of the black and stringy nosebleeds, swollen and bleeding tongue, bleeding gums, and the vomiting of blood. Other symptoms of Crotalus include retinal hemorrhages, headache with pain in the occiput and center of the forehead. The headache is accompanied by vertigo. There is also liver destruction with hemorrhage, and eventually, hemorrhaging from every orifice of the body.

GELSEMIUM SEMPERVIRENS *Gelsemium seems most useful for the very early stages, and in the recovery or convalescent stages of the flu with other remedies needed in between.* Gelsemium is useful for preventing NSS (never the same since) situations and in creating full and complete recoveries

A keynote of Gelsemium is great fatigue; the fatigue is so total there is often great trembling and drowsiness deep enough to be considered a stupor. Sometimes the person becomes delirious. The pulse is weak and slow, with pain in the heart region and a feeling of oppression in the chest. With Gelsemium the face is usually hot and has a flushed appearance—unlike Arsenicum whose picture is blueness. In spite of the flushed face and heat, Gelsemium's picture includes chills running up and down the spine.

Intestinal symptoms include a feeling of emptiness in the stomach and bowels accompanied by cramping, diarrhea, and very little appetite or thirst. There is gnawing or spasmodic pain in the transverse colon with painful contractions and tenderness in the right iliac region.

Respiratory symptoms include pain running from the throat to the ear with the feeling of a large lump in the throat that cannot be swallowed. There is much mucus in the bronchial tubes that cannot be coughed up. This creates a continuous violent cough that results in retching, dizziness, and blurred vision. Almost any illness that would benefit from Gelsemium has muscle soreness.

VERATRUM ALBUM The major keynote of Veratrum is that all symptoms are sudden and violent. The symptoms are often accompanied by fainting and the face is pale, bluish, and cold with the tip of the nose being very cold and a cold sweat on the forehead. The person looks, from the very beginning of the illness, as though they are about to collapse and if the illness becomes more severe, a total collapse state with blueness will exist.

Respiratory ailments will include heart palpitations with audible respiration and a lot of mucus in bronchials and throat. In intestinal or stomach flu the vomiting is violent and profuse with diarrhea that often becomes violent purging. An **unusual keynote** is voracious appetite and thirst, even when ill, but eating and drinking, particularly cold things, causes immediate vomiting. The nausea and vomiting are worse with even the slightest movement. Also there are large hard stools followed by watery diarrhea, then more hard masses.

With influenza, it is important that your response be quick, intense, thorough, and that you follow up all the way through the recovery and the convalescent stages. Many remedies have never the same since influenza in their symptom pictures, and you do not want the people you work with to have that story to tell. Remember Arsenicum album for relapses of the same, or similar, virus or bacteria.

There are nosode remedies being made available of various strains of the flu. Remember, a nosode needs to be given concurrently with another remedy which matches the current symptom picture of the disease and that this picture may change as the course of the illness progresses. Of course, herbal remedies, essential oils, and excellent nutrition should also be employed.

While nosodes are important remedies, it should be remembered that the first rule of homeopathy is "the law of similars" not "the law of exacts." The very best remedy, generally, is the remedy that matches the symptoms—the person when they are as well as they ever get combined with the symptoms of this ailment they are experiencing right now. The nosode will cover the "now" symptoms but will not touch the other half—the person they are. Nosodes, when used, require an intercurrent remedy and, many times, something else altogether may be a better choice.

MORE CONTAGIOUS AND EPIDEMIC DISEASE

DIPHTHERIA

Diphtheria is bacterial in nature and affects the tonsils, throat, nose, and sometimes the skin. Diphtheria, like all contagious diseases, can manifest quite differently from person to person. In some, the throat will be excruciatingly sore. In others the membrane, which is adhering to the pharynx, larynx, and trachea is the scariest and most uncomfortable symptom. There is generally fever and fatigue. Heart and nerve damage are not uncommon. Diphtheria is passed by droplet transmission when a sick person has coughed, sneezed, or even laughed. This disease can also be spread by handling used tissues or drinking from the same glass as an infected person. Worldwide statistics on diphtheria show it in decline at the moment.

SUGGESTED REMEDIES

Arsenicum album, Apis mellifica, Bromium, Kali bichromicum, Kali chloricum, Kali permanganicum, Lachesis muta, Lycopodium clavatum, Mercurius cyanatus, Mercurius solubilis, Nitricum acidum, Phosphorus, Phytolacca decandra, Rhus toxicodendron and Thuja occidentalis.

ARSENICUM ALBUM is generally given at the first sign of illness, before the symptoms have really defined what is going on. Often it is all that is needed. In diphtheria some keynote symptoms are a very swollen throat—inside and out, dark colored membrane, edema, thirst, fever with flushing of the face, and the feeling of being very tired and worn down.

APIS MELLIFICA is keynoted by edema and scanty urine. The throat is glossy red and swallowing is difficult. The membrane of Apis-type diphtheria (will likely respond to Apis) is greyish, dirty-looking and tough. Apis is always nervous and fidgety.

KALI BICHROMICUM is most useful when the throat has deep ulceration. The accompanying membrane is yellow looking and often streaked with blood. There is pain in the chest, often moving out to the shoulders and neck when coughing. There is swelling in the glands that is not seen when other remedies are needed instead of Kali bichromicum.

LACHESIS MUTA is a true polycrest for diphtheria; probably no other remedy has been used with good result as often. Indications for this remedy include great sensitivity and pain in the throat, usually beginning and remaining worse on the left side. The throat is purplish, swelling is pronounced, and it is difficult to breathe unless sitting up. Other snake remedies, such as Crotalus and Naja, should also be looked at and considered.

LYCOPODIUM acts in a very different manner from Lachesis. The pain usually begins on the left side of the body and then moves to the right, remaining more pronounced on the left side, however. Like Lachesis, the person is worse when waking from sleep and the throat feels worse for drinking, particularly cold drinks. With Lycopodium, there is a general aggravation from 4 to 8 pm. Flaring of the nostrils is also seen.

NITRICUM ACIDUM The two outstanding keynotes of Nitricum acidum in diphtheria are 1) nausea and the vomiting of all food, and 2) a greyish membrane in the nose along with the throat symptoms. The nose also fills with sores that are quite painful. The pulse is intermittent and the throat is so sore and painful that swallowing is difficult.

DIPHTHERINUM is, of course, the nosode. Nosodes, generally, are not usually effective by themselves. The remedy that most closely matches the symptoms should be used intercurrently with Diphtherinum.

MERCURIUS CYANATUS (an odd choice, in some ways) has been used successfully in the Children's Hospital in Paris for diphtheria. Higher potencies are used in this hospital. Diphtherinum is also used if there is any post-diphtheria paralysis.

TUBERCULOSIS

Tuberculosis (also called consumption, especially in previous centuries) is an ancient disease—as ancient as man's recorded history. Once thought to have been eradicated in the United States, there have been yearly increases in cases in recent years. These emerging strains are increasingly more resistant to antibiotics.

Since tuberculosis was one of the major causes of death in the 1800's when homeopathic hospitals were more common, we have a fairly substantial base of knowledge about possible homeopathic treatments. Homeopathic remedies have an excellent record in slowing the progress of the disease and providing an improved quality of life, sometimes for many years, and there are an impressive number of recorded cures.

Diocletian Lewis began his studies in an orthodox medical school and then later converted to homeopathy. He cured his wife of tuberculosis in 1851, and his "Consumption Cure" became famous throughout America. Unfortunately, I could find no record of exactly what homeopathic remedies this medicine contained. In 1852, Emily Dickinson, an American poet, was cured of suspected tuberculosis by William Wesselhoeft (a German orthodox physician who converted to homeopathy).

A very famous homeopathic physician named James Kent, as well as many other homeopathic practitioners both today and in the past, believed that the bacillus was not the real cause of tuberculosis. They found that the tuberculosis came first and then the bacillus moved in as a scavenger of dying lung tissue. They list the Psoric miasm, with a possible tandem presentation with the sycosis miasm, as the underlying, genetic cause.

SUGGESTED REMEDIES

Agaricus phalloides, Arsenicum album, Arsenicum iodatum, Bryonia alba, Calcarea carbonica, Hepar sulphuris calcareum, Iodum purum, Kali carbonicum, Kali iodatum, Lachesis muta, Lycopodium clavatum, Medorrhinum, Phosphorus, Psorinum, Pulsatilla nigricans, Senecio aureus, Silica terra, Stannum metallicum, Sulphur, and Theridion curassavicum. Tuberculinum is the nosode of Tuberculosis, and Bacillinum is often also employed.

Please note that once again that great polycrest remedy, Arsenicum album, is found on the list of homeopathic remedies that have been used successfully in the treatment of a dreaded contagious disease.

POLIO

Polio is one of the most dreadful and dreaded of all the epidemic diseases. Paralysis was so total that breathing was compromised and kidney damage resulted for approximately 2% of sufferers in the epidemic of the late 1940s early 1950s. (I was born in 1951.) Death is very uncommon from polio, but certainly possible.

The onset of polio very much resembles the common cold. Following the cold-like symptoms, there is a high fever and pain in the affected muscles. The muscle pain is not much different from the achiness that often accompanies the high fever you might get with a particularly virulent cold or flu.

Homeopathic physicians around the world treated everyone they could find with Lathyrus sativus, especially if they had cold symptoms with fever coming on as is described in the materia medicas under Lathyrus sativus. They speculated that they probably treated many cases of incipient polio since they saw almost no cases of polio itself (only numerous summer colds) in children that they had treated, even when surrounding hospitals were inundated with serious cases.

Polio, its possible causes and cures, were mentioned a bit during our discussion of the polio miasm—although, as I hope you remember, the disease and the miasm are not the same thing. Just as the poliomyelitis virus is not the cause of the miasm named polio, it is certainly not the *only* cause of polio-like paralysis.

POLIO AND PESTICIDES

There is an interesting body of statistics that links polio epidemics to pesticides. I will cite just a few from among the long list of research papers by referring to the work of only one researcher on this topic. I am indebted to Jim West, HARpub, for the charts and statistics bearing his name which follow. When I contacted him by phone to obtain permission to copy and quote his work, he was delighted that what he had learned was of interest to someone and that word of it was being spread to others. Much of the next few pages, and both of the charts, are part of his research.

(a) The first patent for a pesticide sprayer occurred in 1874. This was followed by a large amount of pesticide development and an intense marketing effort. By 1887, when the first polio epidemic hit, pesticides were a major portion of the profits of many companies who manufactured chemical pesticides.

(b) In 1908 a polio epidemic in Massachusetts occurred in three manufacturing towns that were located within a 20 mile radius of each other. These towns were involved with the production of carbon tetrachloride. This chemical was used as a fumigant, insecticide, herbicide, cleaning solvent, and in the extraction of cotton seed oil. The highest polio rates in this 20 mile area were in a town with three cotton mills, giving this town a double whammy of the fumes—once during production of the tetrachloride and again when the tetrachloride was used during the cotton oil extraction. *An interesting side note: No exclusively breast fed infant acquired polio during this epidemic.*

(c) In 1915, Hooker Chemical and DOW Chemical began the first high-volume production of chloral benzene in the United States at Niagara Falls. This chemical is used in herbicides, insecticide, moth control chemicals and polymer resins. This sudden surge of chloral benzene production coincides in time and place with and is considered by many statisticians to be the probable cause of the epidemic of central nerve system diseases that followed the next year all across the region between Niagara Falls and New York City. Strangely, the epidemic lasted only six months, June to November, with 82% of cases occurring in just 8 weeks.

(d) 1921 President Roosevelt acquired polio in the Bay of Fundy, off the coast of Canada. This bay is downstream from several major industries that dumped these same chemicals into the rivers during the previous months. This bay was the site of a study of the horrible effects of high levels of DDT on porpoises.

(e) 1942-1962 was the great polio epidemic in the United States. This era is known as the "Pesticides as a Panacea" era. In other words, if you have a problem of any kind, dump a pesticide on it—won't hurt and it might help and, besides, your neighborhood chemical company will make some money.

(f) In 1945 U.S. troops in the Philippines experienced polio epidemics where casualties from the disease were very high. These soldiers were routinely doused with DDT. The notable thing about this statistic is that the surrounding populations, not doused with DDT, were unaffected by the epidemic.

(g) Another very interesting statistic occurred in the 1958 polio epidemic in three New Jersey counties. These counties include the Gayonne and Linden petroleum refineries. Lab work conducted on the victims indicated that only 65% of them had the poliomyelitis virus in their blood. Although the other 35% had identical symptoms their cases were re-categorized as other things, thus driving the polio statistics for the area way down. (Please note that the name change did not change the nature of the suffering experienced.)

It needs to be remembered that the polio virus and the polio miasm discussed previously are not the same thing. Apparently, it is possible to have many of the nasty symptoms of polio without exposure to the virus. The poliomyelitis virus manifests in different ways in different people and can cause paralysis and death. It would seem from studies and statistics, that a similar condition (referred to by homeopathic physicians as a polio miasm) can be created by exposure to certain chemicals. It, too, can result in paralysis and death.

The majority of the soldiers in the Philippines—statistic (f) above—did not have blood work done, so there are no statistics available on whether or not the virus was present in their systems. In 1952, and again in 1964, there were major rabies outbreaks in the Philippines. These outbreaks corresponded with mosquito abatement programs undertaken by the government. Rabies is a paralytic disease that is physiologically and symptomatically similar to polio but believed to be caused by a different virus. The Philippines continue to this day with agriculture and antimosquito campaigns that include the use of DDT.

(h) In the United States, DDT was outlawed for use as a pesticide in 1972. This followed the presentation to Congress of scientific evidence of the toxic effect of DDT on people and animals. T***he EPA was created as a result of this testimony and one of the first acts of this new governmental agency was to begin a phase-out and eventual ban of this pesticide.*** DDT was linked to the thinning of the egg shell of birds, both domestic and wild, with the bald eagle population being particularly hard hit. Bald eagle populations made dramatic recoveries following the banning of DDT.

(i) In 1983, legislation allowed the return of DDT for use in insecticide blends. In March of 1984, post-polio was recognized as an emerging epidemic in former polio victims. Post-polio victims in the United States, by the end of 2004, were estimated to be 600,000.

(j) One last statistic: In 2003-2004, Nigeria recorded the highest post-polio case count worldwide. WHO (World Health Organization) conducted the largest DDT anti-malaria campaign ever in that country in 2003. These campaigns were not in effect in the previous years in this country and the polio case count was very low. Once again, the rise in post-polio cases happened simultaneously with the DDT anti-malaria campaign.

Please see the two very interesting charts provided by Jim West following the list of possible homeopathic remedies.

The purpose of these statistics is to bring to your attention two facts. These are:

1) The world of Samuel Hahnemann, with only three basic miasms, no longer exists today. Because of our world-wide love affair with chemicals and medical interventions and, perhaps, changes in the basic structure of society, we have many more miasmic patterns to deal with.

2) When you are in pain and cannot accomplish what you want to accomplish or have the quality of life that you want, it is the cure and not the cause that matters most. This is especially true if the cause is chemically-based poisons over which we have so little control in our environment today. Pesticide programs go forward in counties all over this fine nation year after year.

There are other forms of paralysis besides those being labeled as polio. Originally polio was called infantile paralysis. It was considered a problem of childhood and caused entirely by the poliomyelitis virus. Subclinical polio, as mentioned earlier, resembles a cold at its onset. As the virus, or the chemical poison, advanced, muscles were affected. If the brain and spinal cord became involved, paralysis of the lungs, intestinal tract, and/or heart muscle occurred.

Paralysis in old age is often the result of either a rupture or a blockage of one or more blood vessels of the brain. The question in my mind is whether these ruptures are a normal part of aging or the result of the myriad of drugs our older people are encouraged to take.

HOMEOPATHY—WHERE DEEP HEALING OCCURS

Of all the modalities of alternative medicine that I know and use, I find homeopathy at deep levels the most effective at eradicating really serious problems and strengthening the system against the onslaught of bacteria, viruses, and chemical poisonings of any kind. I love essential oils and I use herbal remedies every day, but homeopathy is, so many times, where the really deep work gets accomplished. This seems to be true no matter what the cause of the malady.

SUGGESTED REMEDIES FOR POLIO-LIKE PARALYSIS

Aconitum napellus, Belladonna, Causticum, Dulcamara, Gelsemium sempervirens, Lathyrus sativus, Nux vomica, Opium, Phosphorus, Plumbum metallicum, Rhus toxicodendron, and Veratrum album

ACONITUM NAPELLUS Aconitum is characterized by the suddenness of the attack and by the extreme restlessness, mentally if not physically, of the patient. There is much anguish and fear, with this symptom worsening towards evening. The person feels like death is iminent and they mention this frequently. Other keynotes are dry, hot skin and unquenchable thirst for very cold drinks.

ARSENICUM ALBUM Once again this amazingly versatile remedy is seen. This is a remedy everyone should become very familiar with. It should be used as a first response/preventative remedy whenever several of its keynote symptoms are seen. In polio, the keynote is paralysis of the legs with atrophy of the muscles following very quickly. There will be burning pains.

BELLADONNA Sudden paralysis on the right side with a severe burning sensation—all the symptoms related to Belladonna come on suddenly. If the attack of paralysis is severe enough there may be semiconsciousness or delirium. The face is usually bright red and the eyes are dilated.

CAUSTICUM The picture of this remedy includes burning pain in the stiffened joints and congestion in the lungs. Causticum is keynoted by its mental symptoms which include intolerance for any kind of injustice, becoming angry at hearing bad news, and obsessive attachment to various causes.

CHINA OFFICINALIS There will be terrible pain in the lumbar region. Paralysis begins as trembling and numbness, progressing to paralytic stiffness in all joints, especially on rising.

GELSEMIUM SEMPERVIRENS With Gelsemium, the symptoms include the legs feeling aching, tired, and incredibly heavy. There will be a steadily increasing lack of muscular coordination accompanied by trembling. The keynote that sets Gelsemium apart from other remedies is the gradual nature of the onset of the paralysis—unlike the suddenness of the Belladonna picture. A person needing Gelsemium is thirstless, and in spite of the seriousness of their illness, seems quite apathetic about it and overly anxious about other things of lesser importance.

LATHYRUS SATIVUS The ingestion of this plant causes serious damage to the spinal cord which result in spasms and possible paralysis of the lower limbs. This is the picture of the homeopathic remedy. Interesting note: when lying down the legs can be moved from side to side but cannot be lifted. Legs are cold during the day but become hot and burning at night.

NUX VOMICA The paralysis of Nux vomica is mostly of the lower limbs, forcing the patient to drag his feet while walking. There is often involuntary drawing-upward motions of the right hand. Other keynotes of the distinctive Nux vomica remedy should also be seen.

OPIUM The paralysis of Opium is almost painless. There will be deep sleep with heavy, stertorous breathing. Preceding and accompanying the paralysis will be involuntary twitching and jerking of limbs. There is unusual perspiration over the upper body and obstinate constipation.

PHOSPHORUS Paralysis starts with the toes and fingers and then spreads over the entire body. Like Causticum, there is burning in the affected parts. For Phosphorus to be effective, there should be a worsening of symptoms when lying on the left side and a craving for cold foods. The Phosphorus personality includes a very sensitive nature.

PLUMBUM METALLICUM With Plumbum there is progressive paralysis, usually of single muscles or parts of the body. The extensor muscles are affected first and more drastically, so that the person will suffer from hand or foot dropping. Other keynotes of Plumbum are excessive depression, ringing in the ears, and distinct blue lines in the gum margins very near the teeth.

RHUS TOXICODENDRON The paralysis of Rhus toxicodendron comes on gradually, with the early attacks following overwork or exposure to dampness. The stiffness centers in the joints but there will be tearing pains in the tendons, ligaments, and tissues. The back, neck, and sacrum are also often involved. The pain and stiffness is usually a little better for motion.

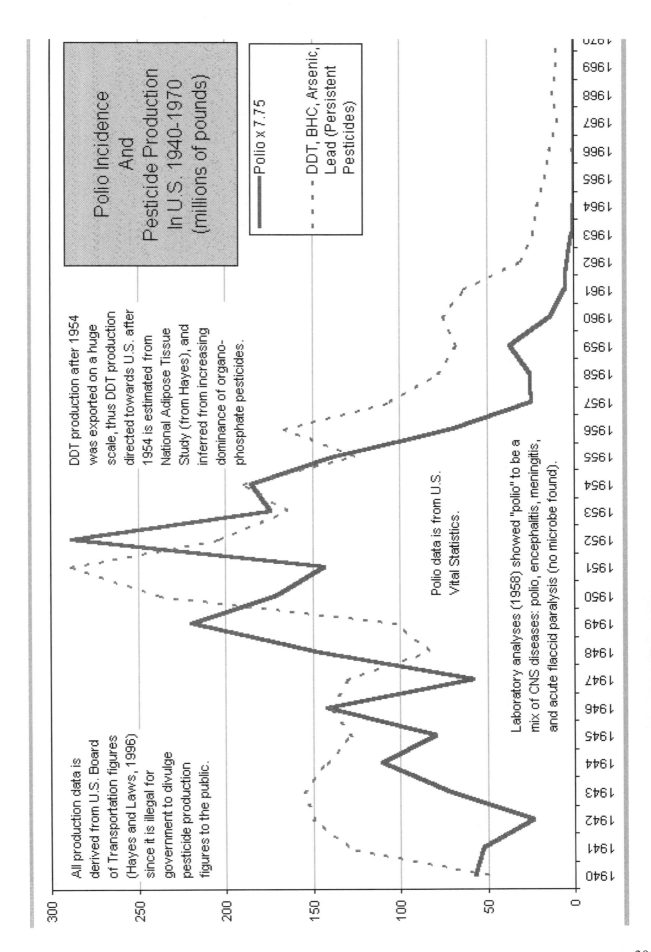

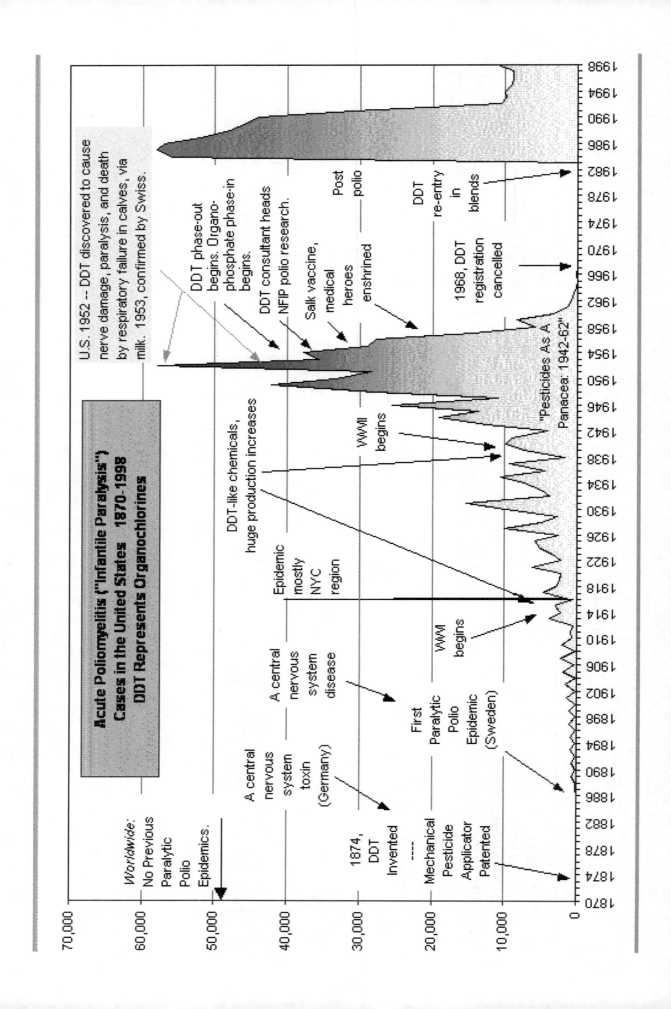

VACCINATIONS AND THE POLIO EPIDEMIC

I have many pages of information—statistics, mostly—about various vaccines, their side effects, and their role in the disappearance of childhood diseases and epidemic diseases. I am going to limit myself to a few statistics from only two or three sources, notable among them are the publications of the U.S. Vital Statistics and statistical compilations by New York City Health Commissioner, Haden Emerson, concerning the polio epidemic that occurred during my very early childhood. (Paragraphs (1) and (2) below.)

If you set aside the rhetoric found in medical publications and newspaper reports and use statistics alone, some interesting facts emerge.

(1) The great polio epidemic actually occurred from 1942, with gradually increasing cases in the following years through 1962. Polio was firmly entrenched in the United States **before** the troops returned home, and was **not** a post-war epidemic at all, as some would have us believe. Since the United States led the world in polio cases just before the end of the war, the returning troops obviously did not bring it home with them, although they certainly did their share of suffering from it.

(2) The epidemic declined dramatically (took a nose dive, really) in the early 1950's, a full 3 years before the Salk vaccine was approved for sale, and 4 years before vaccine programs got underway. In other words, the Salk vaccine enters the picture only **after** polio's dramatic decline. The evidence points **away** from the Salk vaccine as a factor in the decline of polio, and certainly cannot be reasonably construed as proof for the victory of vaccines over the poliovirus, as we have so often been told.

In fact, according to renowned researcher and author Neil Z. Miller (quoting information from government sources published as early as 1956).

> When national immunization campaigns were initiated in the 1950's, the number of reported cases of polio *following* mass inoculations with the killed-virus vaccine was significantly greater than *before* mass inoculations, and may have *more than doubled* in the U.S. as a whole.

For example, Vermont reported 15 cases of polio during the one-year reporting period ending August 30, 1954 (before mass inoculations), compared to 55 cases of polio during the one-year period ending August 30, 1955 (after mass inoculations)—a 266% increase.... and in Massachusetts they swelled from 273 to 2,027—a whopping 642% increase (see table below).

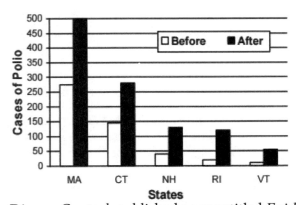

The CDC, Center for Disease Control, published a paper titled *Epidemiology of poliomyelitis in the U.S.* **one decade after the last reported case of indigenous wild virus associated disease** (bolding is mine) in which they stated that "the live-virus vaccine had become the dominant cause of polio in the United States." According to figures published by the CDC, every case of polio in the U.S. since 1979 was caused by the oral polio vaccine. This vaccine was eventually banned.

One last statement: As reported by the Washington Post, Dr. Jonas Salk, creator of the killed-virus vaccine used in the 1950's and used almost exclusively in the U.S. from the early 1960's to the year 2000, testified that the vaccine was the "principal if not sole cause" of all reported polio cases in the U.S. since 1961.

DR. SHEPHERD ON VACCINATIONS

It was Dr. Shepherd's belief, based on her vast experience, that when travelers or soldiers were forced to have multiple vaccinations against several diseases at, or near the same time, the effect on the body and the cells was devastatingly confusing.

She found that when soldiers who had these multiple inoculations later developed influenza, it was generally a particularly virulent type and did not respond either to the usual conventional or homeopathic treatments. Interestingly, according to her reports, their flu responded to Pyrogenium (in high potency). Pyrogenium is recognized as a major remedy for the ill effects of vaccines and the vaccinosis miasm. (Please see pages 131 and pages 282-3 for further mention of Dr. Shepherd.)

VACCINE SAFETY

The Vaccine Adverse Event Reporting System—VAERS—conducted an independent study using the government's own vaccine database for the early 1990s. They reported (OPV Vaccine Report Doc #14) that during a period of less than five years there were 13,641 *documented* adverse reactions to the oral polio vaccine. 6,364 of these were serious enough to require hospital emergency room visits. 540 people died.

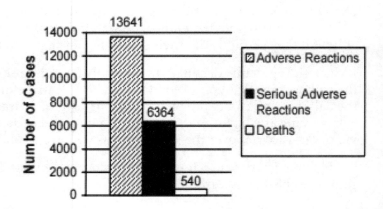

Have I checked these sources rather than just take Mr. Miller's word for them? Of course I have. That is what I do—and anyone can do with a little bit of time and effort. A good place to start looking for Mr. Miller's sources is his website, *thinktwice.com*. He puts source references at the end of his articles better than anyone else I have ever known.

TO VACCINATE OR NOT TO VACCINATE

What caused the decline of polio? More importantly, what caused polio and what was the cause of the decline in the number of polio cases? Just as importantly, what has caused the rise of post-polio syndrome in the last few years? And most important of all, are vaccines safe and effective and should my child be vaccinated?

Neil Z. Miller, despite the overwhelming research and statistics that he has uncovered, does not presume to tell parents to reject vaccinations out of hand. He says

> Every year, more than 12,000 people in the United States file vaccine-damage reports with the FDA documenting serious adverse reactions to mandated immunizations (children are mainly affected). The FDA estimates that this represents just 10 percent of the true rate. Yet, even these figures pale in comparison to the number of cases of new diseases scientifically linked to inoculations. MMR and autism, polio vaccines and cancer, the hepatitis B vaccine and multiple sclerosis, the Hib vaccine and diabetes, to name just a few.

> For these reasons, among others, I am opposed to *mandatory* vaccines. I do not recommend for or against the shots. I want everyone to think through this enigmatic and controversial subject on their own. I believe that parents are capable of obtaining the facts and making knowledgeable choices regarding the care and welfare of their children.

I whole-heartedly agree with the above statement—even with my own grandchildren! But please, parents, do your "homework" and do it with an open mind, looking at all sides of the issue using government and other research reports and statistics!

GROUP A STREP

Strep A (also known in the medical community as group A strep) has several strains, one of which is referred to as the flesh-eating bacteria. It is estimated that 10% of the world's population are carriers of group A strep but experience nothing more than a nasty case of seemingly ordinary strep throat.

According to Eileen Nauman, DHM, in her book Homeopathy for Epidemics, the statistics for strep in the United States show 20 to 30 million cases every year. (That is quite a range for a statistic, but it is the best I could find since strep is often diagnosed by symptoms, not by a blood test.) The CDC estimates that 15,000 of these cases are invasive strep A and 5% to 10% are of the necrotizing, or flesh-eating, variety. Eileen Nauman has an excellent description of what these strains of bacteria do to the proteins of the body.

Are these bacteria alarmingly deadly? Yes. Jim Henson, the famous Muppeteer, died of a strep A infection when his blood pressure dropped too low to sustain his life. Even if the blood pressure can be stabilized, group A strep stimulates the overproduction of T-cells and cytokines (usually the good guys of our immune responses). Too many cytokines damage the cells lining the blood vessels allowing fluid to leak out. This reduces blood flow, and organs and tissues begin to die due to lack of oxygen.

Another protein in this deadly bacteria goes directly to work on other body tissues by breaking down the proteins from which they are made.

Group A strep seems to like the extremities of the body. After the bacteria has entered the blood stream, it finds an area where circulation has been compromised (such as a bruise) and begins to churn out its distinctive toxins. The toxins create an even larger area of dead cells, giving the bacteria an ever increasing area in which to grow. Increased growth results in even more dead tissue until amputation of the infected parts becomes the only way to halt the destruction of this life-threatening infection.

SUGGESTED REMEDIES

Aconitum napellus, Crotalus horridus, Lachesis muta, Pyrogenium, Rhus toxicodendron, and—once again—Arsenicum album. Lachesis muta has proven particularly effective and should be considered first, especially if the characteristic mental and emotional symptoms fit.

Can homeopathy be effective against such deadly killers? I believe so, but I also know that a lifelong habit of dealing with any symptom the minute it arises is necessary to give you the running start needed in a serious battle. If you wait until some invader has a foothold, there is a good chance that the remedies you use will be too late to be of much use. If you see in yourself any trace of a miasm rearing its ugly head, deal with it today, and you will most likely spare yourself the trouble of a truly life-threatening invasion.

HEPATITIS

Hepatitis (A, B, C, D, E) are all viral liver diseases. Another form, toxic hepatitis, is the result of chemicals, injections, and the ingestion or absorption of environmental toxins. The symptoms of hepatitis include fatigue, poor appetite, nausea, pain in the abdomen above the liver (upper right side), and a slight fever. The urine becomes dark and jaundice (a yellowish discoloration of the skin) appears.

Hepatitis (especially the B, C, D & E varieties) can result in lifelong infection, cirrhosis (scarring) of the liver, liver cancer, liver failure, and death. The western medical world has no known cures, although they do claim to have vaccines which are effective preventatives, and are, supposedly, relatively risk free. The homeopathic Materia Medica lists over 100 remedies for hepatitis and liver disease.

Hepatitis A is a highly contagious, but rarely fatal, disease. It is extremely common in developing nations where unsanitary conditions and contamination of food or water supplies spread the virus very rapidly.

Hepatitis B is the best-known form of viral hepatitis. This strain can be severe and can lead to chronic hepatitis and cirrhosis of the liver. Hepatitis B is spread by close personal contact with an infected person, or by exposure to infected blood. Hepatitis B was commonly transmitted through transfusions of contaminated blood in past years. New blood tests and stricter screening have largely eliminated this threat.

Hepatitis C also frequently results in chronic hepatitis and cirrhosis. Some experts believe that body piercing and tattoos are the major source of exposure to this strain.

Hepatitis D is the most serious, and thankfully, the rarest form of viral hepatitis. Hepatitis D is only seen in people who have hepatitis B and occurs primarily among intravenous drug users. Hepatitis D is often fatal.

Hepatitis E occurs most often in epidemic form and is linked to poor hygiene and contaminated water supplies. This strain often leads to serious illness in pregnant women. This strain of hepatitis is seen almost exclusively in developing nations, and occasionally, as the result of a major natural disaster.

SUGGESTED REMEDIES

Aconitum napellus, Arsenicum album, Belladonna, Carcinosin, Carduus marianus, China officinalis, Crotalus horridus, Hepar sulphuris calcareum, Humulus Lupulus, (listed as Lupulus humulus by Murphy) Hydrastis canadensis, Lachesis muta, Lupulus humulus, Lycopodium clavatum, Myrica cerifera, Natrum sulphuricum, Nitricum acidum, Phosphorus, and Podophyllum.

ACONITUM NAPELLUS This remedy is generally used in the beginning stages of all types of hepatitis, but is used especially for new born babies suffering from jaundice brought on by toxic conditions in the mother that have created stress on the baby's liver. A keynote of Aconitum, even in infants, is extreme restlessness.

ANDROGRAPHIS PENICULATA This little known remedy is useful for jaundice that has resisted other remedies and treatments. It has been successful against both hepatitis B and C when the polycrest remedy, Chelidonium majus, had proved unsuccessful.

ARSENICUM ALBUM Once again we see Arsenicum album as the first response remedy. Keynotes of Arsenicum album are weakness, rapid weight loss, and coldness with lack of vital heat. A 1M, or even a 10M, remedy is recommended.

CARCINOSIN is mentioned here because it is indicated for Hepatitis B developing after a blood transfusion. The person usually has a history of recurrent attacks of bronchitis, pneumonia, or repeated viral infections. Carcinosin has also proven effective for relief of chronic relapsing hepatitis.

CARDUUS MARIANUS is specific to inflammation of the left lobe of the liver. The symptoms will be worse for lying on the left side.

CHAMOMILLA VULGARIS This remedy is most often used in cases of infant jaundice. The baby will be irritable and fussy with bilious vomiting.

CHELIDONIUM MAJUS The keynotes of this remedy are pain under the right rib cage and abdominal pain after eating. The pain comes from hepatic and gallbladder obstruction. In cases where Chelidonium would be most effective the symptoms will worsen when the person lies on their right side and there will be strong desires for hot food and drinks.

CHINA OFFICINALIS The keynotes of China in hepatitis are sensitivity to touch of the right side of the abdomen and abdominal bloating that is not in the least relieved when passing the copious amounts of gas.

CROTALUS HORRIDUS Crotalus is not a common remedy for hepatitis, but is very useful if the disease is manifesting any hemorrhagic symptoms. This type of hepatitis seems to be limited to cases that originated with a contaminated blood transfusion.

LACHESIS MUTA is indicated mostly for hepatitis due to alcoholic liver failure.

LUPULUS HUMULUS Lupulus, like Chamomilla, is indicated for jaundice in infants. Keynote is profuse sweating.

LYCOPODIUM CLAVATUM This remedy is keynoted by shooting pains across the lower abdomen. The pains move from the right side to the left. There is excessive flatulence and the symptoms are aggravated by breads.

MYRICA CERIFERA is indicated for carcinoma of the liver from chronic hepatitis and for metastasis into the liver from prostatic carcinoma.

PHOSPHORUS This is a remedy for acute, extreme hepatic conditions such as fatty degeneration of the liver, with associated jaundice and cirrhosis associated with pancreatic disease.

PODOPHYLLUM PELTATUM This remedy's leading indication is a history of repeated (chronic) jaundice. There is pain in the right hypochondrium. Another keynote is that the person has never been completely well since the first attack of hepatitis. Mental keynotes are an irritable temperament with suicidal thoughts.

For chronic hepatitis of either toxin or environmental origins the suggested remedies are: Carduus marianus, Carcinosin, Lachesis muta, Natrum sulphuricum, Phosphorus. Psorinum is considered to be the leading nosode.

SMALL POX

Small pox was declared eradicated by the World Health Organization in 1980. The last known case of small pox occurred in Somalia in 1977. There are 2 clinical forms of small pox, variola major and variola minor. Variola major had severe symptoms and a high mortality rate of between 20% and 40%. Variola minor had less severe symptoms with a low mortality rate of about 1%. The virulent form was responsible for the death of millions of people and the blinding and scarring of millions more.

SUGGESTED REMEDIES

Historically, small pox is said to be prevented with the nosodes, **Variolinum** and **Malandrinum**. Both of these nosodes are also used in the aftermath of cancer and for treatment of the vaccinosis miasm.

Historically effective homeopathic remedies for the treatment of small pox include Antimonium tartaricum, Arsenicum album, Belladonna, Bryonia alba, Hepar sulphuris calcareum, Kali bichromicum, Mercurius solubilis, Pulsatilla nigricans, Rhus toxicodendron and Thuja occidentalis.

MALARIA (AND OTHER INTERMITTENT FEVERS)

Malaria is caused by a parasite called plasmodium, which is transmitted via the bites of infected mosquitoes. The parasites multiply in the liver, and then infect red blood cells. The plasmodium carrying mosquito is indigenous to tropical areas.

Symptoms of malaria include fever, headache, and vomiting. These symptoms usually appear between 10 and 15 days after the mosquito bite. Malaria can quickly become life-threatening by disrupting the blood supply to vital organs. In many parts of the world, the parasites have developed resistance to commonly used malarial medicines and mosquito abatement sprays.

There are books and web sites that claim both cures and ways to prevent malaria. As always, repertorizing by symptom and using common sense are advised. Don't forget to work with any NSS that may appear.

SUGGESTED REMEDIES

Abrotanum artemisia, Artemisia annua, Arsenicum album, Belladonna, China officinalis—also known as Cinchona, Chininum arsenicosum, Eucalyptus globulus, Eupatorium perfoliatum, Gelsemium sempervirens, Helleborus niger, Ipecacuanha, and Natrum muriaticum. The nosode is called Malaria Co. and is a combination nosode of all four strains of malaria.

TYPHOID FEVER

Typhoid fever is a life-threatening illness caused by the bacterium Salmonella typhi. In the United States, approximately 400 cases occur each year—most of which are brought in by travelers from developing nations. In considering homeopathic remedies for the treatment of typhoid, it must be remembered that there are four distinct symptom pictures. The basic constitution and susceptibility of the sufferer will give you clues as to which of the types you are dealing with. Of course, there will be symptoms from each group in every case and remedies that will cross over from one list to another. It is the preponderance of symptoms of one type that sets the remedies apart from each other.

The four symptom types of typhoid are 1) usually in the early stages, cases exhibit a large number of brain and nervous system symptoms, 2) typhoid with predominantly abdominal symptoms, and 3) cases in which the abdominal and cerebral symptoms are evenly matched, and 4) more severe cases where the blood becomes deranged and hemorrhagic conditions exist.

Typhoid may begin with trembling, great heaviness and weariness, exhaustion and debility, and pain in the forehead that deteriorates into delirium. The source of these symptoms is in the brain and in the nerves. If the face is red and the eyes are bright, **Belladonna** should be considered as the first remedy. There will also be red spots like flea bites or blood stains on the chest, face, neck, and abdomen.

SUGGESTED REMEDIES
WHEN BRAIN/NERVOUS SYSTEM SYMPTOMS DOMINATE
Belladonna, Hyoscyamus niger, Lachesis muta, Opium, and Stramonium. When one or more of these remedies has accomplished all that it can, follow up with Arsenicum album, Bryonia alba, or Sulphur.

SUGGESTED REMEDIES
WHEN ABDOMINAL SYMPTOMS DOMINATE
Arsenicum album, Carbo vegetabilis, China officinalis, Colchicum autumnale, Mercurius solubilis, Nux moschata, Secale cornutum, and Sulphur

CHOLERA
Cholera is an acute, diarrheal illness caused by infection with the bacterium Vibrio cholerae. Symptoms, in addition to severe watery diarrhea, include nausea, vomiting, muscle cramps specific to the abdominal area, dehydration, and eventually shock. Cholera ranges from mild, almost symptomless attacks in a few people to a sudden onset illness that can lead to hypovolemic shock and death in only a few hours. Homeopathy has been used in many epidemic situations with good results. (Statistics about cholera and homeopathy are found elsewhere in this book. Please see Cholera in the Index.)

Homeopathic remedies have a unique way of dealing with contagious epidemic diseases. They do not kill the bacteria outright, leaving the body to cope with the dead bacteria as well as the remaining live ones which continue to multiply and mutate, becoming stronger and more deadly. Instead, homeopathic remedies strengthen the body's own defenses and support the eliminative channels at the same time. But even with the best homeopathic care, cholera (and other severe and acute contagious diseases) are going to take some intense fighting and recovering from.

It is homeopathy's great statistical record with cholera in the previous 2 centuries that gives me hope that in the event of major epidemics we might have some good statistics similar to those experienced by homeopaths in previous centuries—at least among the alternative community.

In epidemics in the last two centuries, homeopathic hospitals consistently showed a far greater survival rate than surrounding hospitals. It is estimated that untreated, cholera has a mortality rate of 50% to 60%. The mortality rate in both England and the United States in the 1800's and 1900's, under conventional treatment, was between 40% and 55%. The worst homeopathic hospital statistics came in at 9%, with some hospitals turning in mortality rates of 3%. (Yes, these were documented cases, complete with names, addresses, and outcomes that were verified by government officials.)

SUGGESTED REMEDIES
Aconitum napellus, Arsenicum album, Calcarea carbonica, Camphora, Carbo vegetabilis, Cuprum metallicum, Hydrocyanicum acidum, Laurocerasus officinalis, Phosphorus, Podophyllum peltatum, Veratrum album.

ACONITUM NAPELLUS This is another excellent first response remedy. Keynotes are the suddenness of the onset of the illness, burning and cutting pains in the abdomen, and nausea usually accompanied by sweating. The Aconitum person usually feels great fear and shows great anxiety. There is restlessness from the anxiety and worry.

ARSENICUM ALBUM Once again we see this great polycrest remedy in the list of possible remedies. Arsenicum would make a good first response remedy whenever a person is showing cramping or violent pains in the bowels, nausea with vomiting, and sudden great weakness with restlessness.

CALCAREA CARBONICA A major keynote of Calcarea carbonica is that all symptoms are aggravated by milk, fruit, and anything containing even small amounts of sugar. In cholera, there is great flatulence which has an overpowering offensive odor before the diarrhea and vomiting set in. It is during this stage that Calcarea can be employed with great effectiveness.

CAMPHORA has achieved fame in homeopathic circles for its efficacy in cholera epidemics. The keynote symptoms are, of course, vomiting and diarrhea, but the diarrhea, when it finally comes after much cramping and feeling of fullness and distention is extremely violent. There is stiffness in the muscles and dry skin that feels cold to the touch. There is great fatigue, chilliness, shock, a bluish tint to the skin, and a state of collapse from the intensity of the attack on the nervous centers and immune system.

CARBO VEGETABILIS With Carbo veg there is debilitating weakness and a rapid pulse. The diarrhea almost always comes first, followed by frequent vomiting after the diarrhea has improved. The lips have a blue tinge and the respiration rate slows.

CUPRUM This remedy is known mostly for the intensity of the muscle spasms and abdominal cramping which are accompanied by cold sweats. Like Camphor, there is a bluish tint to the skin and great coldness.

HYDROCYANICUM ACIDUM has the same coldness and blueness of other remedies. The keynote is that the vomit is very dark, almost black.

PODOPHYLLUM PELTATUM There is vomiting, of course, but the keynote symptom is the watery diarrhea. There is a distinct lack of appetite, and everything eaten, no matter how mild, aggravates. The vomit is hot and frothy and belches smell like rotten eggs.

VERATRUM ALBUM Violent and continuous vomiting with a cold feeling in the stomach keynote this remedy. There is general coldness with extreme cold feeling in the abdomen and profound prostration, blueness, and weakness. Cold perspiration on the forehead is another unusual symptom.

Q FEVER

Q Fever is caused by the Coxiella burnetii bacteria and is distributed globally because cattle, sheep, and goats are the primary carriers of the tick that harbors this bacteria. Infection has also been found in a wide variety of other domesticated animals.

Bacteria organisms are excreted in milk, urine, feces and are shed in high numbers in the amniotic fluids during birth. These organisms are resistant to heat, drying, and many common disinfectants, making it possible for the bacteria to survive for long periods of time.

Infection of humans occurs by inhalation of these organisms from contaminated air such as barnyard dust. Humans are very susceptible to the disease, and very few organisms may be required to cause infections. Farmers and others who work with animals on a daily basis, and especially, people who work on the killing floor of slaughter/meat packing houses are at higher risk for becoming infected with this bacteria.

Acute cases of Q fever begin with the sudden onset of one or more of the following symptoms: high fevers (up to 104-105 F), severe headache, general fatigue, myalgia, confusion, sore throat, chills, sweats, non-productive cough, nausea, vomiting, diarrhea, abdominal pain, and chest pain. The fever stage usually lasts for 1 to 2 weeks but weight loss and other symptoms can occur and persist for a long time. Many patients will develop pneumonia and some will develop hepatitis. Most people recover within a few weeks without any treatment.

The symptoms of Q fever, as you can see from the above description, are similar in many ways to those of influenza. You will find many of the same remedies on this list as you have found on previous pages for influenza type illnesses.

Chronic Q fever is characterized by infection that persists for more than 6 months and is a much more serious disease. Q fever may become chronic as soon as 1 year or as long as 20 years after the initial infection. Heart valve problems are a serious complication of chronic Q fever, and heart valve problems seem to be an indicator of susceptibility to Q fever. Transplant recipients, cancer patients, and those with chronic kidney disease are most likely to have a Q fever progress to a chronic condition.

The mortality rate of chronic Q Fever is as high as 65%. Q fever is not a common problem in the United States and statistics do not show a rise in cases over the last 10 years.

SUGGESTED REMEDIES

Apis, Arsenicum, Baptisia tinctoria, Belladonna, Carbo veg, China officinalis, Crotalus horridus, Ferrum metallicum, Gelsemium, Hyoscyamus, Lachesis, Nitricum acidum, Phosphorus, Phosphoricum acidum, Rhus toxicodendron, Stramonium and Veratrum album. When cardiovascular symptoms appear the indicated remedies shrink to Crotalus horridus, Lachesis muta and Phosphorus.

WEST NILE VIRUS (AND OTHER FLAVIVIRUS ILLNESSES)

Flavivirus family related illnesses, West Nile virus, dengue fever, and yellow fever, can cause—among other nasty symptoms—encephalitis, which is an inflammation of the brain. Encephalitis can be relatively mild or become very serious. It is the occasional serious symptoms that are cause for alarm (and even panic) among the medical community, the news media, and the public.

DISTRIBUTION OF WEST NILE VIRUS

West Nile is one of the most widely distributed flaviviruses. It is found in most states in America (although in 2010 the Center for Disease Control documented only 1 case in Idaho and 2 in Utah). The Idaho Department of Health and Welfare tells a different story. They claim that mosquito-borne human infections were first seen in Idaho in 2004. In 2006, Idaho led the nation in reports of human illnesses associated with West Nile Virus with 996 cases reported to the department of health.

Although spread by the bite of a mosquito, it is now known that migratory birds serve as amplifying hosts. There is, however, no evidence that a person can become infected by handling dead host birds. Dogs, cats, and other domestic animals may also be amplifying hosts, but here again, there is no evidence that humans can be infected by anything other than the bite of a mosquito.

An infected bird (or animal), dead or alive, is bitten by a mosquito. The virus is sucked up in the blood where the mosquito acts as an incubator for the virus. The incubation period, in the mosquito, is about 10 days, after which the mosquito can transmit the virus to others.

The mortality rate for West Nile Virus is very low. The majority of people bitten by infected mosquitoes develop no symptoms at all. But I have known people, and whole families, become very ill and need a lot of time and care to recover.

The West Nile Virus carrying mosquitoes fly only at dusk and dawn, so a little common sense and caution can go a long way towards prevention.

SYMPTOMS OF WEST NILE VIRUS

When a person has been bitten by an infected mosquito, it takes anywhere from 3 to 14 days for symptoms to appear. Many times West Nile is mistaken for other ailments with similar symptoms. Only a lab test can confirm, with any confidence, that the symptoms are being caused by the West Nile Virus. (With homeopathy, it doesn't matter. The remedy you use, based on the symptoms, will cause the immune system to react against the cause of those symptoms, whatever the cause may be.)

Mild to moderate symptoms include: fever, headache, body aches, a rash on chest and arms that usually lasts about a week, diarrhea, abdominal pain, loss of appetite (anorexia-like symptoms), vomiting, swollen lymph glands, muscle pain, stiff neck, and eye pain.

About 1 in 150 cases of West Nile Virus progresses to more severe neurological diseases. These symptoms appear more often in the elderly than in the general population. Encephalitis (inflammation of the brain tissue) is more commonly reported than meningitis (inflammation of the membrane covering the brain).

Severe symptoms include very high fever, severe muscle weakness, flaccid paralysis, serious gastrointestinal disturbances, disorientation, and even coma. Other severe conditions, with their definitions—thankfully these are quite rare—include ataxia (lack of coordination in the muscles), damage to the cranial nerves, myelitis (inflammation of the spinal cord leading to a variety of symptoms including loss of feeling to parts of the body, loss of bladder control, etc.), optic neuritis (loss of vision, loss of color vision, increased sensitivity to light, and pain when moving the eyes), and polyradiculitis (inflammation of the nerve roots which can lead to just about any horrible symptom you can imagine, including respiratory insufficiency).

With the above list of symptoms, it is easy to see why this virus is one of the most publicized and feared of the viral diseases. An ounce of prevention is really worth a pound of cure in this case. Homeopathy has great potential, especially if symptoms are treated immediately.

SUGGESTED REMEDIES

As you can see from the descriptions of the symptoms, they are many and varied, and some of them are quite unique. It will be necessary to look closely at each suggested remedy to see which one is the best match in the most areas for a particular person.

Ammonium carbonicum, Apis mellifica, Arsenicum album, Belladonna, Bryonia alba, Carbo vegetabilis, China officinalis, Crotalus horridus, Cuprum metallicum, Eupatorium perfoliatum, Hyoscyamus niger, Mercurius solubilis, Phosphorus, Rhus toxicodendron, and Sulphur.

CYTOMEGALOVIRUS

The name, cytomegalovirus, comes from 2 Greek words meaning "large celled." This genus of virus is more commonly known as Herpesviridae (herpes viruses) and includes the subfamily HCMV (also known as human herpes virus-5, HHV-5, or CMV). Another subfamily of this genus includes the herpes simplex viruses 1 and 2 (HSV-1 and HSV-2). Other subfamilies of the cytomegalovirus genus include the Epstein-Barr virus, which is present in many cases of Chronic Fatigue Syndrome, and the varicella-zoster virus, which is responsible for chicken pox.

All cytomegaloviruses share a characteristic ability to remain latent within the body over long periods of time. Impairment of the immune system by medications or disease can reactivate the virus from a latent or dormant state to an active symptomatic state.

HHV-5, or CMV, is found throughout all geographic locations and socioeconomic groups. Government statistics show that CMV infects between 50% and 85% of adults in the United States by the time they reach 40 years of age, depending on geographic location. (Scary statistic—I wish I thought it was incorrect!) Transmission of CMV occurs from person to person—not through food, water, or animal carriers. This virus may be transmitted by saliva, urine, or other bodily fluids. CMV can be sexually transmitted and can also be transmitted via breast milk, transplanted organs, and from blood transfusions. Exposure through a blood transfusion happens only rarely.

For most healthy persons who acquire CMV sometime during their lifetime rather than at birth, there are few symptoms and no known long-term health consequences. If symptoms are experienced, they are usually a mononucleosis-like syndrome with prolonged fever and a mild hepatitis. Once a person becomes infected, the virus remains alive, but usually dormant, within the person's body for life. The major concern with CMV is the risk of infection to an unborn baby if the mother is infected during the pregnancy.

CONGENITAL CMV

If a pregnant woman is infected with CMV, her developing baby may be at risk for a congenital (meaning from birth) CMV disease. CMV remains the most common cause of congenital viral infection in the United States. The CDC (Center for Disease Control) estimates that about 1 in every 150 children is born with congenital CMV infection.

For infants who are infected in utero by their mothers, two potential problems exist. These are:

(1) Generalized infections which may occur in the infant shortly after birth. Symptoms may range from moderate enlargement of the liver and spleen with accompanying jaundice to serious illness and death. With treatment, most infants with CMV disease survive. However, 80% to 90% will have complications within the first few years of life that may include hearing loss, vision impairment, and varying degrees of mental retardation. For pregnant women and their babies, CMV is a serious threat.

(2) Another 5% to 10% of infants who are infected, but are without symptoms at birth, will subsequently have varying degrees of hearing, mental, or coordination problems.

Many of the remedies suggested for the treatment of this virus are polycrest remedies. If a pregnant woman is treating herself homeopathically for everyday ailments and discomforts, she is likely to eradicate the virus by one of the remedies she is using before it can create problems for her unborn child.

PREVENTION
Basic hygiene habits are all that is required to avoid infection. Everyone, and pregnant women in particular, should be very careful about drinking from another person's glass. Hands should be washed thoroughly with hot soapy water after changing a child's diaper and diapers should be disposed of carefully and properly. Glasses and eating utensils should always be washed in hot soapy water, not just casually rinsed.

SUGGESTED REMEDIES
Homeopathic treatment of herpetic viruses have been shown to stimulate the body to throw off the encapsulated or buried virus so that future infections or compromise of fetal health is avoided.

Remedies that have been demonstrated to be effective against this family of viruses include Arsenicum album, Causticum, Graphites naturalis, Kali chloricum, Lachesis muta, Mercurius solubilis, Natrum muriaticum, Petroleum oleum, Rhus toxicodendron, Thuja occidentalis and Variolinum.

Mononucleosis-like symptoms, enlarged spleen and liver, and the Epstein-Barr virus can be treated using regimens which include the following remedies, as appropriate: Arsenicum album, Causticum, Carcinosin, Gelsemium sempervirens, Kali iodatum, Mercurius solubilis and Phosphorus.

Neurological damage (hearing loss, vision impairment): Causticum, Gelsemium sempervirens, Natrum muriaticum and Phosphorus. Causticum is the leading remedy for viral-caused neurological damage.

HERPES SIMPLEX

HSV-1 and HSV-2 (herpes simplex viruses) are also members of the cytomegalovirus genus. HSV infection causes fluid-filled blisters which form in small clusters and then continue to spread. Fatigue, irritability, low-grade fever, slow healing of cuts, infections around the fingernails, and whitlows (hardened skin around the fingernails) are other signs of infection.

These viruses are carried from person to person in body fluids such as saliva. The initial infection often occurs during childhood when well-meaning relatives subject children to on-the-mouth kisses. Other sources of infection include carelessness in dish washing habits or children being allowed to share drinking glasses and eating utensils. Once the virus has entered the body, it 'creeps' along neural pathways and establishes a home-base.

HSV-1's site of latency preference is the trigeminal ganglion, a collection of nerve cells near the ear. From this spot, outbreaks of blisters tend to occur on the lower lip or face. They occur most often when the body is under stress or the immune system has been compromised or overloaded in some way.

HSV-2 seems to prefer to lodge in the nerves at the base of the spine or sacral area. Symptoms appear in the genital areas. Fatigue, stress, and lowered immune response, as listed above, are usually present with both types of infection (HSV-1 and HSV-2).

One of the main characteristics of Herpes viruses is their resistance to traditional medication and the fact that it can go dormant only to appear again and again. Any treatment targeted only at the eruptions has absolutely no chance of eradicating this virus.

SUGGESTED REMEDIES
BEFORE BLISTERs APPEAR
Apis mellifica, Croton Tiglium, Lachesis muta, Natrum muriaticum, Rhus toxicodendron, Sepia succus, Vaccininum

SUGGESTED REMEDIES
Apis mellifica, Arsenicum album, Borax veneta, Croton tiglium, Graphites naturalis, Lachesis muta, Mezereum, Rhus toxicodendron, Sepia succus, Vaccininum

APIS MELLIFICA Useful at the first sign of burning that indicates an impending eruption of blisters with accompanying herpes symptoms. Constant whining and restlessness are part of the Apis picture.

ARSENICUM ALBUM Eruptions come with a burning sensation and many small blisters. Eruptions on the lips often spread to the inside of the mouth and genital eruptions spread to the anal area. Shortness of breath (this symptom occurs most often when the blisters have been suppressed by allopathic treatment). Once again, please note how often Arsenic album fits the symptom picture of an oncoming disease, especially in the early stage.

BORAX VENETA Thrush in infants is one typical picture of Borax. The baby's mouth feels hot to mother's nipple and the child lets go and cries with pain or refuses to nurse at all. If the mother is also suffering from herpes, either HSV-1 or HSV-2, her milk will be thick and foul tasting.

CROTON TIGLIUM This homeopathic remedy, indicated mostly for women, should be utilized when there is great redness, intense itchiness, and sensitivity in the area. Croton tiglium has vesicular eruptions on both the face and the genitals in its symptom picture. Although the eruptions itch horribly, scratching only makes them worse.

GRAPHITES NATURALIS is often a remedy for people—both men and women—who are overweight. The lesions are large and very itchy and often target the corners of the mouth.

LACHESIS MUTA Lachesis muta is mostly suitable for women who tend to have genital herpes outbreaks just before their periods. The eruptions of a Lachesis nature are particularly open, raw, and burning.

MEZEREUM is indicated if the blisters are filled with a whitish liquid. The blisters, which are found on the insides of the lips and at the corners of the mouth, evolve rapidly into sores with itchy crusts.

NATRUM MURIATICUM Indicated before the blisters have formed when there is nothing more than a characteristic tingling sensation in the area. The eruptions of Natrum mur tend to worsen during the day.

PETROLEUM OLEUM is mostly used for HSV-2 (genital herpes) that has spread to the anus and thighs. The eruptions tend to worsen during the winter months and improve in the summer.

RHUS TOXICODENDRON is indicated and should be taken as soon as the characteristic stinging sensation appears. Eruptions, when present, will be many small blisters that itch intensely at night.

SEPIA SUCCUS is another remedy (like Lachesis) that is indicated when the outbreaks come on just before a menstrual cycle. There should be some of the characteristic signs of Sepia such as heavy feeling in the genital area, laxness of tissues generally, and feelings of being overburdened or bothered by family responsibilities.

ARBOVIRAL ENCEPHALITIS

There are four main virus agents where symptoms may progress to encephalitis in the United States. These are eastern equine encephalitis, western equine encephalitis, St. Louis encephalitis, and La Crosse encephalitis. All are transmitted predominantly by mosquitoes, although they may be carried by bed bugs, ticks, and other such insects.

Most human infections result in symptoms which are difficult to tell from the flu. Onset may be gradual and insidious—just not feeling well and then gradually getting worse. On the other hand, symptoms may come on suddenly with fever, headache, neuralgias, malaise, and occasionally, physical and mental prostration. In either case, infection may lead to encephalitis (defined as inflammation of the brain). Encephalitis is extremely serious, too often progressing to a fatal outcome or permanent neurologic damage. Fortunately, only a small proportion of infected persons progress to encephalitis.

Experimental studies have shown that at least some invasion of the central nervous system generally follows initial virus infection. Problems may include swelling of the brain until there is loss of the centers of the brain which control autonomic breathing. Another complication of viral infection is a simultaneous bacterial pneumonia. There are no commercially available vaccines for humans for these diseases.

Jamestown Canyon and Cache Valley viruses are related to the LaCrosse strain of Arboviral Encephalitis. These two "cousin viruses" rarely cause encephalitis. LaCrosse encephalitis initially presents with fever, headache, nausea, vomiting, and lethargy. Severe disease occurs commonly in children under the age of 16 and is characterized by seizures, coma, paralysis, and a variety of neurological damage after recovery.

In each of these diseases, there are initial flu-like symptoms followed by a small percentage of people getting the much more serious attack to the brain and spinal cord. Here is yet another reason to treat any symptoms, but especially flu-like ones, immediately. Homeopathic remedies are an especially good method of treatment because they are prescribed according to symptom pictures. Whether the cause is bacterial, viral, or something else entirely is not usually relevant to the success of the treatment. This makes it possible to begin treating long before medical tests have discovered the source of the problem. Treatment should begin, every day of our lives, the moment we notice that they don't feel quite right.

SUGGESTED REMEDIES FOR FLU-LIKE SYMPTOMS

Arsenicum album, Apis mellifica, and Gelsemium sempervirens.

SUGGESTED REMEDIES FOR NEUROLOGICAL INVOLVEMENT

Agaricus phalloides, Apis mellifica, Argentum nitricum, Belladonna, Gelsemium sempervirens, Hyoscyamus niger, Natrum sulphuricum, Phosphorus, Rhus toxicodendron, and Stramonium. These remedies could also be useful for spinal meningitis.

AGARICUS PHALLOIDES The abdomen is distended with violent pains that extend through to the lumbar region of the back. Frequent vomiting, with suppressed urine and fatty degeneration of the liver make this a remedy for extreme, sudden, and scary types of flu or flu-like illnesses.

APIS MELLIFICA The Apis picture includes frothy mucus-filled vomiting with diarrhea. The abdomen is extremely tender with rumbling and pain. There are usually heart palpitations of a violent type and inflammation of the kidneys. Apis is a slow acting remedy. It often needs to be continued—**if the symptoms match—for a day or two before improvement occurs; do not give up on the remedy too soon.**

ARGENTUM NITRICUM Symptoms include colic with much gas and abdominal distention, lassitude, and weariness. The cerebral symptoms include headache with coldness and trembling.

ARSENICUM ALBUM Arsenicum is the first remedy I would reach for with flu-like symptoms of unknown origin especially if there was lack of vitality or sudden weight loss. Look for liver and spleen enlargement as further indications for this remedy. The headache often leads to vomiting and the symptoms will alternate between the head and the stomach. There will be extreme nervousness and anxiety with constant changing of position. Please become well acquainted with this remedy's symptoms.

BELLADONNA Symptoms come on suddenly, and usually, violently. Belladonna is a remedy that acts upon the brain and nerve centers. Symptoms include twitching and trembling. The face will be unusually red and the eyes very bright. Abdominal symptoms include extreme sensitivity to touch, tenderness, and swelling.

GELSEMIUM SEMPERVIRENS The picture of Gelsemium includes great fatigue, trembling, dullness of thought, and various degrees of motor paralysis. Gelsemium is renowned as a remedy that strengthens the nerves.

HYOSCYAMUS NIGER The Hyoscyamus picture is one of a brain and nervous system in serious disorder. There will be weakness and nervous agitation, confusion and even delirium. The behavior can become mania of a particularly quarrelsome and even obscene nature. Nausea will be accompanied by burning pain and vomiting which leads to vertigo and convulsions.

NATRUM SULPHURICUM In the classical homeopathic literature, Natrum sulphuricum is thought of as a remedy for the consequences of head injury. In the case of encephalitis, the symptoms would be the result of the inflammation in the brain brought about by the viral attack.

Symptoms include periodic attacks of mania, with sensitivity and suspicion. There is often depression and suicidal impulses. The stomach and abdominal symptoms, while present, are quite general and are not as important to the choice of remedy as the mental and emotional symptoms, especially with this remedy.

PHOSPHORUS A keynote of Phosphorus is ravenous hunger during a fever, great hunger just before an attack of sickness, hunger soon after eating, and low blood sugar with headaches when going too long without food. The brain feels tired and there is loss of memory. The mind wanders off; there is a pronounced inability to keep the mind focused on any one thing. This spaciness comes with irritability and occurs when a meal is missed. Every aspect of the Phosphorus picture shows mental and emotional sensitivity.

RHUS TOXICODENDRON has a large and varied symptom picture. Some keynotes, as they relate to flu-like symptoms and encephalitis, are dullness of mind, mild delirium, incoherent speech, forgetfulness of both recent events and names, and inability to hold the mind on one subject. There is almost always an anxious sureness that some terrible thing is about to happen to themselves or someone close to them. Physically there is pain in the ascending colon and soreness around the navel. There is a feeling of a lump in the abdomen. Vertigo often accompanies the other symptoms.

STRAMONIUM This remedy, somewhat like Hyoscyamus, shows cerebral/spinal cord damage to a great extent. Symptoms include paranoia, manic depression with rapid changes from joy to extreme sadness. There is a lot of terror, dread of darkness, and desire for light and company. There is no relief even in sleep because sleep is filled with frightful dreams. There will be nausea and vomiting of mucus and green bile accompanied by diarrhea. This remedy antidotes Belladonna, so be careful of taking them as part of the same regimen.

EBOLA (FILOVIRUS STRAINS)

Among virus strains is a particularly nasty family called Filovirus, so called because they all look like long snakes or worms (filaments) under a microscope. I mention it here in this book, even though the United States has so far been spared an outbreak, because it is virulent and it is posed in a perfect position to be the next epidemic of historic plague proportions. The panic of 2015 concerning Ebola, although blown out of proportion by the media, did give the public some idea of what is only too possible where epidemic diseases are concerned.

HISTORY OF THE VIRUS

In 1967, simultaneous outbreaks of this new strain of virus occurred in two German cities and in Yugoslavia. 38 people were infected with 7 deaths. The commonality in the blood streams of all of the victims was that this was a substrain of filovirus that was named Marburg, after the first city where an outbreak occurred. The other common denominator was a Ugandan green monkey being processed in labs in all 3 cities.

The virus then disappeared until 1975 when 3 cases of this horrible hemorrhagic fever were reported in Johannesburg, South Africa. The first case was a man who had just returned from Zimbabwe.

In 1976, the next attacks erupted, again simultaneously in two locations—Zaire and the Sudan. It was much more severe with a total of 550 cases, 430 of which resulted in death—a 78% kill rate. The strain of virus common to these attacks was given the name Ebola. It was some time before the scientific community realized that Ebola was the same strain called Marburg in 1967.

In 1979 there was another small outbreak in the Sudan with 34 cases and 22 deaths. A year later the virus was identified in a Kenyan man who had recently visited Uganda, in the same area where the 1967 green monkeys had been captured. The green monkey seemed to be the culprit carrier and thousands of specimens were taken from Uganda, Zaire, and the Sudan. No filovirus, or antibodies to them, were found!

Scientists and virologists are completely mystified. Only one thing is certain. This strain of virus, called Ebola around the world now, is the most lethal killer the world has ever seen. It makes the black plague of Europe look like child's play, in comparison.

There is no traditionally accepted medical treatment available for filoviruses, no vaccine, no antibiotics that have proven even vaguely helpful, and no homeopathic remedies that have ever been tried against it.

SPREAD OF THE EBOLA STRAIN

In 1990 Ebola cases were discovered on the docks in Philadelphia. All cases were quarantined and an epidemic prevented. In April of 1995 another Ebola epidemic broke out in Zaire. An infected man took an airplane trip from Africa to Canada. Fortunately, he was symptomatic by the time he reached the Canadian airport and airport officials had him quarantined while tests were run.

Quarantine of travelers displaying symptoms is the only protection we have from this virus which has a 7 to 21 day incubation period.

It seems amazing to me—in this time of traveling around the world by plane—that some world travelers have not returned, asymptomatic at the time they passed through airport checkpoints, and started epidemics simultaneously around the world, even here within our own borders.

The Ebola virus is distantly related to the viruses that cause measles, mumps, and rabies. It is also related, in a general way, to the parainfluenza virus (which causes colds in children) and to the respiratory syncytial virus (which causes RSV in infants and proves fatal to AIDS patients). Symptoms of Ebola include the overall body rash that is typical of measles, psychosis and mania similar to rabies, and severe respiratory and cold symptoms.

The incubation period for Ebola is 3 to 21 days. This disease causes devastating destruction throughout the body within 10 days. Typically the AIDS virus takes 10 years to accomplish this type of complete destruction.

A FEW LAST FRIGHTENING STATISTICS
There are 4 known strains of Ebola at this time.
Ebola Zaire—overall fatality rate is 90%
Ebola Sudan—fatality rate, overall, is 50%
Ebola Marburg—fatality rate, 25%
Ebola Reston—similar to the other Ebola strains and finally identified in monkeys. There have been no known human infections. In fact, it does not seem able to cross over into humans. Baffling!

HOMEOPATHY AND EBOLA

A study group in Arizona has made an extensive and detailed search for specific symptoms of the various Ebola strains. Without their itemization and detailing of symptoms it would be impossible to identify remedies that might prove useful.

General symptoms of all strains (This is only a partial list. See Homeopathy for Epidemics by Eileen Nauman, DHM (UK) for more information.)

- The abdominal wall lining sloughs off into the bowel which fills with blood and the whole mess is expelled with hemorrhagic bleeding.
- The blood thickens, circulation slows, and clots form, causing stroke and grand-mal seizures.
- The kidneys, filled with clots and dead cells, fail.
- The liver swells, turns yellow, and begins to liquefy.
- The spleen becomes large and hard with huge clots.
- Kidney and liver failure cause the blood stream to become toxic.
- Proteins created by the virus attack collagen throughout the body causing, first off, the connective tissue throughout the body to turn to mush.
- The skin shows a rapidly moving spotty necrosis produced by dying cells. Eventually the skin simply liquefies or forms tears which then hemorrhage horribly.
- Gums and salivary glands hemorrhage and the eyes fill with blood.
- Cells of the throat, the tongue, and the lining of the trachea begin to sluff off until hemorrhage occurs.
- The heart, as it comes under attack, bleeds into itself and the heart muscle softens
- There is eventual bleeding from every body orifice and from tears in the skin and muscle tissues.

The Zaire strain is by far the most lethal, Sudan is next, with the Marburg variety being the gentlest—if such a term can even be applied to these viruses. (See statistics on previous page.)

SUGGESTED REMEDIES

The remedies whose symptom picture contains the hemorrhagic symptoms that kill with this virus are those remedies which are derived from snake venom. There are 21 of these remedies, as near as I can determine, 7 of which are fairly commonly used remedies.

CROTALUS HORRIDUS most nearly matches the symptoms of Ebola Zaire, according to the symptoms collected and collated by the study group in Arizona. In fact, the symptom picture of Crotalus horridus and the list of symptoms of Ebola Zaire very nearly match each other.

OTHER SNAKE REMEDIES INCLUDE

Bothrops lanceolatus, Cenchris contortrix, Elaps corallinus, Lachesis muta, Naja tripudians, and Vipera berus.

LACHESIS MUTA seems to most closely match the symptoms of the Sudan and Marburg varieties of Ebola filovirus.

To pick up all the symptoms of Ebola from the beginning through the recovery stages, it may be necessary to use Mercurius solubilis, Phosphorus and/or Pyrogenium, one right after another.

PLAGUE

Plague is a disease that has been around since ancient times. It still occurs in an irregular pattern in enough numbers to be counted as an epidemic in parts of Asia, the Middle East, Eastern Europe, Africa, South America, and to some extent, in the United States. The last rat-borne epidemic of plague in the United States occurred in Los Angeles in 1924-25. All plague cases in the United States since then have been confined to wild rodents and their fleas.

There were, and still are in this day, three forms of plague. All forms are caused by infection from the bacteria Yersinia pestis and are distributed by rodent (not necessarily rat) populations. The three types of plague are Bubonic Plague, Pneumonic plague, and Septicemic plague.

The first type, called bubonic plague, is the most common form. Bubonic plague does not pass directly from person to person. It occurs when an infected flea bites a person or when the person with some sort of open break in their skin is exposed to materials that have been contaminated by Y. pestis. The symptoms are swollen, tender lymph glands (called buboes), fever, headache, chills, ugly black sores, mass hemorrhaging, bloody saliva, nausea, vomiting, diarrhea, and lung tissue that simply dissolves away. The strain is extremely virulent and not easily killed. Death usually occurs within two days.

The second type, pneumonic plague, occurs when the primary target of the bacteria is the lungs. This type of plague can spread from person to person as one person breathes in Y. pestis in respiratory droplets from a person or animal with pneumonic plague. Person to person infection usually requires close contact. Pneumonic plague can also be the result of bubonic or septicemic varieties of plague left untreated.

The first signs of this illness begin about 6 days after exposure and include fever, shortness of breath, chest pain, headache, cough that sometimes contains blood, and it also has a very high mortality rate unless intervention is successful, estimated at between 98% and 100% in untreated cases and 40% if treated aggressively in the first 24 hours *A vaccine has been developed but even its proponents admit that it takes several weeks in the body to achieve effectiveness, so would be of little use in an epidemic situation.*

Plague is bacterial in nature and when exposure is known to have occurred, a 7 day regimen of antibiotics is advised. Statistically, this has proven to be a quite successful prophylactic program.

In some persons, for reasons unknown, this bacteria invades the bloodstream instead of the lymph system. Septicemic plague can be a complication of either bubonic plague or pneumonic plague. As the bacteria circulates through the body in the blood, the extremities (fingers, toes, and nose) become gangrenous and turn black. Without appropriate and constant treatment septicemic plague has a 100% mortality rate.

SUGGESTED REMEDIES FOR BUBONIC PLAGUE

Arsenicum album, Arsenicum iodatum, Bromium, Lycopodium clavatum, Mercurius solubilis, and Tuberculinum bovinum (nosode).

SUGGESTED REMEDIES FOR PNEUMONIC PLAGUE

Arsenicum album, Bufo rana, Hepar sulphuris calcareum, Kali iodatum, Kali bichromicum, Mercurius solubilis, Nitricum acidum, Phosphorus, Sulphur and Carcinosin (a nosode).

SUGGESTED REMEDIES FOR SEPTICEMIC PLAGUE

Aconitum napellus, Apis mellifica, Arnica montana, Arsenicum album, Baptisia tinctoria, Belladonna, Carbo vegetabilis, Crotalus horridus, Echinacea angustifolia, Lachesis muta, Phosphorus, Pyrogenium, Sulphur, Veratrum album, and Anthracinum (nosode).

AIDS / HIV

Other than the Ebola virus strains AIDS/HIV is potentially the most serious of all of the pandemic/epidemic diseases. It is predicted by those who study these things that AIDS will impact every person in the United States either directly or indirectly in the coming years. The miasm certainly is impacting us all. AIDS is an insidious disease with a very long incubation period (10 - 12 years) in an otherwise healthy adult. During this time there may be gradually deteriorating health that does not get linked to the AIDS/HIV viruses.

The virus appears to be made from parts of several other lethal diseases. This has led to the speculation that it is somehow related to vaccinations. A less well known aspect of this disease is that it can be spread by mosquitoes, bed bugs, ticks, horse flies and other insects. In one monastery in Thailand, every Buddhist monk was found to be carrying HIV; investigation showed that bed bugs in the monastery were all carrying the virus. One epidemiologist stated that AIDS could become the black plague of the 21st Century.

There are two distinct phases to this disease:

1) The person has the virus but no active symptoms. Suggested remedies are Carcinosin and Psorinum.

2) The active AIDS state.

In the second stage, the immune system is under drastic attack and serious secondary diseases have begun to show themselves. The most common secondary diseases are tuberculosis, hepatitis C, pneumonia, and leukemia. With the horribly compromised immune system of AIDS, absolutely anything is possible from day to day. Living with AIDS means facing multiple diseases—usually life threatening of themselves—while trying to fight the original virus.

The rule is still, as always, treat the presenting symptoms and characteristics. The secondary diseases must be treated simultaneously with the basic AIDS. Two or more remedies will need to be used in tandem—something that is new to the world of homeopathy, except when using nosode remedies. Do not forget the use of the nosode remedies listed above, Carcinosin and Psorinum. Other nosodes may also be appropriate.

GONORRHEA

Gonorrhea holds a special place in the study of homeopathy because Samuel Hahnemann, who founded this system of healing, discovered and reported the debilitating, long-term effects of gonorrhea as the basis of the sycotic miasm. The miasm, or predisposition to symptoms similar to Gonorrhea, can be passed generationally. (See sycosis miasm in the index at the back of this book.)

Symptoms of gonorrhea in women include painful or frequent urination, abnormal vaginal discharge, abnormal vaginal bleeding during or after sex or in between periods, general itching, irregular menstrual bleeding, lower abdominal pain, fever, general fatigue, swollen and painful glands in the genital area with pain during sex, sore throat, and pinkeye.

Symptoms of gonorrhea in men include abnormal discharge from the penis. This discharge will be clear or milky at first, then yellow, creamy, excessive, and sometimes, blood-tinged. Other symptoms are painful or frequent urination, anal itching with pain, bleeding, or discharge, sore throat, and pinkeye.

In both men and women symptoms of gonorrhea that has spread to sites other than the genital areas will include rash, joint pain or arthritis, and inflamed tendons.

HOMEOPATHIC REMEDIES
NAMED BY HAHNEMANN FOR MIASM AND THE DISEASE ITSELF

Nitricum acidum and Thuja occidentalis.

SUGGESTED REMEDIES

Calcarea sulphurica, Cantharis vesicatoria, Cochlearia armoracia, Hydrastis canadensis, Kali chloricum, Kali iodatum, Kali sulphuricum, Mercurius solubilis, Natrum sulphuricum, Petroselinum sativum, Phosphorus, Pulsatilla nigricans, Terebinthiniae oleum, and Sulphur.

SYPHILIS

Syphilis is a complex, sexually transmitted disease. The primary stage of syphilis begins with a sore on the skin at the site of initial exposure—usually the genitals, rectum, or mouth. The sore feels like a button: firm, round, and usually measuring about 1/2 inch across and is not tender to the touch. There are usually no other symptoms at the early stage and the sore heals by itself after 4 to 6 weeks. The disappearance of the sore does not indicate the disappearance of the syphilis, which is continuing to spread throughout the body.

When syphilis moves into the second stage several weeks later there will be symptoms such as headache, general achiness, loss of appetite, and perhaps a rash. The appearance of the rash can vary dramatically. The rash can last for several weeks or months. Other symptoms of this stage are sores in the mouth, nose, throat, genitals, and in the folds of the skin. Lymph node swelling and patchy hair loss can occur. All the signs of this stage will also disappear without treatment, but the syphilis is not gone.

The third stage of syphilis, described as the latent stage, can last from a few years to 50 years. There are no symptoms and for the first approximately 2 years an infected person may be contagious to others. During this latent stage a pregnant woman can transmit syphilis to her unborn baby.

If the syphilis moves into the final stage, symptoms will include fever, painful skin ulcers that will not heal, bone pain, liver disease, and anemia. This stage of syphilis, called quarternary syphilis, can damage internal organs, including the brain, nervous system, eyes, heart, and blood vessels.

Syphilis and the syphilitic miasm are believed by homeopathic practitioners to be at the root of all diseases that cause organ destruction. Hahnemann believed that inherited syphilis energy underlies this miasm. (*Please see the chapter on miasms—and the Index at the back of this book for further page number choices*).

Mercurius solubilis was considered by Hahnemann to be the chief antisyphilitic remedy and is still considered today to be effective against both active cases and generational problems.

SUGGESTED REMEDIES

Arsenicum iodatum, Aurum metallicum, Kali iodatum, Kali sulphuricum, Lachesis muta, Mercurius solubilis, Mercurius iodatus flavus, Nitricum acidum, Phytolacca decandra, Silica terra, and Stillingia sylvatica. Generational syphilitic conditions (did not contract syphilis in their own lifetime) are often treated with Arsenicum album, Thuja occidentalis, and Tuberculinum bovinum.

SOME ENVIRONMENTAL DISEASES

LYME DISEASE

The spirochete bacteria that causes Lyme disease is carried by ticks and was first discovered in Lyme, Connecticut, from which it got its name. There are other illnesses that are also carried by ticks. Not every tick carries Lyme disease, but every tick poses risk as it leaves some sort of toxin behind.

Ticks are small creatures, as many of you probably know. It is easy to have one and not know it for a while because they like to hide in your hair or beneath an item of clothing. When removing a tick it is very important not to leave the appendages in the body. One good way to do this is to light a match, blow it out and immediately place the match head on the tick. It withdraws from the body in an attempt to get away from the heat. I was interested to read in Eileen Nauman's book that this method, which was taught to me by my grandmother, was also used by her father who was born in the hills of Kentucky.

The above method for tick removal may save you from rocky mountain spotted fever but is not really very helpful with Lyme disease. It is the saliva that is largely responsible for the infection, and the saliva enters the capillaries and then the blood stream almost immediately.

SYMPTOMS

The first symptom of Lyme disease, appearing 3 to 12 weeks after exposure to the tick, is a large, hot, red spot on the skin that continues to grow in diameter. Soon after the first red spot appears, many people develop multiple, smaller spots. The spots usually lasts for several weeks.

The next stage of the illness, which may occur in just a few days or may wait several years to appear, will include some or all of the following symptoms: abnormal fatigue and exhaustion, chills, fever, headache, a stiff neck, nausea, sore throat, lymph gland swelling, spleen enlargement, tenderness or pain in muscles, and muscular rheumatism. Because these symptoms appear long after the tick bite, they are sometimes misdiagnosed and not properly treated.

In severe cases, the nervous system also comes under attack. Meningitis, which is characterized by irregular low-grade fevers, loss of appetite, constipation, intense headaches, intolerance to light and sound, contracted pupils, delirium, convulsions, and eventually coma can occur. Chorea (tics, tremors, involuntary muscle spasms, and violent involuntary movements), Bell's palsy (inflammation of facial nerves that causes short-term paralysis of the face), radiculoneuritis (inflammation of the roots of the spinal nerves) or myelitis (inflammation of the spinal cord) are other possible complications. Myocardial abnormalities of the heart occur in approximately 1 out of every 10 patients, which leads to an enlarged heart. Painful swelling in the joints can also occur.

Sometimes chronic fatigue syndrome and general persistent fatigue of no known cause are really Lyme disease. A blood test (or good muscle testing skills) is necessary to determine if Lyme disease is involved. National and medical statistics show a very low rate of infection in the U.S. Except along the eastern coast. However, from everything I can learn, reported cases represent only about 1 out of 4 actual illnesses. The repertories do not list very many remedies for this combination of symptoms. It will be necessary to start with one or two, taken concurrently, and change remedies as the symptom picture changes.

SUGGESTED REMEDIES

ARSENICUM ALBUM: With Arsenicum, the skin will be itchy and burning during the rash stage. It may resemble a nettle rash and will be painful if scratched. There will be burning sensations in the joints, muscles, and nerve endings. Weakness, with difficulty walking and aggravation from movement of any kind. Part of the mental picture of Arsenicum is a vague feeling that something is wrong. This, combined with the intermittent nature of the symptoms often causes people (even doctors) to tell the person that they are being hypochondriacal and advise them to get over it. This remedy is indicated if there is restlessness, heart palpitations, irregular heartbeat, congestion, with burning, or itching in the chest region.

ANTIPYRINUM: The symptoms of this lesser known remedy include a very scarlet rash with swelling and itching, fever accompanied by heavy sweating, an unusual headache located under the ears, and exhaustion with trembling.

BELLADONNA: The rash of Belladonna is bright scarlet and very hot to the touch. There may be a fever that spikes from time to time, during which the face will be bright red. Another symptom is joints which swell very quickly, are hot, and have a bright red color that usually runs up and down from the joint. These joint symptoms will shift from place to place on the body. If there is a headache, it will be intense, throbbing, and come on very suddenly.

COCCULUS INDICUS: may be indicated for the rash stage if the rash resembles a nettle rash and is burning and itching. The joint pain is usually centered in the shoulders and small of the back. There is liver involvement with this remedy along with the irritability and anger at interruptions that characterizes people with liver problems. Headache and heart palpitations with vertigo are also part of this remedy picture.

MERCURIUS SOLUBILIS: The rash exudes a thin, clear liquid when the bumps break. After being broken they clear quickly, so the rash lasts only 1 to 2 weeks. The fever is accompanied by heavy, foul-smelling perspiration. Sometimes there is swelling of the hands and feet, especially at joint sites, and the skin may appear greasy and shiny.

RHUS TOXICODENDRON: The rash of Rhus toxicodendron progresses rapidly to a leaky stage and the sores fill with pus which scabs over. The fever is accompanied with chills. The joint pain and swelling is better for movement—unlike Arsenicum—but stiffness sets in when sitting or lying still. This is especially true of the pain in the lower back. Headaches usually center in the back of the head and are accompanied by stiffness in the neck.

ROCKY MOUNTAIN SPOTTED FEVER

Rocky Mountain spotted fever is a severe tick related illness. The disease is caused by Rickettsia rickettsii, a species of bacteria that is spread to humans by hard ticks. Initial signs and symptoms of the disease include sudden onset of fever, headache, and muscle pain, followed by development of a rash. The disease can be difficult to diagnose in the early stages because it looks like so many other, less nasty, illnesses. Without prompt and appropriate treatment, tick-borne illnesses—this one in particular—can progress to a myriad of unpleasant symptoms that just keep getting worse and worse as time passes. Rocky Mountain Spotted Fever can even cause death.

Some of the symptoms that people who have been diagnosed with RMSF display are vomiting, a ticking sound in their ears, increased sensitivity to noise, twitching muscles, problems with balance, nerve problems in hands and arms, dizziness that results in bumping into walls when walking, and musculoskeletal pain (described as pain between the muscles and the bones, the periosteum). A person does not need to have all of these symptoms (and may even have many others) when suffering from RMSF.

The name Rocky Mountain spotted fever is a bit confusing since this disease occurs in many parts of the United States other than the Rocky Mountain region. It is now recognized that this disease is broadly distributed throughout the continental United States, and occurs as far north as Canada and as far south as Central America, Mexico, and parts of South America. Between 1981 and 1996, this disease was reported from every U.S. state except Hawaii, Vermont, Maine and Alaska.

Rocky Mountain spotted fever remains a serious and potentially life threatening infectious disease today. Despite the availability of effective treatment with antibiotics (if you discount their side effects) approximately 3% to 5% of individuals who become ill with Rocky Mountain spotted fever still die from the initial infection. Many more suffer debilitating symptoms for years or even for the rest of their lives.

SUGGESTED REMEDIES
FOR THE INITIAL STAGE

Arsenicum album (again, take at the very beginning, or even just after any tick is discovered), Belladonna, Rhus toxicodendron, and Sulphur have reported cases where symptoms were eliminated and a great measure of health restored—even after years of suffering.

LEGIONNAIRES DISEASE

Legionnaires is caused by the bacterium Legionella pneumophila and is quite severe. Early symptoms appear 2 to 14 days after exposure to the bacteria. The early symptoms are headache, muscle pain, high fever, and chills. By the second or third day, a cough which will bring up mucus and possibly, blood, will be seen. There will be chest pain, loss of appetite, nausea, vomiting and diarrhea. Legionnaires sometimes progresses to pneumonia, and quite often, kidney impairment. Legionnaires moves very rapidly and can become life threatening in a hurry.

Pontiac fever is a milder form of this disease and is characterized by fever, chills, headache, and muscle aches. Pontiac fever does not affect the lungs and symptoms are usually gone in 2 to 5 days.

Since the initial symptoms of Legionnaires include a high fever with body aches—caused by toxin build-up—as well as diarrhea, a high potency (1M or 10M) Arsenicum album would probably be the first remedy given most of the time. Other remedies used would be similar to the ones used for SARS and pneumonia.

Lachesis muta works with many types of pneumonia and kidney problems and is often the next remedy in the regimen.

SUGGESTED REMEDIES

Antimonium tartaricum, Arsenicum album, Arsenicum iodatum, Bromium, Kali chloricum, Kali iodatum, Lachesis muta, Mercurius solubilis, Phosphorus, Pulsatilla nigricans and Pyrogenium.

HANTAVIRUS

This virus was first seen during the Korean conflict where the very common striped field mouse was identified as the primary carrier of the virus. The virus is spread to humans when they inhale the fine, dry, powdery dust of mouse droppings.

In the 1970's, extensive studies of rat populations were conducted around the world. It was found that virus carrying rats inhabited every port city tested. A few years later it was realized that the virus carrying rats were not limited to port cities. In 1993, following a very rainy summer, there was an outbreak of this deadly virus in the four corners area of the United States (Colorado, Utah, New Mexico and Arizona). That same year there were several cases in my little corner of Idaho. I personally knew two people who died that year, and another who survived. The survivor was treated with homeopathics and other alternative treatments. Her recovery included recovery from the kidney and liver damage that debilitates so many survivors of this very nasty virus.

The first symptoms of this virus are a high fever, headache, flushing of the face and neck with a red rash, quite sudden septic shock to the entire system, nausea, vomiting, diarrhea, abdominal pain, respiratory stress as the lungs fill with blood and fluid, kidney and bladder stress with sudden renal failure from loss of electrolytes and toxin buildup. There is often confusion with inability to communicate simple things like the time or the day. One of the keynotes of this virus is the suddenness and seriousness with which it attacks. It often hits so violently that the person is dangerously ill within hours of the virus entering their system. The aftermath of hantavirus, for those who survive, is usually kidney and liver damage and an increased risk for strokes and high blood pressure.

Early statistics in 1993 gave this virus a kill rate of 60%. These numbers fell off slightly as medical people became aware of the symptoms and reacted more quickly and more appropriately.

SUGGESTED REMEDIES

Aconitum napellus, Arnica montana, Apis mellifica, Arsenicum album, Baptisia tinctoria, Belladonna, Bryonia alba, Carbo vegetablilis, Crotalus horridus, Echinacea angustifolia, Gelsemium sempervirens, Lachesis muta, Pyrogenium, and Rhus toxicodendron.

In my one and only treatment opportunity with this symptom pattern following a person's exposure to mouse droppings, we used **Baptisia tinctoria, Arnica montana, Carbo vegetabilis**, and later, **Gelsemium.** We also employed herbal remedies and energy modalities throughout the initial illness and the follow-up rebuilding stages. It was a very scary afternoon and has stood in my mind for years now as a testimonial to the effectiveness of immediate treatment with homeopathic remedies and other alternative treatments.

Other people have reported that **Arsenicum album** is a good first remedy as it will begin to break the bacterial infection, reduce the fever, halt the vomiting and diarrhea, and begin the elimination of the toxins from the body. According to the symptom picture, this would probably have been a better match in the case I worked with but the combination that we used was wonderfully effective. I had not yet discovered the amazing polycrest, Arsenicum album.

The remedies listed above are basic polycrest remedies and useful in many serious situations. It would be a good idea to become familiar with their symptom pictures, and especially what makes one remedy different from another. When you look at the person that is becoming ill, you should immediately be able to key in on a few basic characteristics of theirs when they are well, observe the changes that the illness is making, and then match these symptoms to the key symptoms of a remedy. This should be done on physical, emotional, and spiritual levels all at once. As the first remedy kicks in and they stabilize, you will have more time to determine a perfect match for the next stage of the illness.

BEING PREPARED

I thought about calling this section something like ***Biological Warfare*** or some other such thing, but I am less concerned about the source of potential problems than about giving you information that will help you cope with various chemical-based situations and poisons. I have always believed that if you are prepared, you need not fear anything that may come into your life. With the Lord's help, we can handle anything (if we have followed his previous instructions and made proper preparations). With that in mind, let's discuss some possible responses to a few of the toxins that may find their way into our world someday.

ANTHRAX

The bacteria Bacillus anthracis is responsible for the disease called anthrax. Anthrax is normally found in sheep, cattle, and horses and can be transmitted to humans by infected animals or their products. When anthrax moves from animals to humans, it is by skin contact or by inhalation of the bacterial spores found in sheep wool. Disinfection of surface areas may be accomplished using chlorine bleach and water.

PULMONARY ANTHRAX (INHALATION)

Early symptoms are very similar to a respiratory flu, making diagnosis difficult. Inhalation anthrax rapidly progresses, within a few days, to pneumonia. Following the initial symptoms, inhalation anthrax has a nasty habit of improving somewhat, only to come back online suddenly with difficulty in breathing, profuse sweating, swollen lymph glands, nausea, vomiting, pain and stiffness, cyanosis (blue tinge to the skin indicating serious oxygen deprivation), shock, and death. Death can occur within 24 to 36 hours. The CDC says that pulmonary anthrax of the most virulent strains, treated medically, has an 80% mortality rate. It should be noted that there are anthrax strains that are absolutely symptomless.

SUGGESTED REMEDIES
FOR STAGE ONE

Anthracinum (anthrax nosode), Arsenicum album, Lachesis muta, Secale cornutum, Bryonia alba

SUGGESTED REMEDIES
FOR STAGE TWO (WITH MEDICAL TREATMENT)
Arsenicum album, Lachesis muta, Carbo vegetabilis, Baptisia tinctoria, Pyrogenium.

CUTANEOUS ANTHRAX (SKIN CONTACT)
The anthrax spores must come into contact with skin that is broken. The first symptoms will look like a spider bite. The spot quickly becomes a black colored, ulcerated sore with dying tissue in the center. By now the person has begun to run a fever and lymph glands near the area may begin to swell. The sore eventually turns reddish brown and breaks open, forming a scab. Chills and fatigue are often seen. This type of anthrax responds well to antibiotics, and according to the literature, to homeopathic remedies as well. Completely untreated, cutaneous anthrax is fatal for 1 in 4 persons; when treated, the mortality rate is less than 1 percent.

SUGGESTED REMEDIES
Arsenicum album, Lachesis muta, Nitricum acidum, Secale cornutum, Carbo vegetabilis.

GASTROINTESTINAL ANTHRAX (INGESTED)
Infection is caused by ingesting contaminated food. Anthrax, if ingested, causes acute inflammation of the intestinal tract. The early symptoms are nausea, vomiting, and fever with abdominal pain, severe diarrhea, and the vomiting of blood following soon after. Diagnosis is difficult because the symptoms so closely match the flu. This business of diagnosis of specific bacteria is not critical in homeopathy as long as the symptoms respond dramatically to the first remedy applied. (I know, I have said this several times already.)

SUGGESTED REMEDIES
Arsenicum album, Ipecacuanha, Phosphorus, China officinalis, Veratrum album. The Bach Flower Combination, Rescue Remedy, should be given every 10 to 15 minutes whenever you are dealing with a life threatening situation.

BOTULISM
Botulism is an extremely serious muscle paralyzing disease that is the result of a nerve toxin being released in the body by the Clostridium botulinum bacteria. Death occurs in about 8% of cases and the seriousness of botulism poisoning—especially with children—should not be underestimated. The bacterium, Clostridium botulinum, which causes botulism is one of the most deadly substances known to mankind. Miniscule quantities are enough to produce illness in humans.

Spores of this bacteria are found in soil the world over. Approximately 110 cases of food-borne botulism occur in the United States each year. Cases of botulism poisoning are most often the result of ingesting improperly prepared home-canned products. We are cautioned constantly about how to prevent botulism with home-canning. A few outbreaks of botulism have also been the result of improperly prepared food in restaurants.

While there are many factors involved in the safe home-canning of food (I have done it for years), there is one factor that too many women in the mountain west region of America are either unaware of or choose to ignore. At sea level, a pressure of 11 pounds per square inch (psi) is required to reach 240 degrees Fahrenheit. As the altitude rises, more pressure is required to achieve a similar high temperature. It is necessary, if you live in a mountain valley, to increase the pressure from the 10 lbs recommended in the canning books to at least 12 lbs in order to be confident that all of the bacteria have been killed. Not factoring this in when canning can increase the risk for botulism.

TYPES OF BOTULISM
Food-borne botulism occurs when contaminated food is consumed. Washing produce thoroughly before eating it just makes good sense.

Infant botulism is presumed to be caused by the infant ingesting, in some way, viable botulism spores which grow and produce toxins in susceptible infants. Since the spores are found in soil everywhere, the possibility of ingesting the spores from garden soil, dust in the air, vacuum cleaner dust, etc. should probably result in more than the 100 reported cases a year.

Wound botulism results when the bacterium enters a wound site. The first cases of wound botulism occurred in 1943. Since 1980 the number of cases has been steadily increasing, especially among drug users. (I wonder if Botox injections should be considered drug injections?)

SYMPTOMS OF BOTULISM

Symptoms of botulism from food begin to occur anywhere from 6 hours to 2 weeks after the consumption of the contaminated food, although the most common time frame is 12 to 36 hours. The symptom picture of botulism, in any form and in any age group, is dominated by the ***devastating neurological symptoms.***

Infants with botulism appear lethargic, do not nurse well, have a diminished and weakened cry, become constipated, and develop abnormal neck and peripheral weakness (described as floppy baby syndrome). The constipation and intestinal problems sometimes precede the other symptoms by many days. Other symptoms include loss of facial expression, paralysis of the muscles around the eyes, and dilated pupils, as well as slowing of deep tendon reflexes. Respiratory failure and death follow, often very quickly, for about 2% of infants.

In adults, it is often difficult to diagnose botulism unless the case is part of a group of people who were similarly poisoned at the same time and by the same product. Unlike a bout of flu, botulism manifests with neurological symptoms such as blurred vision, drooping eyelids, difficulty swallowing, food catching in the throat, a dry mouth, weakness in the extremities, and paralysis or a paralytic type of weakness. Botulism can be fatal and should always be considered an emergency requiring immediate intervention and then appropriate follow-up treatment.

SUGGESTED REMEDIES

Botulinum (nosode), Gelsemium sempervirens, Arsenicum album, Carbolicum acidum, Nux vomica, Phosphorus.

BOTOX INJECTIONS

I think that before moving on from the subject of botulism, I would like to bring to your attention the fact that the serum of Botox injections is made from the toxin produced by the bacterium, Clostridium botulinum. It is this toxin that causes botulism poisoning. Remember, the Center for Disease Control calls this toxin "one of the most potent lethal substances known to man."

I would like to quote directly from the Mayo Clinic site for most of this section on Botox injections. I found what they had to say about these injections extremely interesting. *Double indented (indented both left and right) paragraphs are quoted exactly as they are found on the Mayo Clinic site, except for bolding and italicizing, which I have added for emphasis of specific points.*

The first statement that caught my eye on the Mayo Clinic site was;

> Botox is a well-known brand name for a ***medicinal*** form of botulinum toxin type A, which is also known as onabotulinumtoxinA. ***The toxin is produced by the specific bacterium that causes the food poisoning botulism.***

The specific bacteria which causes botulism poisoning, Clostridium botulinum, is very carefully not mentioned by name and the toxin being used is carefully referred to only by its "also known as" names, but it is at least referred to as a toxin. I find the wording of this sentence deceptive, but not actionable—the question is whether or not the deception is deliberate and intended to mislead the public.

The Mayo Clinic statement calls what they use in their injections a medicinal form of the toxin. I can't find any information about what that means nor can I find any evidence that the Clostridium botulinum makes any toxin other than the nerve paralyzing one that causes botulism poisoning and is also referred to as botulinum toxin type A.

At the Mayo Clinic, Botox injections are used, at least part of the time, to treat neck pain, muscle spasms, lazy eye, stiffness in joints, excessive sweating, and chronic migraines. Botox injections are used *less frequently* for back pain, bladder dysfunction, pelvic floor problems, and other things because, according to the Mayo Clinic site, *there is insufficient evidence that Botox works for these conditions.*

What makes Botox injections a medicinal form of this very toxic substance? Apparently, if you use a toxic substance for medicinal purposes and have it prescribed by a doctor, it becomes a medicinal form. It is still the specific toxin—not quite a case of "a rose by any other name" but you get the correlation, I'm sure!

The Mayo Clinic site continues by saying:

> When injected in small doses into specific muscles, Botox doesn't poison you, but acts as a muscle relaxant, with effects that can last several months.

Let me re-emphasize that the toxin produced by **Clostridium botulinum** is a nerve agent which will paralyze muscles. Referring to it as a muscle relaxant when injected into the body by a doctor is a gross misstatement and requires more faith in a doctor than I could ever muster. If you need more concrete proof for the statement that this toxin is a paralyzing agent, you need only look up the statistics on the side effects that too often occur from Botox treatments.

Again, an exact quote from the Mayo Clinic website (italics are mine):

> Botox injections are *relatively* safe when performed by an experienced doctor. But side effects and complications can occur. Side effects that you should mention to your doctor if they're bothersome or don't go away include: pain and bruising at the injection site, redness, itching, headache, nausea, temporary muscle weakness, and increased body sweat.
>
> Although very unlikely, **there is a possibility that the effect of botulinum toxin may spread to other parts of the body and cause botulism-like signs and symptoms.** Call your doctor right away if you notice any of these effects **hours to weeks** after receiving Botox: muscle weakness all over the body, vision problems, trouble speaking or swallowing, trouble breathing, loss of bladder control, allergic reaction (itching, hives, swelling, chest tightness, trouble breathing), eye pain, bleeding or bruising around your eye, blistering, peeling of your skin or severe rash, chest pain, shortness of breath, uneven heart rate, flu-like symptoms, face or neck pain, seizures. **Doctors generally recommend against using Botox when you're pregnant or breast-feeding, since the effects on the baby aren't known. The benefits of the treatment should exceed the risks.**

The last two sentences in the quote above (taken directly from the clinic's website) really confuse me. Are they saying that if the benefits to the mother outweigh the risks to the baby, it is OK to go ahead with them in spite of the potential harm to the unborn child?

The Mayo Clinic continues with a discussion of this toxin as a way to prevent wrinkles by saying,

> "It is *less desirable* to treat the lines around your mouth because muscles in this area are used for eating and talking."

Sounds to me like they are saying that it is OK to take the risks associated with paralyzing the muscles around your eyes (after all, they are only used for seeing and for facial expressions), but we should think carefully about risking paralysis of the muscles around our mouths.

Why have I included this information here? I guess I just needed to say it somewhere and I find these statements about Botox to be typical of the medical community and prescription drugs in general. If you take a toxic chemical, get a doctor to write a prescription for it, and use it for a medicinal purpose, it becomes a medically accepted medicine. Many people will put almost anything into their bodies if it was recommended by a medical doctor, without a thought for what it is or what its side effects might be.

The assumption that poisons do not cross the placenta to the baby is so out-dated as to be ludicrous. We do not need tests on specific substances to know the risks. Enough tests on enough other substances have been conducted to show us the danger to unborn babies of anything the mother is exposed to.

There has to be a better way, and fortunately, there is! Homeopathy is particularly interesting because it is a way (discovered, I believe, through hard work and inspiration) to take the things that God has made and use them in a manner that has no side effects in order to benefit humanity.

NERVE AND CHEMICAL AGENTS

Make no mistake about this—I am not telling you in this part of the book (or anywhere else, for that matter) that homeopathic remedies, by themselves, will cope with the really nasty stuff. They might, and I and many other people have had some amazing successes using them, but the decision of when and how to seek medical attention must always be determined by you. It seemed appropriate, however, to provide a little information from the Center for Disease Control (CDC) about the agents that are being developed around the world, and then to provide a list of homeopathic remedies to consider—based on the symptom pictures.

The possibility of nerve and chemical agents being employed against us by an enemy is not as farfetched as you might think. Nerve agents can be manufactured by fairly simple techniques and the raw materials are both inexpensive and readily available. Nerve agents are relatively stable, easily dispersed, and highly toxic whether absorbed through the skin or breathed into the body.

Nerve agents cause changes in the transmission of nerve impulses in the body in specific ways. These chemicals affect the nerves related to the smooth muscles of the body, or the nerves related to the skeletal muscles, or they attack the central nervous system.

There are basically three types of muscles in the body. These are skeletal (fibrous), smooth muscles (example: bowel and stomach), and cardiac muscle. When muscles come under attack, there may be a plethora of symptoms simply because there are so many muscles, of one variety or another, in the body.

SMOOTH MUSCLE ATTACKS

There may be pain and cramping in the abdomen, involuntary urination and bowel movements, excessive perspiration and saliva, difficult breathing with asthmatic cough, tightness and oppression in the chest, nausea and vomiting, to name just a few possibilities.

SUGGESTED REMEDIES

Apis mellifica, Arsenicum album, Belladonna, Digitalis purpurea, Nux vomica, Gelsemium sempervirens, Mercurius solubilis, Phosphorus, Pulsatilla nigricans, Veratrum album.

SKELETAL MUSCLE ATTACKS

Twitching, cramping, and weakness of various muscles, hypertension, problems with the heart and heart muscle, constricted breathing, and coughing up a mucus from the lungs, blurry vision, eye inflammation and watering, headache, hypertension. A high level of exposure may result in loss of consciousness, seizures, paralysis and muscle flaccidity, and breathing may become erratic or stop altogether for short periods of time.

SUGGESTED REMEDIES

Belladonna, Cuprum metallicum, Phosphorus, Arsenicum album, Sulphur.

CENTRAL NERVOUS SYSTEM ATTACKS

Nerve agents cause psychological and behavioral pattern changes in people. Symptoms may include irritability, quarrelsomeness, over sensitivity, restlessness, nervousness, anguish, fear, impatience, loss of memory, poor concentration, poor short-term memory, delirium, and dementia. There may be sadness, despondency, brooding, discouragement, inconsolable grief with sighing and weeping, foolish and uncharacteristic behavior, stupor, unconsciousness, and coma.

Physical symptoms include weakness, flabbiness of muscles, desire to lie down, convulsions and convulsive movements of muscle groups, disconnected speech, respiration that sounds like snoring (even when awake). There may be a very slow heartbeat but the pulse may be racing or feel faster than normal. The lungs may fail to bring enough oxygen to the organs of the body. Hypertension usually becomes a problem. When the attack seems to be centered in the heart and circulatory system there are a few additional remedies that should be considered.

SUGGESTED REMEDIES

FOR HEART/CIRCULATION

Digitalis purpurea (bradycardia—slow heartbeat), Veratrum album, Phosphorus, Aconitum napellus (bradycardia), Crataegus oxyacantha.

AFTER EXPOSURE

Central nervous system effects such as, fatigue, irritability, nervousness, and memory problems may persist for many weeks after the worst of the effects have gone away. These longer-term effects need to be treated with homeopathic remedies, according to the current symptom picture, until all of the symptoms have disappeared.

The After-Effects of Serious Disease
and
Suggestions for Treatment

When a person has survived a serious, life-threatening disease, exposure to chemicals in whichever of the many forms we are exposed to chemicals in our world today, or has survived a traumatic accident or illness, complete recovery may take a long time and seem almost beyond reach. Long-term compromises to the immune system, the neurological system, or a general "collapse state" are common. Homeopathy, over the last 200 years, has identified many remedies and solutions for what they term "never the same since" (NSS) conditions. These solutions apply equally well to the aftermath of serious contagious diseases and to the effects of chemical agents and pollutants.

The after-effects of serious disease generally fall into one of the categories mentioned above. Below are some of the basic issues with some suggestions of remedies.

Compromised immune system: Some people are susceptible to everything that "goes around the neighborhood." This increased susceptibility seems to date back to, and be a result of, a serious contagious disease that they have otherwise recovered from or it appeared with exposure to toxic chemicals. It could be said that they were just "beaten down" by whatever happened to them. The two principal homeopathic remedies that are used to restore the vital force are **Carciosinum** and **Psorinum.** In the literature "never the same since" issues are most often covered by one or both of these remedies, regardless of the cause.

Some examples of conditions that have been treated by one of these remedies are:
- Never the same since chronic fatigue—**Carcinosin, Psorinum**
- Never the same since whooping cough—**Carcinosinun, Tubersulinum**
- Never the same since influenza—**Psorinum, Gelsemium sempervirens**
- Never the same since pneumonia—**Psorinum, Tuberculinum, Phosphorus**
- Never the same since hepatitis—**Psorinum, Lachesis, Phosphorus**
- Never the same since mononucleosis—**Carcincsinum**
- Never the same since tuberculosis—**Psorinum, Thuja occidentalis, Nitricum acidum**

Using Psorinum in tandem with the best "symptom picture" matching remedy should also be considered. Neurological impacts: Some diseases directly impact the nervous system and other diseases can leave neurological damage behind because of the high fevers. Diseases like meningitis, encephalitis, and polio, as well as poisons from biologicals such as botulism can leave after-effects of paralysis, paresis (loss of voluntary movement), tremors or palsy. The principal remedies used to combat these after-effects are Causticum, Cocculus indicus, Gelsemium sempervirens, Phosphorus, Phosphoric acid and Plumbum metallicum. Natrum muriaticum has also been used effectively with some people. Use the remedy that is most similar to the symptoms that are remaining and most suited to the person's nature and personality.

Collapse states: Often a person will come through the illness, seem to be doing fine, and then enter a state of debilitating fatigue or complete physical collapse—sometimes with a lot of emotional and mental vulnerability also. The principal remedies for a state of utter collapse are:

- **Ammonium carbonicum:** Lack of physical endurance is often the chief symptom signaling the usefullness of this remedy.
- **Calcarea carbonicum:** Useful for "cold" modalities (symptoms are brought on by, or made worse, by cold) with sluggish metabolism and emotional vulnerability.
- **Acid remedies:** All remedies with "acid" in their names have fatigue as part of their symptom picture.

Chapter Twenty-Five - Homeopathics and Cancer

Dr. A.U. Ramakrishnan is an M.D. and has been a practitioner of classical homeopathic medicine for the past 40 years; as near as I can determine. The following material has been taken from class notes and from Dr. Ramarkrishnan's web page and articles. In the 10 years prior to 2000 he treated over 3,120 cancer cases, 240 of which were stage one and 2,110 of which were stage four (considered untreatable - in fact, almost dead). The rest of the cases were intermediate.

Dr. Ramakrishnan says that he has had poor results using constitutional treatment alone, and has specialized in a lesional approach with much better results.

He believes that classical constitutional treatment is ideal for other circumstances, but is not as effective in cancer for the following reasons:

- There is a race against time. Constitutional treatment may require more time than the person, untreated, has left to them.
- The primary lesions have adverse side effects for other parts of the body.
- The person may be receiving other treatment such as chemotherapy or radiation which may interfere with a homeopathic regimen.

Dr. Ramakrishnan believes that it is important to discuss spiritual matters with the patient and get the patient to see the totality of his/her life situation.

Cancers Dr. Ramakrishnan finds most responsive to homeopathic treatment:

- Cancer of the cheek
- Cancer of the tongue
- Cancer of the esophagus
- Cancer of the head of the pancreas
- Cancer of the breast
- Cancer of the colon and rectum
- Cancer of the ovaries
- Cancer of the cervix
- Cancer of the bladder
- Cancer of the prostate
- Cancer of the skin (epithelioma)
- Cancer of the bone

Note the number of usually fatal cancers that have made this list of ones treated successfully!

POSSIBLE TREATMENT PROTOCOLS

Dr. Ramakrishnan's personal philosophy is to treat stage one cancers with homeopathic remedies alone for 3 to 4 weeks. (Stage one cancers are those that are not immediately life threatening but have the possibility of growing to that level). Even in this short 3 to 4 week period he has frequently seen observable shrinkage of tumors. If, after 4 weeks, the tumor is not shrinking substantially, he recommends that a surgeon or oncologist be consulted for evaluation and possible surgery.

Dr. Ramakrishnan has been quoted in class notes, posted on the web, as saying "Chemotherapy is never the best choice of treatment." Of course, this would have to be the personal choice and opinion of the cancer sufferer.

Treatment is usually given using two remedies alternately, following a protocol similar to the way nosode remedies are usually administered. Use each remedy for a one week period with ***the first remedy being organ specific to the location of the cancer.*** The second remedy is Carcinosin or, occasionally, another cancer nosode. These remedies are usually given at the 200C potency although, if the overall vitality is good, 1M potencies may be used. Follow your own best judgement, your intuition, and the muscle test (if you can) for the specifics.

When improvement is happening at a stable rate the localized organ specific remedy is replaced with the person's constitutional remedy. This constitutional remedy is still taken in an alternating manner with the cancer nosode in a manner more nearly consistent with normal nosode remedy protocols. The typical nosode protocol is to take the nosode once and then, at the appropriate interval, take the constitutional remedy. This pattern may need to be repeated more than once.

Dr. Ramakrishnan gives the remedies in a "plussing" protocol that he has devised. He believes that plussing gives improved results and enables a remedy to work faster with less chance of any aggravation of symptoms along the way.

Plussing: Dissolve three to five globules (or place a few drops of the liquid remedy) in eleven teaspoons of pure water. One teaspoon is taken every 15 minutes for a total of ten doses. One teaspoon is reserved to take the following day. This works best in a 1M or deeper potency. 200C remedies are usually taken without plussing, although I have found this plussing method to be gentler, yet very effective, especially with particularly debilitated patients even at this lower potency.

STAGES OF TREATMENT

Precancerous	Homeopathy alone
Detected at an early stage	Homeopathy alone
A small lump—operable	Surgery and homeopathy
Primary lesions which are not operable	Homeopathy, initially, and if not successful, the radiation followed by homeopathy
Late stages—widespread	Homeopathy for palliation and pain relief

POTENCY GUIDELINES

- In precancerous stages, or when the cancer is in remission, plussing is not required but may prove advantageous. Dr. Ramakrishnan's suggestion is a 200C remedy, one dose a week for a few weeks and then, upon improvement, taking the remedy once a month. It has been my experience that following the muscle test sets the dosage intervals up much differently from the protocol used by Dr. Ramakrishnan, usually much more frequently

- In more advanced stages and in the higher potencies, plussing is always recommended.

- When the cancer is well under control, use a single dose once a week and later once a month—or, more appropriately, follow the protocol as established by the muscle test.

SPECIFIC CANCERS AND SUGGESTED REMEDIES

- *Brain Cancer:* Plumbum metallicum with Plumbum iodatum if infection is present.

- *Prostate cancer:* Conium maculatum or Thuja occidentalis with Sabal serrulata (homeopathic form of Saw Palmetto) used alternately.

- *Leukemias:* With high fever, low white blood count and collapse: Kali arsenicosum 200C, Chinum arsenicosum 200C and Ferrum phosphoricum 6x together as a cocktail, three times a day for two weeks.

- *Hodgkin's disease:* With high fever and infection: Pyrogenium 200C, and Arsenicum iodatum 6x together two to three times a day.

- *Cancer of the Cheek and Tongue:* Aurum muriaticum

- *Cancer of the Maxillary Antrum or the Sinuses:* Phytolacca decandra works well for the face, sub-mandibular nodes, and mucus membranes.

- *Mucus Membranes, Breasts and polyps of the Colon:* Phytolacca decandra (Poke Root) works well for any of these

- *Esophagus, Breasts, Lungs, and Mediastinum:* Conium maculatum, Carcinosin, Lachesis muta, Phytolacca decandra

- *Cancer of the Head of the Pancreas:* Ceanothus americanus worked well with the spleen in 60% of the pancreatic cases. Pancreatic cancer spreads so fast that there is often no time for the homeopathic remedies to have an effect.

- *Cancer of the Rectum:* Graphites naturalis if there is also constipation. Nitricum acidum when there is any involvement of the mucus lining, and if there are hemorrhoids or ulcers, Hydrastis canadensis (golden seal) for lesions of the stomach, liver, duodenum, large intestine and spleen.

- *Internal Cancers in General:* Arsenicum album often works well for these.

- *Ovarian Cancer:* Lachesis muta for left or right ovaries. Also Lilium tigrinum, Conium maculatum, Terebinthiniae oleum. Also use Cantharis vesicatoria for the management of dysuria and bleeding.

- *Skin Cancer:* Arsenicum iodatum if the cancer is infected. Calcarea arsenicosa. Arsenicum album has a strong affinity for the skin, especially epithelioma or mesothelioma.

- *Stomach Cancer:* Cundurango, Cadmium sulphuratum.

- *Skin Cancer:* Euphorbium officinarum.

- *Bone Cancer:* Lachesis muta.

- *Non-Cancerous Fibroid Tumor:* Epiphysterinum.``1111111111

Section Five

APPENDICES

HOMEOPATHIC TREATMENT MODEL

The basics of this model apply to any type of homeopathic treatment and may be helpful in determining an overall treatment plan. As you read and study the following protocol you will probably think that this is daunting and nearly impossible. It is complicated and can take time and a familiarity with homeopathic remedies, but it is possible to do and to do it well, even without muscle testing. Homeopathic physicians spend many years studying and gaining experience, but if you know and love your people and follow your intuition, you can do a very good job—and you will do no harm.

For the lay person who is just beginning, dependable muscle testing skills are **very** helpful. With a little study, it is possible to use the muscle test both to analyze the case and to determine the correct remedy, or remedies. If, every time you muscle test a case and a remedy, you will take the time to study and analyze why that remedy was the best choice, you can become very competent at homeopathic prescribing very quickly. I have witnessed a high level of competence among members of the classes that I have taught time and time again—many times in a period of only a few weeks.

STEP 1 DIAGNOSTIC

- Determine the totality of symptoms presenting by looking for:
    - physical symptoms
    - mental/emotional symptoms
    - general characteristics of the person and the illness
    - times of aggravation or amelioration
- modalities (what makes it better or what makes it worse)
- Determine the miasms—if any—responsible for symptoms.
- Note deep impact issues (NSS) and list those symptoms separately.
- Note generational issues by discussing family history and commonalities.
- Note separate psoric issues. To note them you must be familiar with them—please study the psora miasm in depth!
- If there are no major miasmic, deep impact, generational, or psoric issues presenting symptoms at the present time, the general type (plant, animal, or mineral) of the indicted constitutional remedy can be determined.

STEP 2 SELECT 1ST REMEDY

You do this by asking yourself what symptoms are presenting most dramatically right now?

It would be nice if I could tell you that the presenting symptoms will all fit nice and neatly into categories. People are human and they do not fit into little boxes. Some symptoms might be easy to categorize, but it isn't very likely that all of them will, and it doesn't really matter. The categories are to help you think, analyze, and understand. You will choose a remedy that most nearly matches the person's symptoms based on the entire person (as listed above in Step 1 Diagnostic, the first bulleted section, above).

If there is nothing life threatening and no acute situation presenting at the moment, you will begin with the constitutional remedy. Beginning with the constitutional remedy is unlikely. If they are looking for a remedy it is usually because there is something unusual, painful, or chronic going on.

If you are working constitutionally and progress halts, give the remedy that most closely matches the deep impact issue or generational issue that is presenting at the moment. Generational issues are often treated first because they have, and are, weakening the person and causing them extreme pain or distress. If the generational issue, although recognized as being present at times in the person's life, is lying quiet at the moment, treat the more pressing needs. Remember, in homeopathy the treatment is based on the symptoms presenting ***most dramatically at the present time.***

STEP 3 DETERMINE THE POTENCY—CHOICE WILL BE BASED ON THE FOLLOWING:

- Vitality of the patient. With very sensitive people, the elderly, infants, and children, the use of lower potencies—but at more frequent intervals—is generally recommended.

- Depth of the problem. If the problem is deep and has been around for a long time, a higher potency remedy may be indicated.

- Past history of suppression by the use of antibiotics and other drug therapies. This is a confusing thing. It is best to begin with lower potency remedies, if possible. On the other hand, the drugs may block the homeopathic remedy and it will require a higher potency remedy to get any results at all. The presence of drugs <u>always</u> complicates homeopathic treatment, but it is also the norm for most people so that situation is what we are usually working with.

STEP 4 TIMING THE FIRST DOSE

- **Patience** is the key to avoiding discomfort. Do not go too quickly unless the person is willing to suffer some discomfort or the seriousness of the situation gives you no choice.

- Acute or life-threatening situations require desperate measures. I have seen several 1M remedies administered as rapidly as possible (to stop the action of a poisonous spider bite and in injury and serious burn situations). In each situation, anything less than very deep remedies applied quickly would have been "too little and too late."

The remedy acts as a trigger to the person's vital energy (immune system). The improvement comes from the eradication of the problem. The deeper into the system the remedy has reached (usually determined by the height of the potency) the more time must be given to allow for completion of this process.

In the situations mentioned above, the healing produced by one remedy was completed very quickly (to save the person's life or limb) and a new remedy was called for to work on the remaining symptoms. Perhaps if the perfectly matching remedy had been available, it would have taken only a remedy or two.

Unless you have hundreds of remedies on hand, you will probably resort to giving several in quick succession. If you give several high potency remedies quickly, you may need to antidote some of them (or some portion of their symptom pictures) a little later. This is a complicated thing and is the reason why these life and limb threatening situations, in the literature, are recommended to be left to very experienced practitioners. Competent muscle testing changes the parameters of what can and cannot be treated at home dramatically. The responsibility for these types of choices must remain with the person being treated, of course. I have seen amazing results by fairly inexperienced muscle testers, many times.

If there was nothing dramatic presenting and you have started with the constitutional remedy, the literature will tell you to follow, as nearly as possible, the following protocol. This will be discussed in depth later in this book.

1M every 3 weeks to 1 month for 3 - 4 times

10M every 6 weeks to 2 months for 2 - 4 times

50M every 3 - 6 months for 2 - 3 times

Remember, just as above, the higher the potency the deeper will be the impact on the energy system. A longer period of time between doses must be allowed. Here again, the recommendations in classical homeopathy and where the muscle test leads are often quite different.

STEP 5 ASSESS RESULTS FROM FIRST REMEDY

The following things, listed in the order they will most likely appear, are what you want to see. They indicate that the body is responding properly, and is systematically throwing off the problem.

WITH A DEEP IMPACT ISSUE
- An improvement, emotionally, on some level or levels will occur first, with a possible aggravation of the most recent symptoms.
- A return or aggravation of the primary symptom; the vital energy (immune system) then corrects it.
- Elimination of the specific deep impact issue. Symptoms they have lived with since the original accident (or whatever it was) go away.
- With the eradication of the deep impact issue, the surfacing of clearer generational or miasmic issues may occur. Treat according to symptoms being presented.

TREATING A PREDOMINANTLY GENERATIONAL OR MIASMIC ISSUE
- An improvement emotionally will occur first, with a possible short-lived and mild aggravation of symptoms.
- Improvement in overall vitality.
- Elimination of generational symptoms in reverse order of their appearance.
- The surfacing of clearer constitutional issues to be treated according to symptoms.

CONSTITUTIONAL TREATMENT
- An improvement in the way they feel within themselves (emotionally).
- A reduction of the most recently acquired symptoms.
- A return or aggravation of the primary symptoms. These long-standing symptoms are brought briefly online and the vital energy eliminates that pattern wherever is it occurring in the body. This will begin with the emotional symptoms, then progress to the physical symptoms.
- An improvement of the physical symptoms following the rules governing the progression of cure outlined on page 90.

SOME OTHER POSSIBLE RESULTS FROM THE FIRST REMEDY

NO CHANGE
- You have chosen the wrong remedy. You will need to get more information to complete the symptom picture and find a remedy that matches more closely.
- You may have chosen the correct remedy but have not given it in a high enough potency to accomplish the desired result.
- The healing process is being blocked by the emergence of the psora miasm.

NEW SYMPTOMS EMERGE
- If this was a symptom that the person had previously at any time, you have a positive indication that you are on the right track. The symptom has surfaced so that the vital energy can throw it off. Symptoms should appear according to the usual progression of homeopathic healing (refer to page 90).
- If this is an entirely new symptom, but not one listed for the remedy you have just given, re-examine the remedy selection based upon the new entire symptom picture that is presenting. Give a follow-up remedy based on your evaluation.

If the newly emerging symptoms are listed in the symptom picture of the remedy you just gave but are not symptoms that the person has experienced before, the person is proving the remedy. The remedy you gave did not match the totality of symptoms that were presenting closely enough. This is not a good thing. Discuss, examine, re-evaluate, and consider antidoting if the symptoms are severe enough to warrant it. Antidoting will probably prevent you from using any other homeopathic remedy for a few days. At the appropriate time, give another remedy that more closely resembles the presenting symptoms. Note: proving does not usually happen with nosode remedies.

PROGRESS IS POSITIVE BUT DOES NOT LAST VERY LONG

- The right remedy was chosen but a higher potency (deeper) remedy is needed to maintain the improvement.
- The person has inherited a weak constitution; you will need to treat for this generational weakness with the appropriate, usually miasmic, remedy before returning once again to the remedy and treatment protocol that you had previously chosen.
- The psora miasm is present. It may have been there all along and you didn't realize it, or it may be coming online as the result of the treatment. In either case, the psoric symptoms being presented are now the most dramatic—said to be *in the forefront of the case*. Treat them and then re-evaluate.

PROGRESS IS POSITIVE BUT STALLS OUT

- A psoric miasm blocking progress is suspected; a regimen of an antipsoric remedy at deep levels is indicated before progress will resume. When psora has gone back to sleep, it will be necessary to continue treating for the remaining symptoms.

(This is similar to the previous situation except that repeats of the remedy, even at higher potency, do not result in progression of the cure.)

PROGRESS ON THE PHYSICAL LEVEL WITHOUT POSITIVE MENTAL/EMOTIONAL SHIFT

This is almost always an indication that the only symptoms evaluated were physical. Too often homeopathics are prescribed in this way. While it may appear to be progress, it really isn't. The underlying emotional disturbances will simply manifest in a new way and have to be dealt with again later. Always pay attention to the emotional symptoms. In fact, they are your most important guide because they are the original source of the problem.

> *Progress on a physical level alone is not an indication of the positive progress toward health.*
> *Do not mistake it for progress.*
> *You have most likely given the wrong remedy and no real healing has occurred!*

Note: When dealing with multi-miasmic situations, improvement emotionally may happen with the first miasmic remedy; thereafter, you will see improvement mainly in physical symptoms. This is acceptable and you are still going in the right direction.

STEP 6   SELECT A SECOND REMEDY

When using nosode remedies (and occasionally with other remedies) it is necessary to use an intercurrent remedy. This remedy will be very specific to the organ, gland, or body system that is under attack. This is most common when working with cancer or other horrendous attacks on a specific area of the body.

STEP 7   PROCEED TO OTHER ASPECTS OF THE PERSON'S HEALTH

The steps listed above are a description of the way homeopathic practitioners who do not muscle test work. If you are muscle testing for a remedy, these three pages will assist you in analyzing why the muscle test led you where it did. This will make you better at what you do and less likely to make a mistake with your muscle testing.

THE PROCESS OF CURE

AFTER TAKING THE REMEDY A PERSON SHOULD FEEL AS FOLLOWS:

- Signs of increased physiological resistance to disease. This sounds better than it feels. When our bodies are responding properly to outside attacks from pathogens, we will produce a fever to aid in killing the pathogens. We may experience diarrhea, an inflammatory response of some kind, and increased mucus discharges. These symptoms may make us think that we are less resistant to disease and are catching everything that comes around. This is far from the truth. These symptoms are usually mild reactions and pass quickly. They are really an indication that the vital force is strong and is responding appropriately to attack.

- A reduction or total disappearance of the symptoms of the illness. This is a welcome phase of the healing process.

- A return of more normal behavior on all levels—physical, emotional, mental, etc.

- A return of old symptoms that were previously suppressed in some way. This can be discouraging unless one focuses on the fact that these suppressed diseases and imbalances are being cleared from the system completely. They are no longer lying there dormant, waiting for a time of stress or lowered resistance to come back online and create real havoc.

- A brief return of symptoms. This will occur 5 - 7 days after a 200C potency was taken, 3 - 4 weeks afterwards when taking a 1 M potency. This indicates that the reaction to the remedy is wearing off. This is an indication that it is time to take the next dose or that it is time to move on to the next higher potency of the same remedy.

- **Total elimination of the symptoms with no aggravations or suppressions coming on.** This is the goal of homeopathic treatment.

The symptoms listed above will follow, in some unique form, the patterns of the progression of cure discusses on page 90.

It should be noted, and remembered, that when treating homeopathically, the first improvement that is accomplished from the right remedy is an improvement in *mental and emotional outlook*. The person often feels that they are on their way to a resumption of health and normal functioning before there are any physical signs of improvement.

KINESIOLOGY

Kinesiology uses the relationship between thoughts and the muscles of the body to access knowledge. The relationship between thoughts and muscles has been studied, recorded, and utilized by medical science in the rehabilitation of muscles for many years. There is nothing of voodoo or magic in this simple relationship and the use of it. Kinesiology is often referred to as muscle testing, bio-kinetic testing, energy testing, etc.

ENERGY

When discussing muscle testing, you will often hear the term subtle energy or just energy. To what do these terms refer, exactly? That is difficult to answer because what is being referred to is such an insubstantial thing with a multitude of characteristics.

Some kinesiologists describe energy as an extension of the electromagnetic energy produced by the body. Donna Eden, in her book Energy Medicine, describes it as wavelengths, rates of vibrations, and patterns of pulsation that are "the common vocabulary of the body, mind and soul". Whatever it is and however you describe it, energy is something as real and as definite as magnetism or gravity. This energy is identified, measured, and quantified in the world every day. This energy is being measured whenever a doctor orders an EKG or many other tests.

There are many branches, or fields, of kinesiology and they are as varied as the people who have developed and are practicing them. There are some beliefs, however, that are common to all. Among these is the fundamental assumption, borne by experience, that each of us possesses a complete knowledge of the basic blueprint of our own creation. In addition, it is assumed that we always know the status of our body mind, and soul at a given time. This is certainly not always a conscious knowing. Sometimes we even seem to hide this knowledge from our conscious mind deliberately. Even so, it is always reflected very accurately in our energy field. Muscle testing is a simple, effective tool that allows us to bring this useful information to our conscious attention.

It is my personal belief that muscle testing is a simple—no more than grade school level—method of accessing the knowledge available in the universe. In other words, muscle testing is a very rudimentary method of tapping into God's knowledge. Are there better ways? Of course. They are intuitions, inspiration, and prayer.

I have found, over many years, that the development of good muscle testing skills can sharpen our perceptions, give us confidence and trust in the intuitive feelings that we have, and teach us to walk more closely with Heaven. I hope that this will be your experience also. After a while, you should find yourself using muscle testing less and less as you learn to trust the things that you just know to be true.

LEARNING TO MUSCLE TEST

How do you learn to muscle test? First; read the information on the next two pages and get your body into a state of basic balance. Then have a good talk with yourself. I mean this quite literally. Tell you mind/body complex what you want it to do. For example; say to yourself "I want to sway forward when the thing I am saying, or thinking, or about to put into my body is right and true, and sway backward when it is not."

Then practice a few times by saying "yes" (sway forward) and "no" (sway backward). If you need to make yourself sway consciously. You are working with muscles, and just like when learning to ride a bike, they may need to be taught what is expected of them and what they should do.

When simple yes and no is testing strongly, move on to making basic statements. It is always better and less confusing to make a statement rather than to ask questions.

SOME EXAMPLES OF BASIC QUESTIONS

To Sway Forward	**To Sway Backward**
My name is (state your name).	My name is (state a fictitious name).
Say words such as "love," etc.	Say words such as "hate" or "anger."
Think of something pleasant.	Think of something unpleasant.
Thing of a food or activity that you like.	Think of a food or activity that you dislike.

Other phrases might be:

"I enjoy my work."

"I need time alone."

"I am married."

Keep practicing and balancing, using the techniques on the following page, until you can feel the difference in the energy and are testing accurately.

MUSCLES TO TEST

Any muscle may be tested. When you are reasonably comfortable with the sway, try testing other muscles. Once again, talk to yourself firmly and clearly. For example: make a circle with the thumb and index finger of your left hand. Tell your left hand that these fingers are to hold firmly for accurate and true things and **break** or release (the equivalent of swaying backward) for inaccurate statements. Put the index finger of your right hand in the circle made by your left hand. Make a statement and then put pressure against the circle with the finger of your right hand. You can test absolutely any muscle of the body with practice.

Making statements and then testing a muscle is one common way to muscle test. Another simple use for this skill (after giving your body instructions) is to hold an item in your hand (or place it on your chest) and see if you sway forward or backward. I like to teach this skill to children, even very young ones, with food allergies. They can quickly determine whether or not a food that is being offered them is going to be a problem or not. I find that children learn to muscle test very easily and usually test very accurately almost immediately.

Often muscle testing is done by having a person hold their arm up and away from their body, make a statement, and another person applies pressure to the muscle. Very little pressure should be applied to a muscle, in any scenario. A good rule is to use no more than 2 pounds of pressure (the weight of a bag of powdered sugar) for no more than 2 seconds.

SURROGATE TESTING

Kinesthetic testing (muscle testing) is sometimes done using another person as a surrogate. For example, a mother may hold an infant or small child on her lap and test, using her own muscles rather than those of the child, to determine the response. When testing small children, a very weak or sick person, or a very elderly one, it is often necessary to test this way. In the early stages of your developing muscle testing skills, it is best to make sure that the person being tested and the surrogate are touching each other in some way.

It is possible, when you have become skilled at muscle testing, to test very accurately for a person across the room or even someone who is far away. This is an advanced skill. It is easy to miss little pieces of the puzzle and obtain inaccurate answers with this form of testing. As you become more confident and better at your statements you will probably find yourself doing this from time to time.

VERY BRIEF INFORMATION AND TIPS ON MUSCLE TESTING

BALANCING FOR ACCURATE MUSCLE TESTING:

In order for your attempts to muscle test to be accurate and successful, there must be a minimum degree of balance within your own body or the body of the person you are testing. Different healing modalities accomplish this in different ways. Here are a few of my favorites.

- **Thymus Thump:** There are many ways to do this. My favorite is to tap with my fingertips in a clockwise direction (place right hand over the heart and tap, moving upward) for 2 or 3 rounds and then place the hand over the navel.

- **Sideways Figure Eights:** Lock both hands together, extending the index fingers to make a pointer for your eyes to follow. With your eyes following and your head motionless, draw figure 8's lying on their sides. Making the 8's both large and small will bring small and large motor centers into play, as well as get your energy crossing the midline of the brain so that information being accessed is coming from both sides.

- **Cross Crawls:** Begin by simply walking in place; then touch the left knee with the right elbow and then the right knee with the left elbow.

- **Water:** Sometimes when you are getting opposite or confused responses a glass of water is all that is needed.

- **Essential Oils:** Often oils such as Sandalwood, LeUnity, LeTranquility, LeLetting Go and others, (sold by Butterfly Express, llc) diffused or applied to the thymus area brings balance and accuracy.

- **Chakra/Central Meridian Zipper:** Bring your hand up the midline 3 or 4 times.

CONFIRMING BASIC BALANCE BEFORE BEGINNING

This is accomplished by making both positive (accurate) and negative (inaccurate) statements and then muscle testing. I would recommend that you set your parameters for a strong (or forward) test on the positive/accurate statements.

TYPES OF MUSCLE TESTING

- **Response Testing:** Place an object on the thymus or just below the navel and determine whether the tested muscle stays strong or goes weak.

- **Verbal Statement:** It is recommended that you make statements instead of ask questions. This requires both knowledge and skill. Your statements/questions will be only as good as your understanding and education make them. Experience is the only way to get good at figuring out all the nuances of a situation and including them in your statements. The better you get at your statements and the more consistent you are about follow-up statements and the double check and rechecks that we talk about here, the more accurate the information you obtain will be.

- **Testing From a List or Book:** With a little bit of practice it is possible to become very accurate at testing what is needed from a list, whether or not you have personal knowledge of the items on the list or in the book. This is an amazing and useful skill. Homeopathic lists, a list of herbal remedies, and the information found in anatomy books make good things to test from.

POSSIBLE USES FOR MUSCLE TESTING

- Muscle testing can help us identify substances, circumstances, and thought patterns that are harmful to us. Muscle testing can also aid us in choosing substances and lifestyles that help us achieve our goals, have more energy, and maintain better health. It should be remembered that, sometimes, it is only the perception of a situation that makes it stressful to us. Careful use of muscle testing can help us ascertain if our perspectives are as clear as they should be.

- By allowing muscle testing to help guide our choices of alternative methods, modalities, and products, we can deal with our discomforts and ailments in the best possible manner.

- Muscles testing can, occasionally, aid us in solving the mysteries of the causes of our illnesses, anxieties and pains. At the very least, muscle testing can aid us in identifying important contributing factors to problems that develop in our lives.

INAPPROPRIATE USE OF MUSCLE TESTING

There are occasions and circumstances when the use of muscle testing is completely inappropriate. Certainly there are questions that should not be asked using a muscle test and there are ways of using muscle testing that are inherently wrong! Using muscle testing in these ways will cause harm—sometimes irreparable harm—in your life and, particularly, in your relationships with friends and family. This warning cannot be overemphasized! It is extremely important that you think through the following suggested taboos (and, probably, others I haven't thought to mention here) very carefully, establish your own parameters, and never violate them no matter how much the situation tempts you!

Muscle testing is inappropriate, or just plain wrong, when:

The person doing the testing has no right to the information being tested for, or the person would not want us to know that information. Invading another person's privacy by reading their mail is wrong; it is so much worse to read another person's mind or access their personal stuff without permission or without their knowledge using muscle testing.

I believe that it is wrong, and usually damaging to a relationship, to muscle test for a person without being asked specifically by that person. Their mother, brother, aunt, or cousin asking you to test for someone does not count as permission! There are few things in life as annoying as a person who gives us a back or neck massage that we do not want, or a person who speaks up with unsolicited advice. It is even more annoying to give people comments or answers, arrived at through muscle testing, without them asking. Muscle testing for a person who has not requested that you do so is almost always inappropriate.

Even when the person has asked for your help and is willing to have you test for them, be very careful about using the muscle test to say things that you wouldn't dare say to them without muscle testing to back you up. It is easy to let your opinions sway the muscle test, especially if there are things you would like to tell them (your children or others) that they have been unwilling to hear. Using the muscle test in this way should only be done under the firmest directive of Heaven, even with (or especially with) family members.

Always find someone else to do the testing if you are so involved in the situation or with the person that you cannot test from a clear, objective space. Try to never let your prejudices color your testing.

Never use muscle testing to predict the future! This should need no further explanation.

If your intuition, or the whisperings of the Spirit, tell you not to test a particular thing or situation, don't test for it! On the other hand, there will be occasions when the Spirit will send you places where all of the above parameters have not been met. If this happens, you will have to find your own way, using prayer and inspiration. Always be very careful in these situations, but don't fail to do the good that Heaven has called upon you to do, either.

A Few Basic Rules of Kinesthetic Testing

(I know that I am repeating myself here. I think it is important.)

First: Always obtain permission. Verbal permission first, if that is possible, and energy permission always. Energy permission is of vital importance! Never, never continue when you don't have it! If energy permission is denied, it is sometimes possible to establish through muscle testing the exact cause of the refusal. The refusal can be coming from either the client or the practitioner and can be as simple as a need for a drink of water by one or the other. A common reason for lack of permission is that the person is already doing something "energetically," such as a homeopathic, essential oil, or energy procedure and it would be overwhelming to their energy system to make further changes at this time.

Second: Remain objective. Test with an open and curious mind, being willing to put your own expectations and prejudices aside. If you do this you will be far more effective and more accurate, and you will learn some interesting things. Bear in mind, though, that there are many ways to accomplish an energy task. I have often had the experience of saying, "There is something else that would be easier or less time-consuming that would be of equal value" and been given several alternative choices, all equally valid. Your intention or opinion can substantially affect the test.

Third: Value your intuition. This intuition is an inspired hunch (or Heaven's directions) and can be a very valuable skill to possess. Everyone I have ever worked with, as they became adept at energy testing, began to exhibit a high degree of intuition. They simply 'know" as they test what the answer will be, and when time is short or nonexistent (an emergency situation) they know, intuitively, what to do and what herb, or something else, to reach for.

Fourth: use cross-checks to validate your testing. Whenever possible, make a statement, test and then make the statement in reverse (if it was positive, phrase it negatively) and test again. If an answer goes against common sense, wait a while and test again after some thought and study. You, or the person you are working with, have gone this long without that piece of information. Chances are they can make it another hour or another day until you are sure of your answers.

Fifth: Be very clear in your statements. The energy system is much like a computer. It takes you very literally. You must be sure what information you are trying to obtain and you must state it clearly. If you are testing for quantity, always say, "At least one, at least two," and so forth.

Sixth: Set parameters for the test. Learn to talk to yourself! Tell your energy system what information you are trying to obtain and let it know that you intend to keep testing until all the pieces are in place. If the muscle test can't trust you to keep looking until you have found the best possible answer, it may give you something less than optimum early on, thinking that you might not keep testing long enough to find the right answer.

Seventh: Always remember the follow-up questions. These are statements such as "anything else", "anything different that would be better in some way", "any reason not to do this or use this at this time", "anything in addition" The use of these statements will make you far more effective and certainly save you a lot of grief and mistakes.

Eighth: Never violate privacy. There are some questions you should never ask and some information you are not entitled to. This can vary from person to person, situation to situation. Your intuition and your conscience should be your guide. Do not ask for any information that you are not willing to admit to having obtained. This is not a problem if you always test out loud, but can be a temptation when working quickly and quietly to yourself. Please trust me on this one—do not violate agency or privacy in any way. The harm it will do—to them and to you—cannot even begin to be measured. Just don't go there!! The end does not justify the means.

If you haven't been invited in—your are trespassing!

HOMEOPATHIC REMEDIES—A RENEWABLE RESOURCE

MAKING HOMEOPATHIC REMEDIES

Homeopathic remedies of all types have historically been made by methods similar to that used by Samuel Hahnemann 200 years ago. These methods involve the systematic dilution and succussion of substances and transfer agents into usable homeopathic remedies. As explained in chapter one, the ratio of dilution and the number of times the remedy is diluted and succussed determines potency.

Eventually, this dilution and succussion process results in a remedy that has no discernible molecules of the original substance. Nevertheless, the newly made remedy has a very distinct energetic imprint which is unique to all homeopathic remedies made from that substance.

This energetic imprint can be transferred to, and carried by, an endless variety of transfer agent materials. The most common transfer agents in use today are milk sugar (saccharum lactose), sucrose, alcohol, distilled water and rice papers. Milk sugar and sucrose are used in tablet, pellet, or powder form. The transferring of this energetic imprint from a homeopathic remedy to the body, by whatever means, sets the healing process in motion.

THE PRACTICAL APPLICATION OF HOMEOPATHIC PREPARATION

Once you have an energetic imprint of a particular substance—a homeopathic remedy, in other words—it is possible to make another bottle of the remedy from the original. This can be done with either a liquid homeopathic or with the more solid forms. The requirements for this process, and the steps to accomplish it, are very simple. You simply place a few drops, pellets or tablets of the original homeopathic remedy into the new bottle. ***You must be careful not to contaminate the energetic pattern of the original with anything else while doing so.***

There are some basic guidelines that various people have discovered by trial and error over the years. I will instruct as though using liquid forms of the remedies in my explanations but the same principles apply to homeopathics in other forms such as pellets or tablets.

- When making a new homeopathic you must always use a *new* bottle. The bottle cannot have contained, previously, any other homeopathic or an essential oil. A new bottle is the best way to guarantee that your new remedy remains uncontaminated by other energies.

- Liquid homeopathic remedies require the additions of a preservative and antibacterial agent. Alcohol is commonly used. I use vodka, mixed with the distilled water at an approximate ratio of 1 part vodka to 6 or 7 parts distilled water. Even with alcohol added, care should still be taken not to touch the dropper.

- Homeopathic remedies may be made in distilled water without the alcohol in certain situations. Making a remedy without adding a preserving and antibacterial agent is occasionally done if the remedy is going to be used in the eye or on some other delicate tissue. Homeopathic remedies made in distilled water with no alcohol are meant to be used immediately. You must be especially careful not to touch the dropper or the mouth of the bottle with your fingers or to contaminate the remedy in any other way. The remedy needs to be discarded, bottle and all, after about 10 days. If you still have need of the remedy (this is unlikely) you will need to make a whole new batch in a *new* bottle.

- If you wish your remedy to remain at the same potency as the original, **do not** succuss (shake or tap) the new bottle after adding the drops of the original remedy. Simply let the energy of the original suffuse the new batch. (This is somewhat similar to the process used to make a new batch of sourdough. The time this process takes depends on the potency of the original. Lower potencies seem to take a bit longer than higher potencies. Two or three days is adequate for any potency.

- If you wish to raise the potency of your new remedy (or you need the new remedy more quickly and don't mind raising the potency a bit) you will need to succuss the new remedy after adding the drops of the old one. Approximately 100 shakes seems to be the optimum number. Remember, when you shake the remedy you have increased the potency. For example, if your original remedy was a 6X your new one will be a 7X. If your original remedy was a 30C the new one will be a 31C. This small increase is not usually a problem if only done once or twice with any homeopathic remedy.

- Most homeopathic practitioners keep a separate bottle of each remedy just for making additional copies of that remedy. This bottle is called a "mother" and is always used to make the new remedies. The alcohol content of the "mother" is generally higher than is necessary for everyday use.

- The purpose of a "mother" is two-fold. First, the "mother" is less likely to become contaminated if it is only taken out of the cupboard once in a while to make a new remedy and is never actually used to administer the homeopathic. Second, every new remedy made from it, even if shaken, only goes up 1 more level in potency. (Remember, when you make a new bottle from a 6X and succuss it, you get a 7X; when you use that 7X to make a new bottle, and succuss it, you will have an 8X.)

CREATING ORIGINAL HOMEOPATHICS

Theoretically it is possible to make a homeopathic from any substance that you like. Some people have done this with various herbs, herbal preparations, or essential oils. I suppose it could be done using any substance at all. To do so you would dilute and succuss the chosen substance according to whichever dilution ratio you choose. The first dilution would be a 1, the second time you dilute and succuss would result in a 2 of whatever dilution ratio that you started with. Continue in this manner until you arrive at the desired potency.

I am not advising that you run about making homeopathic remedies from every substance you think necessary. Scientific methods of testing and homeopathic methods of proving and recording symptoms should be followed whenever possible. Of course, carefully following the results of muscle testing can result in amazing remedies and equally amazing results.

The Original Bach Flower Remedies

Agrimony	Clematis	Honeysuckle	Pine	Vervain
Aspen	Crab Apple	Hornbeam	Red Chestnut	Vine
Beech	Elm	Impatiens	Rescue Remedy	Walnut
Centaury	Gentian	Larch	Rock Rose	Water Violet
Cerato	Gorse	Mimulus	Rock Water	White Chestnut
Cherry Plum	Heather	Mustard	Scleranthus	Wild Oat
Chestnut Bud	Holly	Oak	Star of Bethlehem	Wild Rose
Chicory		Olive	Sweet Chestnut	Willow

North American Flower Essence Remedies

Aloe Vera	Deerbrush	Mallow	Sage
Alpine Lily	Dill	Manzanita	Sagebrush
Angel's Trumpet	Dogwood	Mariposa Lily	Saguaro
Angelica	Easter Lily	Milkweed	Saint John's Wort
Arnica	Echinacea	Morning Glory	Scarlet Monkeyflower
Baby Blue Eyes	Evening Primrose	Mountain Pennyroyal	Scotch Broom
Basil	Fairy Lantern	Mountain Pride	Self-Heal
Black Cohosh	Fawn Lily	Mugwort	Shasta Daisy
Blackberry	Filaree	Mullein	Shooting Star
Black-Eyed Susan	Forget-Me-not	Nasturtium	Snapdragon
Bleeding Heart	Fuchsia	Nicotiana	Star Thistle
Borage	Garlic	Oregon Grape	Star Tulip
Buttercup	Golden Ear Drops	Penstemon	Sticky Monkeyflower
Calendula	Golden Yarrow	Peppermint	Sunflower
California Pitcher Plant	Goldenrod	Pink Monkeyflower	Sweet Pea
California Poppy	Hibiscus	Pink Yarrow	Tansy
California Wild Rose	Hound's Tongue	Poison Oak	Tiger Lily
Calla Lily	Indian Paintbrush	Pomegranate	Trillium
Canyon Dudleya	Indian Pink	Pretty Face	Trumpet Vine
Cayenne	Iris	Purple Monkeyflower	Violet
Chamomile	Lady's Slipper	Quaking Grass	Yarrow
Chaparral	Larkspur	Queen Anne's Lace	Yarrow Special Formula
Chrysanthemum	Lavender	Quince	Yellow Star Tulip
Corn	Lotus	Rabbitbrush	Yerba Santa
Cosmos	Love-Lies-Bleeding	Red Clover	Zinnia
Dandelion	Madia	Rosemary	

Range of Light (Sierra Mountain Range) Flower Essence Remedies

"Well may the Sierra be named, not the Snowy Range, but the Range of Light" John Muir

Almond	Dune Primrose	Lady's Mantle	Red Larkspur
Alpine Aster	Explorer's Gentian	Lemon	Red Penstemon
Blazing Star	Fiesta Flower	Lewisia	Redbud
California Peony	Fireweed	Lilac	Redwood
California Valerian	Glassy Hyacinth	Lungwort	Rue
Cassiope	Green Bells of Ireland	Lupine	Scarlet Fritillary
Cherry	Green Cross Gentian	Madrone	Shasta Lily
Chocolate Lily	Green Nicotiana	Monkshood	Sierra Primrose
Columbine	Green Rein Orchid	Mountain Forget-Me-Not	Splendid Mariposa Lily
Corn Lily	Hawthorne	Ocotillo	Spreading Phlox
Desert Lily	Hyssop	Pedicularis	Tall Mountain Larkspur
Downy Avens	Joshua Tree	Pussy Paws	

Alaskan Flower Remedies

- Alder
- Alpine Azalea
- Balsam Poplar
- Black Spruce
- Bladderwort
- Blue Elf Viola
- Blueberry Pollen
- Bog Blueberry
- Bog Rosemary
- Bunchberry
- Cassandra
- Cattail Pollen
- Chiming Bells
- Columbine Comandra
- Cotton Grass
- Cow Parsnip
- Dandelion Fireweed
- Forget-Me-Not
- Foxglove
- Golden Corydalis
- Grass of Parnassu
- Green Bells of Ireland
- Green Bog Orchid
- Green Fairy Orchid
- Grove Sandwort
- Hairy Butterwort
- Harebell
- Horsetail
- Icelandic Poppy
- Jacob's Ladder
- Labrador Tea
- Lace Flower
- Ladies' Tresses
- Lady's Slipper
- Lamb's Quarters
- Monkshood
- Moschatel
- Mountain Wormwood
- Northern Lady's Slipper
- Northern Twayblade
- One-Sided Wintergreen
- Opium Poppy
- Paper Birch
- Pineapple Weed
- Prickly Wild Rose
- River Beauty
- Round-Leaved Sundew
- Shooting Star
- Single Delight
- Sitka Burnet
- Sitka Spruce Pollen
- Soapberry
- Sphagnum Moss
- Spiraea
- Sticky Geranium
- Sunflower
- Sweetgale
- Sweetgrass
- Tamarack
- Tundra Rose
- Tundra Twayblade
- Twinflower
- White Fireweed
- White Spruce
- White Violet
- Wild Iris
- Wild Rhubarb
- Willow
- Yarrow
- Yellow Dryas

Meridians

- Central Vessel
- Gall Bladder
- Governing Vessel
- Heart
- Kidney
- Large Intestine
- Liver
- Lung
- Pericardium
- Small Intestine
- Spleen
- Stomach
- Triple Warmer
- Urinary Bladder

Tissue Salts

- Calcarea fluorica
- Calcarea phosphoricum
- Calcarea sulphurica
- Ferrum phosphoricum
- Kali muriaticum
- Kali phosphoricum
- Kali sulphuricum
- Magnesia phosphoricum
- Natrum muriaticum
- Natrum phosphoricum
- Natrum sulphuricum
- Silica oxide

Color

- Green
- Indigo
- Magenta
- Orange
- Pink
- Red
- Spectrum
- Turquoise
- Violet
- Yellow

Sound

- A
- B
- D
- E
- F
- G
- High C
- Middle C
- The Chord BW

Basic Polycrest Remedies

- Aconitum napellus
- Allium cepa
- Aloe socotrina
- Apis mellifica
- Antimonium crudum
- Antimonium tartaricum
- Arnica montana
- Arsenicum album
- Aurum metallicum
- Baryta carbonica
- Belladonna
- Bellis perennis
- Berberis vulgaris
- Blatta orientalis
- Bryonia alba
- Bufo rana
- Cadmium metallicum
- Calcarea carbonica
- Calcarea phosphorica
- Calcarea sulphurica
- Cantharis vesicatoria
- Carbo vegetabilis
- Carcinosin
- Causticum
- Chamomilla vulgaris
- Cistus canadensis
- Cocculus indicus
- Colocynthis
- Cundurango
- Conium maculatum
- Crotalus horridus
- Cuprum metallicum
- Dulcamara
- Eupatorium perfoliatum
- Euphrasia officinalis
- Ferrum phosphoricum
- Gelsemium sempervirens
- Glonoinum
- Gossypium herbaceum
- Graphites naturalis
- Hamamelis virginiana
- Hepar sulphuris calcareum
- Hydrastis canadensis
- Hyoscyamus niger
- Hypericum perforatum
- Ignatia amara
- Ipecacuanha
- Kali bichromicum
- Kali carbonicum
- Kali chloricum
- Kali iodatum
- Kali phosphoricum
- Kali sulphuricum
- Lachesis muta
- Latrodectus mactans
- Laurocerasus officinalis
- Ledum palustre
- Lycopodium clavatum
- Malandrinum
- Magnesia phosphorica
- Medorrhinum
- Melilotus officinalis
- Mercurius solubilis
- Mezereum
- Muriaticum acidum
- Natrum fluoratum
- Natrum muriaticum
- Natrum sulphuricum
- Nitricum acidum
- Nux vomica
- Opium
- Petroleum oleum
- Phytolacca decandra
- Phosphorus
- Pilocarpinum
- Plumbum metallicum
- Podophyllum peltatum
- Psorinum
- Pulsatilla nigricans
- Pyrogenium
- Radium bromatum
- Rhus toxicodendron
- Ruta graveolens
- Sabadilla officinalis
- Sabina officinalis
- Sambuscus nigra
- Sarsaparilla officinalis
- Sepia succus
- Silica terra
- Spongia tosta
- Staphysagria
- Sulphur
- Symphytum officinale
- Syphilinum
- Tabacum nicotiana
- Terebinthiniae oleum
- Theridion curassavicum
- Thuja occidentalis
- Tuberculinum
- Urtica urens
- Veratrum album
- Viola tricolor

Index of Remedies

Abies nigra 171, 178, 226
Abrotanum artemisia 168, 227, 290, 307
Achillea millefolium 126, 170, 172, 228
Aconitum napellus 119, 181, 184, 185, 190, 192, 226, 228, 231, 236, 239, 240, 242, 243, 246, 275, 287, 288, 289, 290, 294, 299, 305, 306, 308, 309, 319, 324, 329, 348
Actea spicata 186, 226
Adrenalinum 30
Aesculus hippocastanum 175
Agaricus phalloides 190, 297, 314
Agathis australis 171, 226
Agnus castus 175, 227, 228
AIDS nosode 123, 228
Allium cepa 178, 188, 193, 231, 236, 240, 288, 348
Aloe socotrina 166, 167, 184, 177, 181, 228, 348
Alumen crudum 172, 184, 226, 249
Aluminum oxydata 82, 127, 128, 228
Ambra grisea 208
Ammonium carbonicum 151, 155, 226, 272, 311, 330
Anacardium orientale 70, 172, 173, 179, 228, 251, 253, 259
Andrographis peniculata 306
Anthracinum 30, 226, 319, 324
Antimonium crudum 133, 162, 169, 185, 226, 227, 249, 291, 348
Antimonium tartaricum 133, 185, 291, 292, 294, 307, 323, 348
Antipyrinum 322
Apis mellifica 75, 174, 175, 176, 183, 186, 211, 227, 231, 238, 241, 242, 268, 296, 310, 311, 313, 314, 315, 319, 324, 328, 348
Apomorphinum 183
Aqua marina 207
Argentum metallicum 155, 192, 226
Argentum nitricum 152, 164, 226, 227, 228, 247, 248, 260, 267, 268, 315
Arnica montana 118, 166, 169, 170, 176, 177, 181, 184, 185, 188, 190, 191, 195, 226, 227, 228, 231, 236, 238, 239, 240, 245, 247, 251, 252, 259, 270, 272, 276, 279, 287, 289, 292, 294, 295, 296, 297, 300, 305, 306, 307, 308, 309, 311, 312, 313, 314, 315, 318, 319, 320, 321, 323, 324, 325, 326, 328, 333, 348
Arsenicum album 118, 166, 169, 170, 176, 177, 181, 184, 185, 188, 190, 191, 195, 226, 227, 228, 236, 238, 239, 240, 245, 247, 251, 252, 259, 270, 272, 276, 279, 287, 289, 292, 294, 295, 296, 297, 300, 305, 306, 307, 308, 309, 311, 312, 313, 314, 315, 318, 319, 320, 321, 323, 324, 325, 326, 328, 333, 348
Arsenicum iodatum 155, 186, 227, 228, 259, 297, 315, 318, 320, 321, 323, 333
Artemisia annua 307
Asafoetida 182, 191, 227, 228
Asterias rubens 72
Atropinum purum 189, 227
Aurum iodatum 228
Aurum metallicum 155, 191, 228, 251, 320, 348
Aurum muriaticum 333
Avena sativa 33, 183, 270
Bacillinum 30, 297
Baptisia tinctoria 226, 227, 228, 168, 169, 176, 287, 310, 319, 324, 325
Baryta carbonica 227, 228, 151, 348
Belladonna 5, 73, 133, 167, 170, 172, 173, 180, 183, 184, 185, 189, 190, 191, 192, 226, 227, 228, 240, 260, 268, 288, 290, 291, 292, 299, 300, 306, 307, 308, 310, 311, 314, 315, 319, 322, 323, 324, 328, 348
Bellis perennis 168, 227, 232, 237, 241, 242, 348
Berberis aquifolium 166, 179, 228
Berberis vulgaris 166, 226, 270, 271, 348
Bioplasma 38
Bitis arietans 205
Blatta orientalis 195, 348
Borax veneta 226, 313
Bothrops lanceolatus(no listing) 318
Botulinum 325, 326, 327
Bromium 290, 294, 296, 318, 323
Bryonia alba 282, 288, 290
Bufo rana 195, 318, 348
Buthus australis 197
Cactus grandiflorus 167, 178, 180, 181, 226
Cadmium metallicum 155, 348
Cadmium sulphuratum 61, 154, 238, 333
Calcarea arsenicosa 333, 349
Calcarea carbonica 72, 153, 156, 172, 184, 189, 210, 232, 238, 241, 227, 242, 245, 249, 260, 263, 269, 272, 297,

351

Index of Remedies

308, 309, 330, 348

Calcarea fluorata 40, 47, 152, 153, 156, 226

Calcarea iodata 155

Calcarea phosphorica 40, 47, 153, 154, 156, 162, 164, 168, 169, 210, 228, 232, 237, 249, 348

Calcarea silicata 226

Calcarea sulphurica 41, 47, 153, 157, 182, 320, 348

Calendula officinalis 168, 170, 174, 226, 232, 237, 238, 241

Camphora 175, 177, 179, 181, 190, 226, 272, 308, 309

Cannabis indica 173, 174, 176, 227, 228

Cannabis sativa 173, 174, 226

Cantharis vesicatoria 75, 172, 176, 189, 212, 232, 237, 320, 333, 348

Capsicum annuum 189, 251, 226

Carbo animalis 30, 227, 169

Carbo vegetabilis 16, 177, 178, 179, 181, 184, 226, 232, 240, 242, 272, 290, 291, 292, 294, 308, 309, 310, 311, 319, 324, 325, 348

Carbolicum acidum 227, 326

Carcinosin 30, 82, 99, 115, 116, 117, 118, 227, 228, 247, 248, 250, 261, 306, 307, 312, 318, 319, 330, 332, 333, 348

Carduus marianus 306, 307

Caulophyllum thalictroides 167, 170, 172, 180, 186, 227

Causticum 99, 162, 165, 180, 187, 189, 226, 247, 250, 251, 254, 272, 292, 299, 300, 312, 330, 348

Ceanothus americanus 33, 333

Cenchris contortrix 204, 318

Cereus bonplandii 226, 227

Chamomilla vulgaris 20, 169, 178, 190, 192, 193, 226, 227, 260, 263, 288, 306, 348

Chelidonium majus 33, 170, 174, 183, 184, 226, 270, 306

Cholesterinum 30

China officinalis 168, 171, 178, 179, 183, 184, 186, 191, 226, 247, 261, 263, 272, 306, 307, 308, 310, 311, 325

Chininum arsenicosum 226, 307

Cina maritima 162, 169, 170, 226, 248, 257, 258

Chocolate 43, 44, 72, 95, 96, 226, 117, 161, 179, 182, 205, 208, 248, 249, 273

Cicuta virosa 106, 186, 191, 228, 249

Cimicifuga racemosa 109, 167, 174, 181, 183, 186, 227

Cinnamonum ceylanicum 182, 227

Cistus canadensis 192, 227, 348

Clematis erecta 103, 186, 228, 348

Cocculus indicus 177, 179, 192, 193, 232, 240, 242, 272, 322, 348

Coccus cacti 213, 292

Cochlearia armoracia 320

Coffea cruda 184, 185, 227, 288

Colchicum autumnale 177, 180, 226, 308

Collinsonia canadensis 175, 226

Colocynthis 169, 192, 193, 226, 348

Colostrum 30

Conchiolinum 210

Conium maculatum 70, 115, 175, 186, 191, 226, 227, 228, 333, 348

Copaiva 176, 227

Corallium rubrum 72, 209, 292

Coriandrum sativum 191, 228

Cortisone 16, 51, 143

Crataegus oxyacantha 33, 180, 188, 270, 276, 329

Crotalus horridus 173, 202, 227, 228, 280, 294, 295, 305, 306, 310, 311, 317, 319, 324, 348

Croton tiglium 172, 226, 313

Culex musca/pipiens 214

Cundurango 194, 333, 348

Cuprum metallicum 155, 179, 181, 292, 308, 309, 311, 328, 348

Curare woorari 179, 181, 191, 228

Digitalis purpurea 167, 174, 180, 188, 226, 227, 276, 328, 329

Dioscorea villosa 192, 193

Diphtherinum 30, 227, 296, 297

Drosera rotundifolia 292

Dulcamara 73, 181, 190, 226, 291, 299, 348

Echinacea 33, 169, 176, 227, 228, 233, 241, 267, 268, 319, 324, 348

Elaps corallinus 99, 135, 203, 204, 318

Electricitas 53

Index of Remedies

Equisetum hyemale 33, 270

Eschschoizia californica 125

Eucalyptus globulus 307

Eupatorium perfoliatum 169, 226, 233, 239, 282, 287, 307, 311, 348

Eupatorium purpureum 69

Euphorbium officinarum 174, 203, 227, 333

Euphrasia officinalis 188, 193, 226, 233, 236, 240, 290, 348

Ferrums 146, 154, 161, 233

Ferrum iodatum 155

Ferrum metallicum 155, 161, 165, 184, 310

Ferrum phosphoricum 39, 41, 42, 43, 47, 138, 146, 154, 155, 161, 180, 184, 185, 228, 233, 239, 241, 267, 268, 288, 333, 348

Ferrum sulphuricum 154, 155

Fluoricum acidum 152, 228,

Formica rufa 213

Galium aparine 185, 227

Gelsemium sempervirens 99, 121, 167, 176, 180, 188, 190, 227, 228, 233, 238, 239, 240, 246, 273, 276, 282, 285, 288, 290, 294, 295, 299, 300, 307, 310, 312, 314, 315, 324, 326, 328, 330, 348

Glonoinum 240, 276, 288, 348

Glycyrrhiza glabra 270, 271

Gossypium herbaceum 183, 226, 348

Graphites naturalis 101, 162, 174, 226, 312, 313, 333, 348

Grindelia robusta 62

Gunpowder 227

Hamamelis virginiana 169, 172, 174, 175, 233, 237, 241, 348

Helleborus niger 186, 190, 226, 307

Helianthus annus 126

Helium 147

Helonias dioica 176, 178, 227

Hepar sulphuris calcareum 154, 162, 163, 169, 226, 227, 233, 236, 237, 241, 261, 263, 268, 288, 297, 306, 307, 318, 348

Hydrastis canadensis 166, 170, 174, 186, 191, 228, 306, 320, 333, 348

Hydrocyanicum acidum 308, 309

Hydrophis cyanocinctus 206, 210

Hydrophyllum virginicum 62

Hyoscyamus niger 73, 108, 173, 176, 189, 190, 191, 226, 228, 248, 252, 253, 257, 258, 259, 308, 310, 311, 314, 315, 348

Hypericum perforatum 169, 180, 193, 234, 236, 237, 238, 241, 348

Ignatia amara 6, 112, 180, 181, 182, 184, 190, 227, 228, 246, 247, 249, 250, 261, 263, 269, 273, 288, 348

Iodum purum 297

Ipecacuanha 226, 185, 234, 239, 240, 241, 292, 294, 307, 325, 348

Ipomoea purpurea 166, 172, 182

Juglans regia 107, 174, 228

Kali arsenicosum 154, 247, 333

Kali bichromicum 154, 174, 186, 187, 296, 307, 318, 348

Kali bromatum 154, 155, 158, 159, 251, 228, 348

Kali carbonicum 151, 159, 171, 177, 185, 294, 297, 348, 276, 351

Kali chloricum 296, 312, 320, 323, 348

Kali iodatum 154, 155, 173, 297, 312, 318, 320, 323, 348

Kali muriaticum 42, 47, 154, 192, 227

Kali nitricum 152, 159

Kali permanganicum 296

Kali phosphoricum 42, 47, 154, 158, 191, 234, 238, 241, 273, 292, 246, 248, 269

Kali sulphuricum 43, 47, 154, 184, 185, 187, 292, 320, 348

Kalmia latifolia 167, 276

Kola Nut 183, 228

Kreosotum 171, 294

Lac caninum 30, 113, 196

Lac defloratum 30, 196

Lac maternum humanum 30

Lac vaccinum butyricum 196

Lachesis muta 72, 97, 113, 167, 173, 174, 176, 183, 184, 189, 190, 191, 201, 202, 240, 226, 227, 228, 251, 259, 276, 290, 294, 296, 297, 305, 306, 307, 308, 310, 312, 313, 314, 318, 319, 320, 323, 324, 325, 330, 333, 348

Lappa arctium 170, 228

Lathyrus sativus 121, 176, 227, 279, 282, 284, 285, 297, 299, 300

Index of Remedies

Latrodectus mactans 197, 198, 348
Laurocerasus officinalis 308, 348
Ledum palustre 168, 169, 186, 227, 234, 237, 239, 241, 348
Leprominium 227, 228
Leptandra virginica 174, 188, 228
Lilium tigrinum 167, 178, 183, 186, 227, 333
Limentis bredowii 223
Lithium carbonicum 147, 151
Lobelia inflata 33, 190, 270
Loxosceles reclusa 198
Luna 30, 53, 75, 112
Lupulus humulus 306
Lycopodium clavatum 70, 99, 101, 163, 164, 165, 166, 170, 175, 177, 178, 183, 184, 193, 226, 228, 246, 259, 260, 263, 270, 271, 290, 296, 297, 306, 318, 348
Lyssinum 227
Magnesia carbonica 151, 153, 226, 273
Magnesia muriatia 153, 167, 226
Magnesia phosphorica 44, 47, 153, 154, 192, 292, 348
Magnesia sulphurica 153, 226
Magnetis polus arcticus/australis 53
Malandrinum 32, 130, 195, 227, 291, 307, 348
Mandragora officinarum 73, 167, 228
Mancinella venenata 173, 226
Medorrhinum 30, 99, 104, 105, 106, 169, 173, 174, 226, 227, 228, 253, 259, 276, 297, 348
Melilotus officinalis 176, 226, 348
Mephitis putorius 196
Mentholum 175, 226
Mercurius cyanatus 227, 296, 297
Mercurius iodatus flavus 320
Mercurius solubilis 97, 108, 163, 167, 173, 174, 188, 191, 192, 194, 227, 228, 238, 251, 261, 263, 268, 290, 291, 294, 307, 308, 311, 312, 318, 320, 322, 323, 328, 348
Mezereum 227, 313, 348
Morbillinum 289, 290
Morphinum aceticum 183, 226
Muriaticum acidum 273, 348
Myrica cerifera 171, 174, 188, 226, 306, 307
Myristica sebifera 182, 227

Naja tripudians 203, 204, 276, 318
Naphthalinum 294
Natrum arsenicum 153
Natrum carbonicum 37, 72, 151, 153, 160, 187, 226, 240
Natrum fluoratum 37, 72, 152, 348
Natrum muriaticum 6, 37, 44, 45, 47, 70, 72, 99, 112, 153, 160, 162, 168, 169, 175, 180, 184, 187, 191, 196, 228, 230, 246, 247, 249, 250, 251, 259, 270, 271, 273, 289, 292, 307, 312, 313, 348
Natrum phosphoricum 37, 39, 45, 47, 72, 152, 154, 160
Natrum sulphuricum 37, 46, 47, 72, 99, 153, 154, 161, 227, 250, 251, 259, 294, 306, 307, 314, 315, 320, 348
Neon 30
Niobium metallicum 226
Nicotiana rustica 122, 348
Nitricum acidum 99, 152, 169, 172, 174, 176, 190, 192, 227, 249, 296, 306, 310, 318, 320, 325, 330, 333, 348
Nux moschata 226, 182, 308
Nux vomica 163, 164, 166, 167, 168, 169, 170, 171, 174, 177, 180, 181, 182, 183, 184, 187, 190, 226, 228, 249, 260, 263, 270, 271, 273, 299, 300, 326, 328, 348
Ocillococcinum 30
Ocimum sanctum 228
Oopherinum 228
Opium 99, 168, 183, 184, 185, 186, 227, 299, 300, 308, 348
Ornithogalum umbellatum 129, 178, 227
Pancreatinum 30
Parotidinum 290
Pepsinum 30
Petroleum oleum 312, 314, 348
Petroselinum sativum 320
Phosphoricum acidum 99, 227, 228, 248, 250, 251, 273, 310
Phosphorus 40, 99, 113, 148, 152, 153, 154, 158, 159, 160, 161, 162, 169, 180, 182, 185, 190, 227, 228, 232, 236, 238, 242, 247, 248, 273, 276, 292, 294, 296, 297, 299, 300, 306, 307, 308, 310, 312, 314, 315, 318, 319, 320, 323, 325, 326, 328, 329, 330, 348
Physostigma venenosum 177, 247
Phytolacca decandra 173, 186, 194, 270, 271, 290, 296, 320, 333, 348
Pilocarpinum 290, 291, 348
Pinus sylvestris 61, 119, 171

Index of Remedies

Pix liquida 171, 227

Platinum metallicum 172, 189

Plumbum iodatum 155, 333

Plumbum metallicum 33, 155, 299, 300, 330, 333, 348

Podophyllum peltatum 167, 188, 226, 307, 308, 309, 348

Psorinum 30, 98, 99, 100, 101, 102, 105, 118, 164, 166, 189, 226, 227, 297, 307, 319, 330, 348

Pulmo vulpis 30

Pulsatilla nigricans 72, 99, 162, 164, 165, 169, 170, 171, 174, 175, 178, 183, 184, 186, 187, 188, 190, 246, 247, 248, 250, 288, 289, 290, 291, 294, 297, 307, 322, 227, 228, 323, 328, 348

Pyrogenium 30, 131, 168, 169, 176, 182, 227, 228, 304, 305, 318, 319, 323, 324, 325, 333, 348

Radiation 30, 73, 80, 82, 86, 238, 331, 332

Radium bromatum 73, 155, 227, 348

Ranunculus bulbosus 187, 226

Reserpinum 269, 270

Rhus radicans 165, 226

Rhus toxicodendron 6, 70, 125, 165, 166, 168, 169, 172, 174, 175, 176, 182, 185, 194, 226, 234, 236, 237, 240, 241, 242, 290, 291, 294, 296, 229, 299, 300, 305, 307, 310, 311, 312, 313, 314, 315, 322, 323, 324, 348

RSV 293, 294, 316

Rumex crispus 174, 292

Ruta graveolens 166, 168, 194, 234, 236, 237, 238, 239, 241, 242, 288, 348

Sabadilla officinalis 178, 184, 188, 193, 227, 348

Sabal serrulata 171, 172, 174, 183, 227, 348

Sabina officinalis 171, 172, 174, 183, 227, 348

Saccharum lactis 30

Sambuscus nigra 348

Sanguinaria canadensis 183, 184, 185, 227, 292

SARS coronavirus 287, 293, 294, 323

Sarsaparilla officinalis 133, 166, 174, 177 227, 226, 348

Scutellaria laterifolia 273

Secale cornutum 30, 172, 176, 183, 226, 228, 308, 324, 325,

Selenium 175,

Senecio aureus 170, 176, 178, 227, 297,

Sepia succus 72, 99, 162, 167, 170, 172, 174, 175, 176, 178, 183, 184, 190, 202, 208, 209, 212, 226, 227, 228, 248, 269, 272, 294, 313, 314, 348

Silica terra 37, 40, 41, 42, 43, 46, 47, 101, 132, 164, 173, 182, 187, 226, 227, 228, 235, 236, 242, 2465, 249, 260, 263, 297, 320, 348

Sol 30, 53, 75

Spigelia anthelmintica 167, 180, 181, 188, 226,

Spongia tosta 72, 172, 189, 209, 238, 247, 268, 269, 292, 294, 348

Stannum metallicum 178, 189, 227, 297

Staphysagria 227, 178, 189, 297

Stillingia sylvatica

Stramonium 178, 189, 227, 297

Staphylococcinum 30

Streptococcinum 30

Strychninum 181, 226

Sulphur 28, 101, 102, 148, 153, 154, 164, 166, 167, 168, 169, 173, 174, 177, 183, 184, 185, 187, 189, 190, 193, 226, 227, 228, 238, 248, 261, 263, 273, 274, 290, 291, 294, 297, 308, 311, 318, 319, 320, 323, 328, 348

Sulphuricum acidum 154

Symphytum officinale 169, 194, 228, 235, 237, 239, 348

Syphilinum 30, 97, 105, 108, 109, 113, 173, 228, 252, 348

Tabacum nicotiana 227, 228, 348

Tarentula hispanica 199, 227, 253, 258, 258

Taraxacum officinale 170, 226, 268, 269

Terebinthiniae oleum 171, 172, 174, 226, 320, 333, 348

Theridion curassavicum 198

Thiosinaminum 228

Thuja occidentalis 70, 99, 113, 132, 165, 166, 171, 172, 173, 174, 226, 227, 228, 238, 294, 296, 307, 312, 320, 330, 333, 348

Thymus 30, 56, 58, 196, 274, 343,

Thyroidinum 196, 270

Trifolium pratense 194, 270, 271

Tuberculinum aviaire 98, 112, 113, 114, 186, 228, 253, 294, 297, 318, 330, 348

Tuberculinum bovinum 30, 98, 99, 111, 112, 113, 114, 226, 227, 258, 252, 253, 259, 297, 318, 320, 330, 348

Uranium nitricum 73, 146, 148, 152

Uricum acidum 30

Urtica urens 62, 175, 225, 235, 237, 240, 241, 291, 348

Index of Remedies

Vaccininum 30, 99, 132, 133, 227, 313

Varicella zoster 291, 311

Variolinum 30, 99, 133, 227, 291, 307, 312

Veratrum album 177, 179, 181, 190, 226, 235, 239, 248, 258, 287, 294, 295, 299, 308, 309, 310, 319, 325, 328, 329, 348

Verbascum thapsus 227

Verbena officinalis 120

Vespa crabro 75, 176, 212

Viola odorata 107, 122, 167, 192, 193, 227, 248

Viola tricolor 193, 226, 348

Vipera berus 205, 318

X-ray 30, 53, 228

Zincum metallicum 151, 155, 173, 186, 226, 228, 252, 260

Zincum muriaticum 269, 270

Zincum sulphuricum 154

General Index

Abundance 57, 70, 105, 261

Acute disease 15, 32, 117, 164

Addictive behavior 125, 127, 197, 200, 251,

ADHD 96, 216, 218, 220, 223, 225, 253, 254, 255, 257, 261, 262

AIDS/HIV 17, 47, 80, 85, 87, 93, 95, 123, 124, 125, 127, 128, 129, 142, 146, 215, 218, 228, 246, 247, 251, 257, 287, 316, 319

Alaskan Flower Essences 349

Animal kingdom 30, 65, 66, 70

Anorexia 181, 206, 247, 248, 253, 311

Anthrax 287, 324, 325

Antidoting a remedy 339

Anxiety 1, 2, 29, 40, 43, 44, 46, 49, 67, 68, 84, 87, 94, 100, 106, 108, 116, 118, 120, 122, 140, 141, 142, 152, 153, 154, 156, 157, 158, 159, 162, 164, 166, 175, 180, 181, 182, 185, 187, 190, 193, 197, 198, 203, 205, 206, 208, 209, 213, 223, 224, 231, 233, 238, 239, 245, 246, 247, 250, 251, 252, 259, 260, 265, 268, 269, 272, 276, 273, 288, 294, 309, 315

Arboviral Encephalitis 287, 314

Bach flowers 29, 49, 50, 236, 240, 243, 51, 66, 325

Behavioral disorders 79, 96, 113, 115, 245, 248, 257, 261, 348

Berberidaceae 166, 167

Biochemic Cell Salts 29, 40-47, 66

Biochemic remedies 38

Bioplasma 38

Birds 69, 70, 75, 299, 310

Bone 37, 40, 44, 46, 47, 69, 84, 85, 94, 109, 113, 117, 121, 128, 132, 153, 156, 157, 163, 164, 169, 173, 182, 189, 191, 192, 193, 194, 198, 202, 205, 207, 210, 232, 233, 235, 237, 238, 239, 240, 241, 242, 260, 287, 320, 322, 331, 333

Botox 326, 327

Botulism 287, 325, 326, 327, 330

Brain 37, 40, 45, 47, 50, 67, 68, 74, 127, 158, 162, 190, 199, 205, 211, 234, 254, 255, 268, 270, 288, 299, 308, 310, 311, 314, 315, 320, 333, 343

Breast 40, 178, 191, 194, 203, 209, 290, 291, 298, 311, 331, 333

Bulimia 171, 181, 248, 253

Cactaceae 167

Calcium 37, 40, 41, 42, 45, 148, 210, 232, 242, 260, 268, 268, 269

Cancer 17, 34, 80, 82, 85, 86, 87, 93, 95, 115, 116, 117, 118, 119, 120, 123, 125, 127, 128, 130, 141, 146, 148, 165, 168, 172, 175, 177, 178, 180, 184, 185, 186, 187, 190, 192, 193, 194, 201, 202, 203, 209, 211, 227, 246, 251, 265, 271, 272, 274, 304, 305, 307, 331, 332, 333, 339

Case history 25

Cell Salt (See Biochemic Cell Salts)

CFS 265, 266, 267, 268, 269, 270, 271, 272, 273, 274

Cheek/tongue 11, 38, 42, 45, 46, 47, 160, 170, 176, 186, 196, 208, 211, 212, 221 220, 231, 239, 254, 291, 295, 317, 331, 333, 355

Chemical agents 330

Chicken pox , 117, 136, 166, 175,, 287, 289, 291, 311

Cholera 280, 281, 287, 308, 309

Chronic anxiety 2260, 45

Chronic disease 4, 15, 74, 23, 34, 56, 97, 109, 118, 135, 136, 162

Chronic fatigue syndrome 51, 157, 174, 265, 266, 267, 271, 311, 321

Colds 1, 39, 42, 47, 112, 121, 125, 185, 193, 231, 279, 282, 287, 288, 297, 316,

Color remedies 54, 55, 56, 73

Compositae 169

Confidence 56, 67, 74, 79, 94, 106, 107, 116, 119, 122, 138, 140, 147, 149, 153, 162, 164, 196, 198, 199, 205, 218, 221, 236, 243, 246, 247, 254, 255, 260, 261, 266, 311, 341

Congestive heart failure 180, 275, 276

Conifer 171

Constitution 1, 12, 14, 14, 16, 17, 101, 278, 307, 339

Constitutional remedies/remedy 17, 32, 34, 98, 118, 332, 336, 337

Contraries 1, 2

Courage 41, 79, 59, 103, 107, 109, 110, 111, 119, 122, 123, 138, 149, 189, 208, 250, 270, 271, 280, 299

Cure 1, 2, 3, 4, 7, 9, 13, 15, 16, 18, 19, 20, 23, 24, 34, 39, 68, 76, 90, 92, 103, 89, 90, 91, 92, 97, 100, 119, 122, 130, 135, 171, 204, 205, 226, 251, 279, 283, 287, 292, 297, 299, 307, 311, 338, 339, 340

Cytomegalovirus 287, 311, 312

Deep impact 17, 31, 336, 338

General Index

Dilution 3, 4, 5, 49, 346, 347

Diphtheria 96, 206, 281, 287, 296, 297,

Dosage 7, 9, 10, 11, 14, 24, 27, 39, 55, 135, 286, 289, 332

Drug 2, 22, 23, 24, 32, 34, 50, 83, 90, 92, 93, 96, 97, 99, 103, 106, 124, 129, 130, 133, 135, 184, 234, 238, 245, 255, 265, 276, 278, 279, 281, 283, 306, 326, 337

Dysfunction 18, 45, 57, 71, 110, 265, 268, 271, 327

Ebola 316, 317, 318

Elements 1, 3, 25, 29, 30, 66, 87, 125, 145, 146, 147, 148, 151

Emergency 1, 12, 20, 32, 34, 140, 236, 240, 243, 304, 326, 345

Energetic 4, 9, 12, 14, 18, 19, 20, 29, 30, 39, 53, 55, 66, 68, 88, 98, 100, 104, 106, 122, 124, 126, 130, 135, 193, 216, 218, 221, 245, 252, 267, 278, 285, 346

Epidemic 5, 32, 79, 80, 86, 122, 132, 134, 176, 180, 265, 266, 277, 278, 279, 280, 281, 282, 283, 284, 285, 287, 288, 292, 294, 296, 297, 298, 299, 303, 306, 308, 316, 318

Epstein Barr Virus 99

Esophagus 171, 172, 194, 212, 331, 333

Euphorbiaceae 172

Fear 1, 113, 28, 29, 42, 49, 50, 51, 67, 68, 70, 73, 77, 84, 87, 94, 95, 96, 98, 104, 106, 107, 108, 110, 111, 114, 116, 118, 119, 121, 122, 125, 126, 132, 138, 142, 143, 149, 150, 151, 152, 156, 157, 159, 161, 167, 168, 169, 172, 173, 174, 176, 184, 185, 186, 187, 188, 191, 192, 196, 197, 199, 203, 204, 205, 207, 207, 214, 216, 223, 231, 237, 242, 245, 246, 247, 248, 250, 252, 253, 255, 258, 260, 268, 269, 273, 275, 279, 285, 299, 309, 324, 329

Fibroid 203, 205, 206, 333

Flavivirus (See West Nile Virus)

Flower essences 29, 49, 50, 51, 79, 98, 108, 109, 119, 12, 130, 176, 236, 243, 348

Flue 26, 28, 95, 125, 131, 134, 180, 231, 233, 234, 235, 238, 241, 245, 259, 273, 277, 278, 281, 282, 287, 288, 294, 295, 297, 304, 314, 315, 324, 326

Generational 17, 81, 109, 222, 320, 336, 338, 339

Gonorrhea 83, 287, 319

Grief issues 250, 254, 273

Group A Strep 305

Hamamelidae 173

Hantavirus 293, 323

Headaches 1, 10, 42, 44, 47, 50, 53, 58, 91, 93, 95, 96, 109, 122, 124, 161, 164, 166, 168, 170, 171, 172, 175, 177, 180, 184, 192, 196, 198, 199, 201, 202, 207, 210, 217, 218, 234, 240, 246, 265, 270, 276, 287, 288, 315, 321, 322

Hepatitis 99, 184, 265, 287, 304, 305, 306, 307, 310, 312, 319, 330

Herpes simplex 311, 312

Herpes zoster 186, 192

Hodgkin's 333

Influenza 46, 47, 99, 112, 131, 168, 176, 179, 180, 182, 181, 185, 227, 282, 287, 294, 295, 304, 310, 330

Insects 30, 69, 70, 75, 76, 169, 195, 213, 215, 314, 319

Intercurrent 33, 34, 81, 97, 98, 99, 101, 104, 108, 109, 121, 131, 291, 292, 296, 339

Iron 37, 41, 42, 96, 47, 146, 148, 154, 155, 161, 233, 249, 267

Isopathic 33, 97

Kinesiology 341

Labeling laws 13

Labiatae 175

Law of Contraries 1, 2

Law of Similars 1, 2

Learning disabilities 79, 101, 103, 105, 114, 121, 135, 253, 254, 255, 256, 257

Legionnaires Disease 323

Leguminosae 176

Leukemia 319, 333

Liliflorae 177

Loganiaceae 179, 180

Low potency 9, 10, 11, 12, 29, 34, 35, 38, 49, 61, 62, 101, 112, 195, 262, 266, 267, 271

Lyme Disease 287, 321

Magnesium 37, 40, 42, 44, 101, 148, 153, 157, 158, 292

Magnolianae 181

Malaria 2, 3, 46, 47, 85, 140, 141, 146, 148, 166, 167, 169, 174, 175, 177, 181, 183, 184, 187, 189, 192, 226, 251 277, 287, 299, 307

Malvaceae 182

Materia Medica 3, 5, 6, 12, 17, 18, 26, 28, 29, 51, 89, 92, 151, 153, 154, 165, 180, 181, 199, 202, 217, 230, 231, 272, 292, 297, 305,

Maxillary antrum of the sinuses 290, 333

Measles 99, 136, 287, 289, 290, 316

Metals 29, 30, 33, 42, 44, 66, 82, 108, 151

General Index

Miasms 4, 16, 17, 21, 32, 33, 63, 66, 79, 80, 81, 82, 83, 85, 86, 87, 88, 89, 92, 93, 97, 97, 98, 99, 100, 104, 108, 111, 125, 127, 128, 129, 130, 136, 137, 139, 140, 143, 144, 145, 146, 148, 162, 165, 247, 250, 251, 252, 255, 261, 278, 299, 320, 336

Mortality 83, 86, 100, 101, 215, 280, 281, 282, 283, 307, 308, 310, 318, 324, 325

Mother remedy 4, 5, 6, 347

Muscle test (also See Kinesiology) 7, 11, 24, 25, 28, 65, 98, 127, 144, 286, 332, 336, 337, 339, 341, 342, 343, 344, 345

Nerve agents 328

NSS (Never the Same Since) 17, 43, 99, 101, 129, 131, 132, 250, 267, 290, 295, 307, 330, 336

North American Flower Essences 29, 66, 102, 103, 106, 107, 109, 111, 114, 119, 121, 122, 125, 126, 128, 129, 348

Nosodes 17, 29, 30, 33, 36, 83, 96, 97, 99, 100, 104, 112, 118, 129, 131, 151, 250, 290, 294, 296, 307, 319

Organ 33, 72, 73, 87, 118, 131, 162, 166, 176, 185, 238, 265, 273, 278, 293, 294, 320, 332, 339

Ovarian 172, 192, 199, 204, 211, 213, 333

Palliation 16, 332

Panacea 18, 298

Panic attacks 105, 117, 209, 245, 246, 247

Papaveraceae 183

Pathological 34, 89, 116, 124, 180

Pattern thinking 63, 65, 66, 85

Periodic table 30, 81, 145, 146, 147, 149, 151, 155, 207

Pertussis 96, 133, 134, 284, 291, 293

Pica 40, 249

Plague 201, 202, 277, 287, 316, 318, 319,

Plant kingdom 30, 29, 66, 144, 169,

Polio 17, 80, 86, 93, 95, 120, 121, 122, 123, 129, 130, 132, 134, 141, 143, 146, 148, 205, 206, 226, 287, 298, 299, 300, 303, 304, 330

Polycrest 28, 34, 38, 72, 75, 82, 108, 116, 118, 144, 156, 163, 179, 180, 183, 187, 192, 194, 208, 211, 226, 231, 238, 239, 241, 246, 249, 251, 268, 269, 270, 271, 272, 276, 277, 287, 296, 297, 306, 309, 312, 324, 350

Post traumatic stress disorder (PTSD) 253, 255

Potassium 37, 40, 45, 196, 234, 269

Potency 4, 5, 7, 9, 10, 11, 12, 13, 17, 20, 24, 27, 29, 32, 34, 35, 38, 49, 61, 62, 63, 65, 99, 225, 262, 266, 267, 271, 278, 285, 286, 332, 304, 337, 338, 339, 340, 346, 347

Prevention 39, 40, 127, 193, 284, 285, 291, 310, 311, 312

Process of cure 340

Progression of healing 90, 91, 92

Prophylaxis 118, 121, 284, 290

Prostate 72, 170, 194, 331, 333

Proving the remedy 9, 20, 286, 339

Psora 17, 80, 83, 84, 85, 86, 87, 93, 94, 95, 100, 101, 102, 104, 106, 113, 115, 118, 130, 140, 146, 148, 167, 207, 225, 226, 245, 246, 247, 251, 252, 257, 269, 273, 336, 338, 339

Q Fever 287, 309, 310

Rajan Sankaran 81, 83, 88, 112, 137, 140, 145

Range of Light Flower Essences 348

Ranunculaceae 185, 186

Realms 63, 66, 67, 68, 70, 71, 72, 73, 74, 75, 76, 77, 103, 215, 261

Rectum 176, 194, 208, 212, 320, 331, 333

Repertory 18, 26, 28, 32, 105, 139, 236, 243, 252

Respiratory Syncytial Virus (RSV) 293, 294, 316

Rocky Mountain Spotted Fever 321, 322

Rubiaceae 184

Samuel Hahnemann 1, 2, 4, 20, 23, 38, 53, 54, 79, 80, 83, 90, 135, 280, 299, 319, 346

Sarcodes 29, 30, 66, 97, 151, 271,

Schuessler cell salt (See Biochemic Cell Salts)

Scrophulariaceae 188

Self mutilation 252,

Sensitivities 107, 137, 138, 139, 205, 214, 218, 287, 222, 224, 242, 265

Severe Acute Respiratory Syndrome (SARS) 293, 294, 323

Similars 1, 2, 3, 7, 49, 92, 97, 266, 296

Skin 13, 21, 27, 31, 37, 38, 40, 41, 42, 43, 47, 46, 51, 69, 80, 86, 91, 94, 95, 96, 99, 100, 102, 11, 115, 120, 125, 132, 133, 143, 162, 163, 164, 165, 166, 168, 171, 172, 173, 174, 175, 176, 177, 182, 185, 186, 1193, 195, 196, 199, 201, 202, 203, 206, 209, 210, 211, 212, 213, 214, 217, 218, 219, 220, 221, 223, 224, 225, 234, 239, 240, 249, 276, 289, 291, 293, 296, 299, 305, 309, 312, 317, 318, 320, 321, 322, 324, 325, 327, 328, 331, 333

Small Pox 132, 287, 307

Sodium 37, 40, 44, 45, 46, 47, 72, 148, 270

Solanaceae 73, 189

Sound Remedies 29, 55, 56, 57, 58, 66, 329, 340, 349

Spiders 76, 195, 197, 200,

Spirituality 29, 49, 74, 114, 120, 122, 125

Stomach 2, 11, 37, 43, 44, 46, 47, 57, 67, 91, 95, 102, 106, 117, 120, 132, 157, 159, 170, 171, 175, 176, 178, 180, 187, 188, 201, 202, 203, 208, 210, 212, 213, 219, 232, 246, 247, 249, 260, 265, 269, 270, 287, 295, 309, 315, 328, 333, 349

Succussion 3, 346

Suicidal depression 84, 250, 251

Suppression 16, 21, 81, 83, 91, 92, 93, 106, 109, 115, 116, 162, 183, 238, 250, 253, 276, 281, 337, 340

Sycotic (Sycosis) 17, 80, 83, 84, 85, 86, 87, 94, 95, 100, 104, 105, 106, 108, 113, 115, 130, 141, 146, 148, 167, 170, 172, 173, 175, 176, 178, 180, 182, 184, 187, 188, 191, 182, 227, 246, 251, 257, 275, 297, 319

Syphilis 17, 80, 83, 84, 85, 87, 94, 97, 108, 109, 113, 114, 115, 123, 130, 139, 144, 146, 148, 165, 166, 169, 170, 173, 174, 175, 176, 178, 186, 188, 191, 192, 228, 251, 252, 287, 320

Tissue cell salt (See Biochemic Cell Salts)

Trauma 1, 17, 32, 51, 65, 68, 72, 88, 90, 93, 99, 102, 103, 107, 110, 119, 122, 129, 137, 140, 150, 168, 169, 207, 236, 238, 239, 243, 253, 330

Trust 11, 25, 67, 68, 94, 96, 103, 106, 109, 110, 114, 119, 122, 341, 345,

Tuberculosis 17, 80, 85, 86, 87, 93, 94, 99, 100, 111, 112, 113, 114, 117, 125, 128, 129, 141, 146, 167, 171, 189, 192, 207, 227, 252, 287, 297, 319, 330

Typhoid Fever 307, 308

Umbelliferae 191

Vaccines 21, 29, 82, 96, 115, 129, 130, 131, 132, 133, 134, 143, 195, 278, 303, 304, 314

Vaccinosis 80, 82, 96, 118, 129, 131, 132, 140, 143, 145, 169, 172, 227, 251, 255, 261, 304, 307

Vibrational remedies 29, 30, 53, 54, 66

Violence disorder 253, 258

Vital force 10, 14, 15, 23, 24, 40, 88, 90, 91, 92, 93, 97, 98, 130, 135, 151, 230, 262, 271, 274, 278, 279, 285, 286, 330

Vital sensation 137

West Nile 287, 310, 311

Whooping Cough (See Pertussis)

Meet the Author

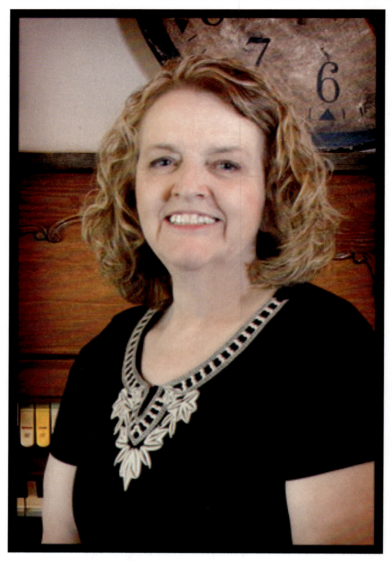

LaRee Westover has been studying and living various natural medicine modalities for over thirty years. Her experience includes the use of essential oils, herbals, and homeopathy, as well as energy work. She has an extensive knowledge of plants, their family groups, and their individual medicinal qualities.

Using this knowledge as a springboard, LaRee has been able to relate the specific energies of each plant and how each is utilized within its specific modality as she has compiled the information for each of her four books. Her practical, no nonsense, hands-on approach has inspired countless people to make the leap to natural healing.

LaRee teaches, "To feel the living spirit and intelligence of each plant is the true foundation of alternative medicine. Just as each plant can exemplify the attributes of our loving Father, so can the plants personify some lessons about the operation of the body and the soul. The possibilities for learning are endless. To think 'alternatively' is to think differently; we must think as nature does—holistically. Nature emphasizes the whole, rather than the precise piece, and nature has an inherent logic and wisdom..

Whether it is through essential oils, herbs, homeopathics, or energy, LaRee's insight into the natural world is precise and helpful to the novice as well as the more advanced practitioner.